USMLE ROAD MAP

Emergency Medicine

SCOTT C. SHERMAN, MD

Assistant Residency Director
M4 Clerkship Director
Department of Emergency Medicine
Cook County Hospital (Stroger)
Assistant Professor of Emergency Medicine
Rush Medical College
Chicago, IL

JOSEPH M. WEBER, MD

EMS Director
Department of Emergency Medicine
Cook County Hospital (Stroger)
Assistant Professor of Emergency Medicine
Rush Medical College
Chicago, IL

Lange Medical Books/McGraw-Hill
Medical Publishing Division

New York   Chicago   San Francisco   Lisbon   London   Madrid   Mexico City
Milan   New Delhi   San Juan   Seoul   Singapore   Sydney   Toronto

USMLE Road Map: Emergency Medicine, First Edition

Copyright © 2008 by The McGraw-Hill Companies, Inc. All rights reserved. Printed in the United States of America. Except as permitted under the United States Copyright Act of 1976, no part of this publication may be reproduced or distributed in any form or by any means, or stored in a data base or retrieval system, without prior written permission of the publisher.

2 3 4 5 6 7 8 9 0   /   16 15 14 13 12

ISBN 978-0-07-146388-1
MHID 0-07-146388-7
ISSN 1938-954X

Notice

Medicine is an ever-changing science. As new research and clinical experience broaden our knowledge, changes in treatment and drug therapy are required. The authors and the publisher of this work have checked with sources believed to be reliable in their efforts to provide information that is complete and generally in accord with the standards accepted at the time of publication. However, in view of the possibility of human error or changes in medical sciences, neither the authors nor the publisher nor any other party who has been involved in the preparation or publication of this work warrants that the information contained herein is in every respect accurate or complete, and they disclaim all responsibility for any errors or omissions or for the results obtained from use of the information contained in this work. Readers are encouraged to confirm the information contained herein with other sources. For example and in particular, readers are advised to check the product information sheet included in the package of each drug they plan to administer to be certain that the information contained in this work is accurate and that changes have not been made in the recommended dose or in the contraindications for administration. This recommendation is of particular importance in connection with new or infrequently used drugs.

This book was set in Adobe Garamond by Pine Tree Composition.
The editors were Jason Malley, Susan Kelly, Jim Shanahan and Karen Edmonson.
The production supervisor was Catherine H. Saggese.
The index was prepared by Pine Tree Composition.

INTERNATIONAL EDITION ISBN 978-0-07-110478-4; MHID 0-07-110478-X
Copyright © 2008. Exclusive rights by The McGraw-Hill Companies, Inc. for manufacture and export. This book cannot be re-exported form the country to which it is consigned by McGraw-Hill. The International Edition is not available in North America.

CONTENTS

To Michelle and Mason.

Scott C Sherman, MD

To my wife, Bridget, for her love and encouragement throughout this endeavor and to my parents, Lois and Bill, whose example I strive to emulate.

Joseph M Weber, MD

USING THE
USMLE ROAD MAP SERIES
FOR SUCCESSFUL REVIEW

What is the Road Map Series?

Short of having your own personal tutor, the *USMLE Road Map* Series is the best source for efficient review of major concepts and information in the medical sciences.

Why Do You Need A Road Map?

It allows you to navigate quickly and easily through your course notes and prepares you for USMLE and course examinations.

How Does the Road Map Series Work?

Outline Form: Connects the facts in a conceptual framework so that you understand the ideas and retain the information.

Boldface: Highlights words and phrases that trigger quick retrieval of concepts and facts.

Clear Explanations: Are fine-tuned by years of student interaction. The material is written by authors selected for their excellence in teaching and their experience in preparing students for board examinations.

Illustrations: Provide the vivid impressions that facilitate comprehension and recall.

PREFACE

We wrote this book because we remember our own experiences rotating through the Emergency Department in medical school. The ED is a unique environment requiring knowledge and skills often not covered in the core third-year clerkships. In this book, we attempt to create a resource for the fourth-year medical student to be used both during their Emergency Medicine clerkship and while preparing for the USMLE Step 2. The book's length and outline format are designed to allow the student to easily digest the broad range of topics inherent to Emergency Medicine. Features including *Procedural Pearls, Key Complaints*, *Clinical Skills Tips,* and *Rule Out* diagnoses help highlight important information for the reader. *Diagnostic Algorithms* are included in each chapter for both quick reference and to give the student a succinct overview of ED management for easier recall. *Case Presentations* and *Summary Points* are used to exemplify the process of medical decision-making and reinforce essential information. We hope this book will enhance the emergency medicine experience of all its users.

Scott C Sherman, MD

Joseph M Weber, MD

ACKNOWLEDGMENTS

We would like to thank our Editor, Jason Malley, for all his efforts on this project. Our developmental editor, Susan Kelly, was outstanding, and this book would not be what it is without her vision and input. Special thanks to Bridget Weber (Figure 6–4) and Susan Gilbert (Figure 10–3) for their illustrations. Patty Donovan guided us through the final stages of the project with a great deal of accuracy and efficiency. Lastly, we would like to thank Ethel Lee, the Cook County EM Student Clerkship Coordinator. Couldn't do it without you Ethel.

Scott C Sherman, MD

Joseph M Weber, MD

CREDITS

Figures 15-2 B and 15-2F from Ferry DR. *Basic Electrocardiography in Ten Days,* 1st edition. McGraw-Hill, New York. 2001

Figures 68-2, 68-3 Furman JM and Cass SP. Benign paroxysmal positional vertigo. New Engl J Med, 1999, Nov 18; 341(21) 1590-96.

Figure 84-1 from Kane KS, Bissonette J, Baden HP, et al. *Color Atlas & Synopsis of Pediatric Dermatology.* McGraw-Hill, New York. 2002.

Figures 36-1; 37-3, 46-1, 46-2, 83-1, 83-2, 83-3 from Knoop KJ, Stack LB, and Storrow AB. *Atlas of Emergency Medicine,* 2nd edition. McGraw-Hill, New York. 2002.

Figures 38-1, 39-1 from Pearlman MD, Tintinalli JE, and Dyne PL. *Obstetric and Gynecologic Emergencies: Diagnosis and Management,* 1st edition. McGraw-Hill, New York. 2004.

Figures 3-3, 37-3, 80-1, 82-1, 82-2, 82-3, 82-4, 82-5 from Reichman EF and Simon RR. *Emergency Medicine Procedures,* 1st edition. McGraw-Hill, New York. 2004.

Figures 7-1, 10-4 A and B, 73-2, 73-3, 73-4, 73-5, 73-6, 73-7, 75-2 from Scaletta TA and Schaider JJ. *Emergent Management of Trauma,* 2nd edition. McGraw-Hill, New York. 2001.

Figure 41-1 from Simon RR, Sherman SC, and Koenigsknecht SJ. *Emergency Orthopedics: The Extremities,* 5th edition. McGraw-Hill, New York. 2007.

Figures 3-4, 3-5, 3-6, 5-2, 7-2, 10-1 from Stone CK and Humphries RL. *Lange: Current Emergency Diagnosis and Treatment,* 5th edition. McGraw-Hill, New York. 2004.

Figures 6-2, 6-3, 6-5, 15-2 E and G, 15-3A, 36-2, 37-1, 40-1, 40-2, 40-3, 49-1, 73-1, 76-1 and Tables 47-1, 51-2, 69-1 from Tintinalli JE, Kelen GD, and Stapczynski JS. *Emergency Medicine: A Comprehensive Study Guide,* 6th edition. McGraw-Hill, New York. 2004.

CONTRIBUTING AUTHORS

John Bailitz, MD
Assistant Residency Director
Department of Emergency Medicine
Cook County Hospital (Stroger)
Assistant Professor of Emergency Medicine
Rush Medical College
Chapters 8, 30, 31, 32, 33, 34

Steven Bowman, MD
Residency Director
Department of Emergency Medicine
Cook County Hospital (Stroger)
Assistant Professor of Emergency Medicine
Rush Medical College
Chapters 38, 39, 40, 59

Sean Bryant, MD
Department of Emergency Medicine
Cook County Hospital (Stroger)
Assistant Professor of Emergency Medicine
Rush Medical College
Associate Medical Director
Illinois Poison Control Center
Chapters 47, 48, 49, 50, 51

Kristine Cieslak, MD
Pediatric Emergency Medicine
Children's Memorial Hospital
Assistant Professor
Northwestern University's Feinberg School of Medicine
Chapters 41, 42, 43, 44, 45, 46

David Harter, MD
Assistant Residency Director
Department of Emergency Medicine
Cook County Hospital (Stroger)
Assistant Professor of Emergency Medicine
Rush Medical College
Chapters 71, 72

Trevor Lewis, MD
Department of Emergency Medicine
Cook County Hospital (Stroger)
Assistant Professor of Emergency Medicine
Rush Medical College
Chapters 15, 16, 18

Jordan Moskoff, MD
Department of Emergency Medicine
Cook County Hospital (Stroger)
Assistant Professor of Emergency Medicine
Rush Medical College
Chapters 61, 62, 63, 64, 65

Lisa Palivos, MD
Department of Emergency Medicine
Cook County Hospital (Stroger)
Assistant Professor of Emergency Medicine
Rush Medical College
Chapters 83, 84

Christopher Ross, MD
Assistant Residency Director
Department of Emergency Medicine
Cook County Hospital (Stroger)
Assistant Professor of Emergency Medicine
Rush Medical College
Chapters 9, 11, 12, 13, 14, 17

Theresa Schwab, MD
Attending Physician
Department of Emergency Medicine
Advocate Christ Medical Center
Chapter 10

Michelle Sergel, MD
M3 Clerkship Director
Department of Emergency Medicine
Cook County Hospital (Stroger)
Assistant Professor of Emergency Medicine
Rush Medical College
Chapters 19, 20, 21, 22, 23

Scott C Sherman, MD
M4 Clerkship Director
Assistant Residency Director
Department of Emergency Medicine
Cook County Hospital (Stroger)
Assistant Professor of Emergency Medicine
Rush Medical College
Chapters 1, 2, 6, 24, 25, 26, 27, 28, 29, 54, 55, 56, 57, 60, 74, 75, 76, 77, 78, 79, 80, 81, 82

Joseph M Weber, MD
EMS Director
Department of Emergency Medicine
Cook County Hospital (Stroger)
Assistant Professor of Emergency Medicine
Rush Medical College
Chapters 3, 4, 5, 7, 35, 36, 37, 52, 53, 58, 66, 67, 68, 69, 70, 73

SECTION I
COMMON PROCEDURES

CHAPTER 1
INCISION AND DRAINAGE

I. Indications and Definitions

A. Incision and drainage (I&D) is the definitive treatment method used for patients with subcutaneous abscesses. An abscess is defined as a collection of purulent material beneath the skin. The overlying skin is swollen, warm, red, and tender (Figure 1–1). It is sometimes difficult to distinguish a localized cellulitis from an abscess unless the overlying skin is fluctuant. The body areas most commonly involved are listed in Table 1–1.

B. Risk factors for abscess formation include summer months, IV drug use, immunocompromise, minor trauma, and poor hygiene.

C. **Sebaceous cyst.** A sebaceous cyst is a small, nontender, subcutaneous fluid-filled structure. The patient will report the presence of the cyst for a long period of time but only recent symptoms when it becomes infected. Removing the capsule when draining an infected sebaceous cyst will prevent recurrence.

D. **Pilonidal abscess.** A pilonidal cyst occurs in the sacrococcygeal area, 5–8 cm above the anus, when pilosebaceous glands become distended with keratin. In an acute infection, an abscess may form that requires I&D. In 85% of cases, these abscesses recur. Definitive surgical excision is usually required.

E. **Paronychia.** This is a common infection of the lateral nail fold (Figure 1–2).

Table 1–1. Distribution of abscesses by body part.

Area of Body	%
Buttocks and perirectal area	25
Head and neck	20
Extremities	18
Axilla	16
Inguinal area	15
Other	6

3

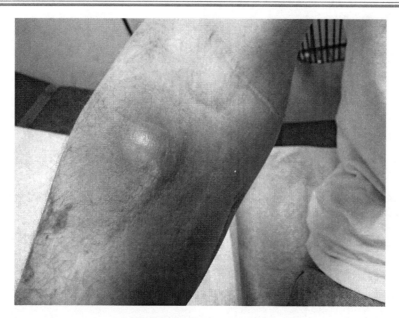

Figure 1–1. A subcutaneous abscess in an IV drug user.

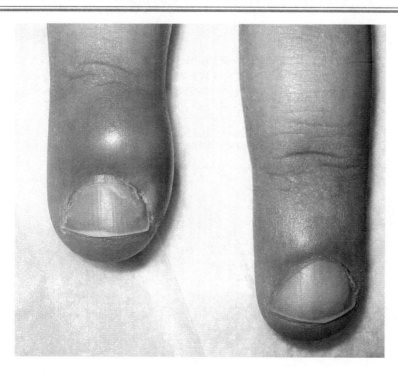

Figure 1–2. Paronychia.

F. **Felon.** A felon is an infection of the closed compartment of the volar fingertip.

G. **Perirectal abscess.** The most common type is the perianal abscess, which is a tender, fluctuant mass palpated at the anal verge. Perianal abscesses are treated with I&D by the emergency physician. Other perirectal abscesses, including the intersphincteric, ischiorectal, and supralevator spaces, are best drained by a surgeon.

H. **Hidradenitis suppurativa.** This is a chronic relapsing inflammatory process affecting the apocrine glands in the axilla, inguinal area, or both. Multiple abscesses can form and eventually lead to draining fistulous tracts that require surgical management. I&D of these abscesses is frequently necessary and performed in the ED.

I. **Bartholin's gland abscess.** The Bartholin's glands are paired glands that provide moisture to the vestibule of the vaginal mucosa. When the opening becomes occluded, either an abscess or a cyst can develop.

II. Contraindications

A. Pulsatile (suggests an aneurysm) or overlying large vessels (anterior triangle of neck, groin, or popliteal fossa).

B. Inability to achieve adequate analgesia (consider drainage in the OR).

C. Proximity to important neurovascular structures or tendons (consult surgeon).

III. Equipment. Povidone-iodine solution, 1% lidocaine, 27-gauge needle and syringe (for local anesthesia), 18-gauge needle and syringe (if aspirating), 11-blade scalpel, curved hemostat, and iodoform packing (Figure 1–3).

IV. Procedure

A. Prepare the area with povidone-iodine solution.

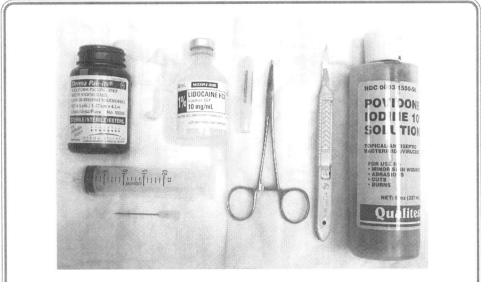

Figure 1–3. Supplies for incision and drainage of an abscess.

B. Use 1% lidocaine to anesthetize the area. Be careful not to inject lidocaine into the abscess cavity itself because this will only increase tension and pain. For larger abscesses, procedural sedation may be necessary.

C. If it is unclear whether an abscess exists, attempt aspiration of pus with a syringe and an 18-gauge needle.

D. Use the 11-blade scalpel to incise the skin. Incision should be at the point of maximal fluctuance and should extend two thirds of the diameter of the abscess cavity (except when draining Bartholin's abscesses, where only an incision 0.5–1 cm should be made).

E. Express pus from the cavity.

F. Use a curved hemostat to break loculations and free any remaining pus.

G. Pack the wound with iodoform gauze and cover the wound with gauze. When treating a Bartholin's gland abscess, a small catheter (Word catheter) is placed in the opening instead of iodoform. The catheter should remain in place for several weeks to allow for the development of a fistula for drainage.

H. The patient is instructed to follow up in 48 hours to have the packing removed. If pus is no longer present and symptoms are resolving, the wound is allowed to heal by secondary intention.

V. **Complications.** Bacterial endocarditis, scarring, neurovascular injury.

CHAPTER 2
ARTERIAL BLOOD GAS

I. Indications

A. A sample of arterial blood is used to determine the partial pressure of O_2 (pO_2), CO_2 (pCO_2), and the pH of blood. Accurate determination allows for the detection of hypoxia, hypercarbia, and complex acid-base disorders.

B. Many blood gas analyzers provide additional useful information to the physician, including electrolytes, glucose, lactate, hemoglobin, carboxyhemoglobin, and methemoglobin levels.

II. Contraindications (Relative)

A. Bleeding diatheses.

B. Possible future use of thrombolytics.

C. Severe peripheral vascular disease.

D. Abnormal skin (burn, dermatitis, infection).

III. Equipment

A. A commercially available ABG kit includes povidone-iodine or alcohol swab, 3–5 cc syringe (heparinized), 22-gauge needle, gauze pad, collection bag, band-aid, and needle cap (Figure 2–1).

B. Additional supplies include gloves, lidocaine (1%), a 25- or 27-gauge needle, a folded sheet or "kidney" basin to extend the wrist, and tape.

IV. Procedure (Figure 2–2)

A. Position the wrist over a folded sheet to extend it approximately 30°.

B. Palpate the radial artery at the proximal flexor crease of the wrist just medial to the radial styloid and lateral to the flexor carpi radialis tendon.

C. Prepare the skin with a povidone-iodine or alcohol swab.

D. Raise a skin wheal with 1% lidocaine over the site. This has been shown to significantly decrease the pain of the procedure and does not affect success rate.

E. Pull the plunger of the heparinized syringe up to 2 cc. (Some ABG kits have syringe plungers that automatically rise with the pressure of arterial blood, making this step unnecessary. This added feature helps distinguish arterial blood from venous blood.)

F. Hold the syringe with one hand like a pencil, while the other hand palpates the radial pulse more proximal to the site of insertion.

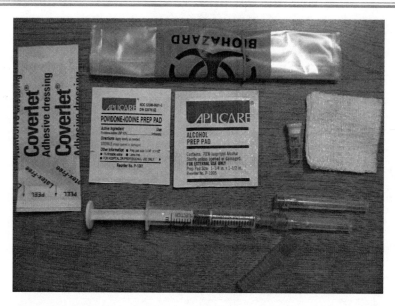

Figure 2–1. An ABG kit.

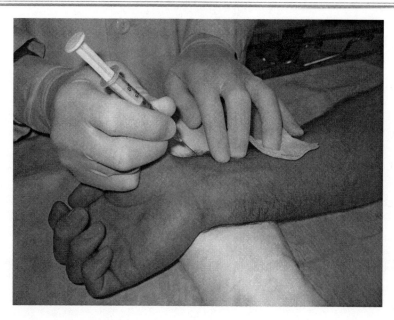

Figure 2–2. Performing an ABG.

G. At a 30–45° angle, and with the bevel of the needle up, insert the needle through the skin wheal and into the radial artery.

H. Blood flow should be brisk (if arterial). The color of the blood will not accurately distinguish arterial from venous blood.

I. If blood does not fill the syringe, withdraw the needle to just below the skin surface and redirect the needle. ***Movement of the needle at any significant depth under the skin should be absolutely avoided because it may lacerate the artery.***

J. After obtaining blood return, withdraw the needle and apply pressure with gauze for 5 minutes to prevent hematoma formation. Placing the gauze on the forearm before the procedure will allow the physician easy access to the gauze.

K. Remove and dispose the needle in a red sharps container.

L. Cap the syringe and carefully expel any air within the syringe.

M. It is necessary to put the sample on ice ONLY if it will take more than 10 minutes to put the blood into the blood gas analyzer.

V. Complications. Infection, bleeding, neuropathy, pseudoaneurysm, arteriovenous fistula.

CHAPTER 3
CENTRAL VENOUS ACCESS

I. Indications

    A. Inability to obtain peripheral IV access.

    B. Need for specific IV medications that may be caustic to peripheral veins (D25, pressors, hypertonic saline).

    C. Transvenous pacing.

    D. Central venous pressure monitoring.

    E. Need for emergent dialysis without previous access.

II. Contraindications

    A. Peripheral access obtainable without other indication for central access.

    B. Cellulitis or anatomic abnormality.

    C. Coagulopathy is an absolute contraindication to subclavian cannulation, as it is a non-compressible site and a relative contraindication to the internal jugular and femoral sites.

III. Equipment

    A. Most of the equipment needed to perform central venous cannulation can be found in commercially available central line kits (Figure 3–1). Kits include povidone-iodine (Betadine) swabs, guidewire introducer needle, J-tip guidewire, multiple 5-mL syringes, 1% lidocaine, 22- and 25-gauge needles for local anesthesia, #11 blade scalpel, dilator, central line, and silk suture on a straight cutting needle.

    B. There are multiple types of central lines. Generally, 1 of 2 types is used in the ED (Figure 3–2). A **triple lumen catheter** is used in patients when there is difficult IV access or those who require multiple different medication drips. A **sheath introducer (Cordis®) catheter** is shorter and wider and is used for the introduction of Swan-Ganz catheters, transvenous pacers, and for rapid infusion of fluid and blood products in the hypotensive patient. These larger catheters can achieve flow rates up to 1 L/min.

IV. Procedure

    A. **Preparation.** Locate anatomical landmarks. Apply povidone-iodine to the area of needle insertion. Place sterile drape with fenestration over the area. Anesthetize with lidocaine.

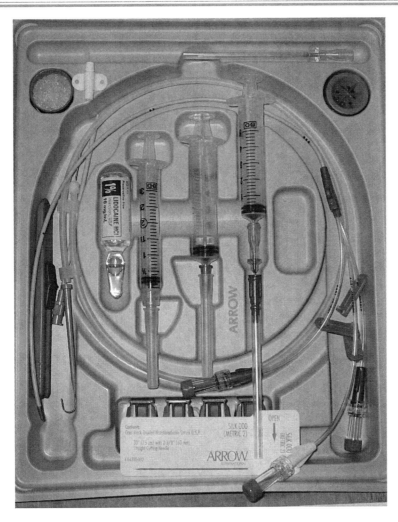

Figure 3–1. Triple lumen kit.

B. **Seldinger Technique**
1. Use large bore needle with syringe to cannulate the vein. There should be free flow of dark non-pulsatile blood into the syringe with traction on plunger (Figure 3–3A).
2. Thread the guidewire through the needle until 3–5 cm of the guidewire remains (Figure 3–3B). If resistance is met, withdraw the wire and confirm that the needle is in the vessel. Attempt to rethread the wire.
3. When the guidewire is in place, remove the needle (Figure 3–3C). *Never let go of the guidewire during any part of the procedure because it can migrate fully into the vessel.*
4. Using a #11 blade scalpel, make a superficial stab incision in the skin at the site that the guidewire enters (Figure 3–3D).

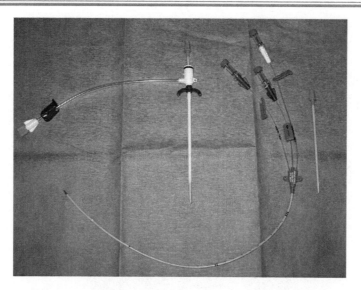

Figure 3–2. From left to right: A, sheath introducer kit (Cordis®) with dilator; B, triple lumen catheter; C, triple lumen dilator.

5. Pass the dilator over the wire and thread into the vessel (Figure 3–3E). (For the Cordis® catheter, the dilator and catheter are inserted together.)
6. Remove the dilator and thread the triple lumen over the wire until it protrudes 2–3 cm out of the brown port.
7. Holding the wire with one hand, thread the line into the vein (Figure 3–3F).
8. Remove the wire and confirm placement with aspiration of blood (Figure 3–3G). Secure the catheter in place with suture.

PROCEDURAL PEARLS

If resistance is met while threading the guidewire, rotate it 90° and attempt to rethread.

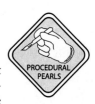

C. **Internal jugular vein** (Figure 3–4). Position the patient supine and in slight Trendelenburg position. Rotate the head 75° to the opposite side. Palpate the triangle formed by the 2 heads of the sternocleidomastoid muscle. Palpate the carotid artery pulse within this triangle. The vein is lateral to the artery in this location. Ultrasound is frequently used to help identify the vein. Insert the needle at the apex of the triangle, aiming toward the ipsilateral nipple with 30° of angulation. The vein should be entered within 2–3 cm of needle advancement.

PROCEDURAL PEARLS

Do not palpate the carotid pulse while attempting to cannulate the internal jugular vein. The slight compression that results can compress the vein, making it more difficult to access.

D. **Subclavian vein** (Figure 3–5). Position the patient supine and in slight Trendelenburg position. Place a rolled sheet or towel between the patient's scapulas to allow the

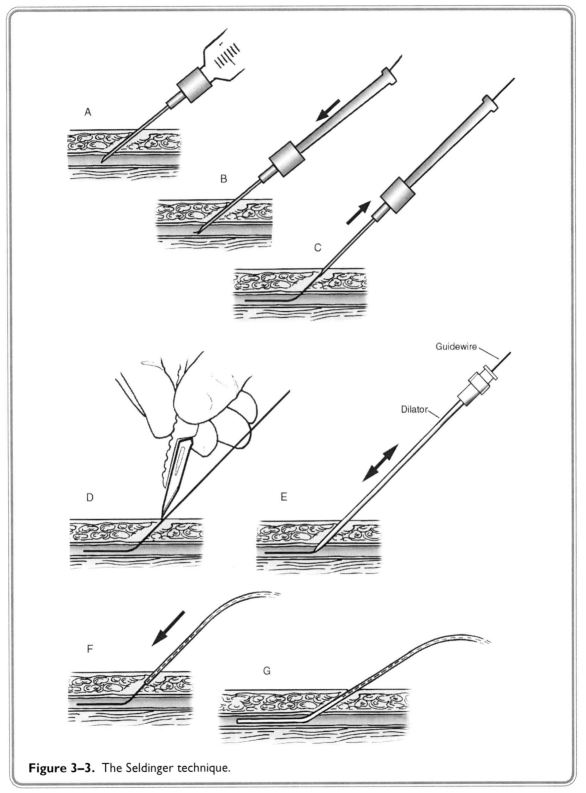

Figure 3–3. The Seldinger technique.

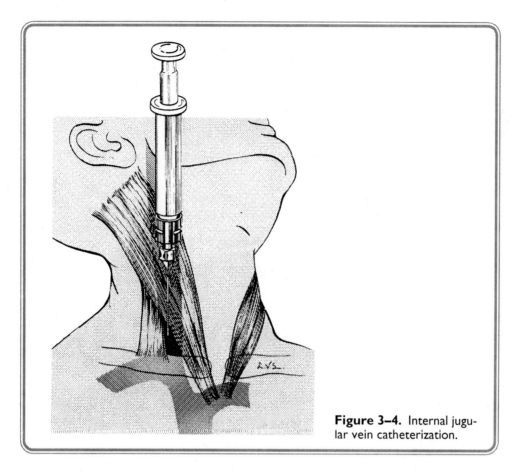

Figure 3–4. Internal jugular vein catheterization.

shoulders to fall backward and flatten the clavicles. Insert the needle 1 cm inferior to the clavicle, aiming towards the junction of the middle and medial thirds. Direct the needle under the clavicle and toward the suprasternal notch, with the needle parallel to the chest wall. The vein should be entered within 4 cm of needle advancement.

E. **Femoral vein** (Figure 3–6). Palpate the femoral artery 2 cm below the inguinal crease. The vein is usually 1 cm medial to the artery at this location. Insert the needle at a 45° angle to the skin, medial to the femoral pulse. In the pulseless patient, palpate the anterior superior iliac spine and the pubic tubercle. Draw an imaginary line connecting these 2 points. If this line is divided into thirds, the vein will be located where the medial and middle thirds intersect.

V. Complications

A. **Internal jugular vein.** Bleeding, airway compression from expanding hematoma, carotid artery dissection, pneumothorax, air embolism, or arrhythmia from cardiac irritation.

B. **Subclavian vein.** Bleeding, pneumothorax, air embolism, or arrhythmia from cardiac irritation.

C. **Femoral vein.** Bleeding, DVT of femoral vein, femoral artery laceration, soft tissue infection, or line sepsis.

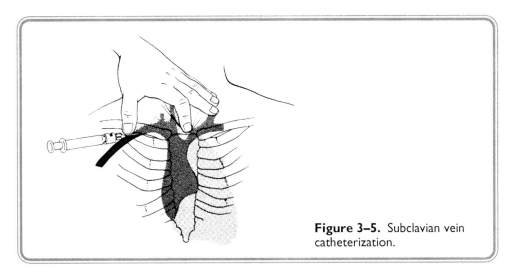

Figure 3–5. Subclavian vein catheterization.

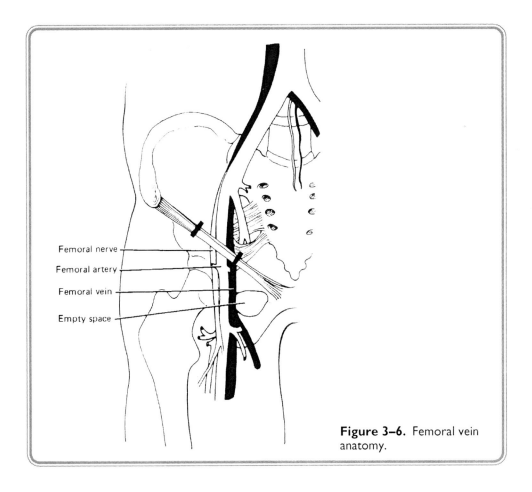

Femoral nerve

Femoral artery

Femoral vein

Empty space

Figure 3–6. Femoral vein anatomy.

CHAPTER 4
PROCEDURAL SEDATION

I. **Indications.** Anxiolysis, sedation, amnesia, and analgesia during potentially anxiety provoking or painful procedures (eg, fracture and dislocation reduction, I&D, burn or wound debridement, LP, pediatric laceration repair, or pediatric diagnostic study).

II. **Contraindications.** Lack of experienced personnel, serious co-morbid pulmonary or cardiac disease (ASA class III-V), lack of proper airway and monitoring equipment, known medication allergy, a meal within 4 hours and liquids within 2 hours (recent data suggests that fasting does not alter the risk of aspiration), and patient intoxication.

III. **Equipment.** Cart with resuscitation drugs and age-appropriate airway equipment, cardiac monitor, O_2 source, nasal cannula (used routinely) and BVM (if hypoventilation), pulse oximeter (and capnography if available), IV access, suction equipment, and reversal agents (naloxone and flumazenil).

IV. **Procedure**

A. Perform a thorough history and physical examination and patient assessment. Assign patients to a physical status classification (Table 4–1). Sedation and analgesia in the ED normally should be limited to patients in classes I and II.

B. Explain the procedure to the patient or guardian and gain informed consent.

C. Connect patient to appropriate monitoring equipment and assemble experienced personnel.

D. Select analgesic, sedative-hypnotic, or dissociative anesthetic, depending on the indication (Table 4–2). Examples include adult procedure (etomidate **or** fentanyl and midazolam); pediatric procedure (ketamine with atropine 0.01 mg/kg to maximum 0.3 mg +/- glycopyrrolate 0.005mg/kg to maximum 0.25 mg for secretions); and pediatric diagnostic procedure (ketamine or midazolam).

E. Have airway equipment and reversal agent (naloxone for opiates and flumazenil for benzodiazepines) at the bedside.

F. Administer medication and titrate to desired effect. Perform procedure while an assistant (MD or RN) is monitoring the patient.

Table 4–1.

The American Society of Anesthesiologist's Physical Status Classification
I.   Healthy patient
II.   Mild systemic disease—no functional limitation
III.   Severe system disease—definite functional limitation
IV.   Severe systemic disease—constant threat to life
V.   Moribund patient—not expected to survive without the operation

Table 4–2. Common medications used for procedural sedation in the ED.

Drug (Class)	Dose	Effects	Onset	Duration	Side Effects	Reversal Agent
Midazolam (benzo)	0.02–0.1 mg/kg IV	Sedation, amnesia, anxiolysis	2 min	20–30 min	Apnea, hypotension	Flumazenil
Morphine (opioid)	0.1–0.2 mg/kg IV	Analgesia	2 min	3–4 hr	Histamine release	Naloxone
Fentanyl (opioid)	0.5–1 mcg/kg to total dose of 2–3 mcg/kg IV	Analgesia, mild sedation	2 min	30 min	Respiratory depression and rigid chest syndrome"	Naloxone
Ketamine (PCP derivative)	0.5–1 mg/kg IV	Sedation, amnesia, analgesia, anxiolysis	1 min	1–2 hr	Increased secretions, tachycardia, increased ICP	None
Etomidate (imidazole derivative)	0.1–0.2 mg/kg IV	Sedation, amnesia, anxiolysis	30 sec	10–30 min	Myoclonus, apnea	None

G. Allow time for patient recovery from medications. Observe patient until level of alertness is equal to that of pre-sedation and patient is able to tolerate oral liquids.

PROCEDURAL PEARLS

Reversal agents. *When using opiates, always have naloxone available. The initial dose is 0.2–0.4 mg IV. It should be used with care in patients who are chronically using or abusing opiates because it may precipitate opiate withdrawal. When using benzodiazepines, have flumazenil available for reversal. The initial*

dose is 0.02 mg/kg maximum 0.2 mg over a 15-second period. Additional 0.2-mg doses may be repeated every minute, with a maximum dose of 1 mg over a 15-minute period and 3 mg in 1 hour. Flumazenil is contraindicated in the following patients: polysubstance ingestions, prolonged benzodiazepine use, tricyclic antidepressant use, and seizure disorders.

V. **Complications (Table 4–3)**

    A. **Respiratory depression and hypoxia.** Prevent with proper dosing, application of O_2, and if needed, positive pressure ventilation (PPV).

    B. **Laryngospasm.** Give succinylcholine to relieve spasm and then PPV.

    C. **Rigid chest syndrome** is a complication of administration of high doses of fentanyl, which causes difficulty breathing due to chest wall muscle spasm. Use IV naloxone to attempt reversal of fentanyl. If no improvement, use succinylcholine and PPV.

    D. **Vomiting with aspiration.** Have suctioning set up and turn the patient on their side if vomiting occurs.

    E. **Prolonged sedation.** Prevent with proper dosing and avoidance of mixing multiple agents.

Table 4–3. Frequency of adverse events that occur in adult procedural sedation.

Complication	Frequency (%)
Desaturation	8
Vomiting	8
Apnea	1
Laryngospasm	0.1

CHAPTER 5
LUMBAR PUNCTURE

I. **Indications.** Suspicion of CNS infection, SAH, or pseudotumor cerebri.

II. **Contraindications**

   A. **Increased ICP** is an absolute contraindication. A non-contrast head CT scan should be performed to rule out a mass before performing an LP in the following clinical situations: AMS, focal neurologic deficits, signs of increased ICP (papilledema), immunocompromise, > age 60, or recent seizure.

   B. **Coagulopathy** and **thrombocytopenia** are relative contraindications. FFP and platelets should be administered before attempting an LP.

   C. **Cellulitis** over the site of needle insertion is an absolute contraindication.

III. **Equipment**

   A. Most EDs have a commercially available LP kit, which contains all of the essential materials except povidone-iodine (Betadine) (Figure 5–1). Kits include 20-gauge spinal needle, 22- and 25-gauge needles for lidocaine administration, 4 collection tubes, stopcock and manometer with extension tubing, sterile drapes (fenestrated, with hole in center, and unfenestrated), skin cleansing sponges, and lidocaine.

   B. Other helpful equipment: additional spinal needles in different lengths and gauges (22 gauge is the smallest needle that can be used to check an accurate opening pressure) and sterile gloves.

IV. **Procedure**

   A. **Position.** The patient should be properly positioned. Lateral decubitus, if opening pressure needs to be assessed. Sitting upright may be easier in obese patients but does not allow an accurate measurement of the opening pressure.

   B. **Anatomy.** The bony landmarks are palpated before the field is made sterile. An imaginary line is made that connects the iliac crests. This line should cross the L4 interspace in the midline. The spinous processes in this area are palpated and the L3–L4 and L4–L5 interspaces are located. Either of these spaces can be used for the procedure (Figure 5–2).

   C. **Sterile technique.** The kit is opened and povidone-iodine is poured into the empty receptacle on the tray. Put on sterile gloves. Cleanse the area with the 3 sponges soaked with povidone-iodine. Use a circular motion, beginning over the penetration site and spreading outward about 10 cm. Place the unfenestrated drape on the patient's bed and the fenestrated drape on the patient's back.

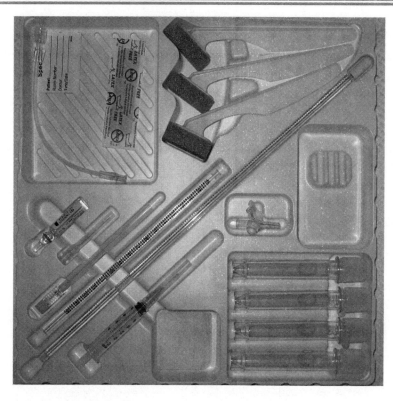

Figure 5–1. Lumbar puncture kit.

D. **Local anesthetic.** Using the 25-gauge needle, raise a skin wheal of lidocaine over the interspace and use the 22-gauge needle to anesthetize the deeper tissues along the approximate line that the spinal needle will pass.

E. **Procedure.** Place the spinal needle between the spinous processes. The needle should be parallel with the bed and directed cephalad about 10°. The bevel should be oriented parallel to the fibers of the dura, which run cephalad to caudad (for lateral decubitus bevel up; for sitting position bevel left or right). By inserting the needle in this fashion, the dural fibers are "spread" apart rather than cut. Theoretically, this will reduce the risk of persistent CSF leak and subsequent post-LP headache. Resistance will be felt as the needle passes through the subcutaneous tissues and interspinous ligaments. A "pop" may be felt as the subarachnoid space is entered. Remove the stylet, and CSF should flow freely. If bone is encountered, remove the needle to the subcutaneous tissues and redirect the needle slightly more cephalad. ***Never advance or remove the needle without the stylet in place.***

F. **Opening pressure** can be assessed by attaching the extension tubing to the needle and then to the manometer. With the base of the manometer and the needle at the same height, the stopcock is opened, allowing the manometer to fill. A normal opening pressure in adults is 10–20 cm H_2O. In adults, 1–2 mL of CSF is col-

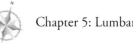

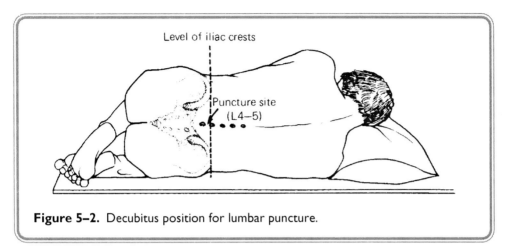

Level of iliac crests

Puncture site
(L4–5)

Figure 5–2. Decubitus position for lumbar puncture.

lected sequentially in tubes 1–4. More tubes may be needed for additional tests or special situations. The needle should be removed with the stylet in place. The patient should remain supine for 1 hour.

V. **Complications**

A. **Bleeding.** Traumatic LP is a common occurrence, with more than half of all LP procedures having from 1 to 50 RBCs in the CSF. The only way to differentiate a traumatic LP from an SAH is noting that the number of RBCs significantly decrease from tube 1, approaching zero in tube 4. Also, the presence of xanthochromia indicates an SAH. Spinal hematomas (epidural or subdural) can form in patients with coagulation disorders.

B. **Herniation** can occur when CSF is removed from a patient with increased ICP from a mass lesion.

C. **Post-LP headaches** are the most common complication of LP, and are thought to be from continued CSF leakage at the puncture site. In most cases, the headache begins within 24–48 hours and is usually postural (worse in the upright position). IV fluids, caffeine (IV or PO), or antiemetics may help improve symptoms. An anesthesiologist may perform a blood patch if the headache has been present > 24 hours, which is helpful in most patients. More serious headaches rarely occur post-LP. Subdural hematomas are due to tearing of bridging veins from decreased CSF volume. This should be suspected when the headache lasts > 1 week, recurs after initially resolving, or if the headache does not have a postural component.

CHAPTER 6
LACERATION REPAIR

I. Indications and Definitions

A. **Wound healing** occurs by primary, secondary, or tertiary intention. **Primary intention** is the most common method of repair and involves the approximation of wound edges soon after the injury with the use of sutures, staples, tape, or tissue adhesive. In **secondary intention,** the wound is cleaned but left open and allowed to heal spontaneously. This method is used when the risk of infection after primary closure is high. **Tertiary intention** (delayed primary closure) decreases infection rate in highly contaminated wounds. It is performed by cleaning and débriding contaminated wounds acutely, then suturing the wound after 3–5 days.

B. Healing wounds contract and reorganize with the deposition of collagen fibrils that gradually increase the strength of the scar. The tensile strength of a wound increases over the following year, never reaching the strength of the skin prior to injury.

C. One week after injury, at a time when most sutures are removed, the wound possesses only 5–10% of its original tensile strength. By the end of the first year, 70–80% is restored.

II. Contraindications

A. The decision to repair a laceration primarily is based on many factors, which can be divided broadly into **host** and **wound** factors.

B. **Host factors** include
   1. **Age** (elderly patients have 3–4 times higher rate of infection).
   2. **Malnutrition.**
   3. **Immunocompromise** (eg, diabetes mellitus).

C. **Wound factors** include
   1. **Timing.** Bacterial counts begin to increase 3–6 hours post-injury, and every attempt is made to close wounds within this "golden period."
   2. **Location.** Wounds of the face and scalp rarely become infected (1–2%) due to an excellent blood supply, and may be safely closed 24–48 hours after injury. Infection rates of upper (4%) and lower (7%) extremity wounds are higher.
   3. **Mechanism.** Lacerations sustained by a blunt, crushing force produce more local tissue damage and therefore have a higher rate of infection than lacerations caused by a sharp instrument (ie, knife). A puncture wound also has a high rate of infection because bacteria are driven into the tissue and are difficult to remove.

4. Contamination. Visible contamination within a wound doubles the likelihood of infection. Bite wounds (eg, dog, cat, human) have a very high rate of infection due to bacterial colonization within the mouth. Generally, bite wounds are not closed primarily unless the wound is gaping or in a cosmetically sensitive area (eg, face).

III. Equipment

A. **Wound preparation.** Povidone-iodine solution, local anesthetic (1% buffered lidocaine with/without epinephrine), 25- or 27-gauge needle, and a syringe. Irrigation with NS or sterile water, 60 cc syringe, and an irrigation shield or 18-gauge angiocatheter.

B. **Wound closure.** Traditionally, sterile gloves are used, although a recent study did not show a decreased infection rate when sterile gloves were used compared to clean gloves in the repair of clean wounds < 6 hours old. Instruments include a needle driver, tissue forceps (pick-ups), and scissors (Figure 6–1). Use the smallest

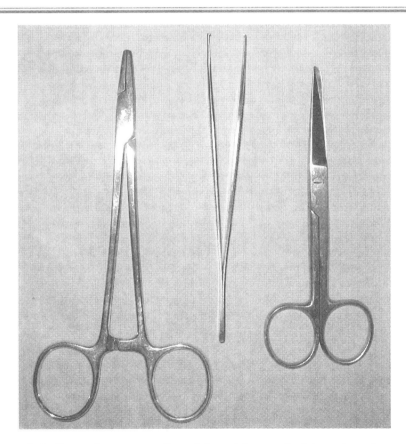

Figure 6–1. Suture instruments. From left to right, needle driver, tissue forceps (pick-ups), and scissors.

monofilament suture available that will adequately appose the ends of the laceration. Usually 4–0 (largest, torso and extremities) to 6–0 (smallest, face) will suffice. Other effective methods to approximate lacerations include staples for scalp lacerations and tissue adhesive. Tissue adhesives should not be used near mucosal surfaces, within the scalp, or over joints (without immobilization).

C. **Wound aftercare.** Antibacterial ointment, gauze, and tape.

IV. Procedure

A. **Wound Preparation**

1. **Examination.** A thorough neurovascular examination is required for all wounds prior to administration of local anesthesia. Tendon function must also be assessed, when appropriate. Wound exploration may detect foreign bodies and diagnose injuries to deeper structures. If the depth of the wound is not easily appreciated and a foreign body is suspected (ie, patient fell on broken glass), then a plain radiograph is recommended. Glass fragments > 2 mm are almost universally visualized on plain radiographs. Plastic and wood foreign bodies are not radiopaque and may require further imaging (CT scan, ultrasound, or MRI).

2. **Local anesthesia.** The edges of the wound are prepped with povidone-iodine solution. Care should be taken not to get the solution in the wound itself, as this inhibits healing. Draw up 1% buffered lidocaine into a syringe using a 25- or 27-gauge needle. Buffering the lidocaine with bicarbonate and using a small needle reduce the pain of injection. Lidocaine is infiltrated within the wound edges and around the entire wound (field block). In contaminated wounds, puncture the skin around the laceration (theoretical lower risk of infection); in clean wounds, puncture the wound edge within the wound itself (decreases pain of injection). Remember, the maximum dose of lidocaine without epinephrine is 4 mg/kg. This equates to 280 mg in a 70-kg (154 lb) man or 28 mL of 1% lidocaine (10 mg per mL). Lidocaine with epinephrine has a maximum dose of 7 mg/kg. The addition of epinephrine is also advantageous, because it decreases bleeding and increases the duration of anesthetic.

3. **Irrigation.** Wound irrigation and debridement of devitalized tissues are the 2 most important ways to decrease the incidence of wound infection. When irrigating a wound, use a commercially available shield to avoid accidental exposure to the healthcare worker and create the required pressure to decrease bacterial counts. If unavailable, an 18-gauge angiocatheter with a 60 mL syringe can be used. Irrigation with a saline bag or bottle with holes punched into the top does not create enough pressure to adequately reduce bacterial counts. The amount of saline required to irrigate a wound is not known, but a basic guideline is to use 50–100 mL for each 1 cm of laceration.

B. **Wound Closure**

1. **Simple sutures** (Figure 6–2). A few principles should be considered when placing simple sutures. Clamp the needle driver in the middle of the needle. (Grasping the end of the needle will damage the cutting edge and make suturing more difficult.) Insert the needle at 90° to help evert the tissue. Eversion permits more rapid epithelialization than inversion and avoids a scar that is depressed after contraction. The tissue forceps are used to lift up the skin on one side of the laceration. Grasping the tissue too tightly (especially when using forceps with teeth) may damage the tissue, and should be avoided. When the nee-

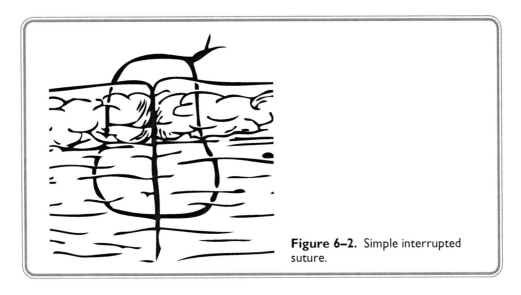

Figure 6–2. Simple interrupted suture.

dle is inserted, maintain the same depth as the other side. Use 4 to 5 instrument ties to secure the knot. Avoid pulling the wound edges too tightly because this may strangulate the wound edges, reducing blood supply. Remember that the tissues will continue to swell after suturing.

2. **Mattress sutures** (Figures 6–3 and 6–4). These sutures can be placed vertically or horizontally. Both provide excellent wound eversion and help to better approximate wound edges that are under tension and difficult to pull together. Vertical mattress sutures are especially useful in lacerations where there is minimal subcutaneous tissue for deep sutures. In addition, these sutures will help stop bleeding from a scalp laceration. The disadvantage of these sutures is that they may strangulate the tissues.

3. **Deep sutures** (Figure 6–5). The deep suture should be placed with absorbable suture material. To get the knot to the depth of the wound, make the first pass of the needle from the deep portion of the wound to the superficial portion. Avoid infection by placing only deep enough sutures to effectively bring the wound edges together and cut the suture as close to the knot as possible.

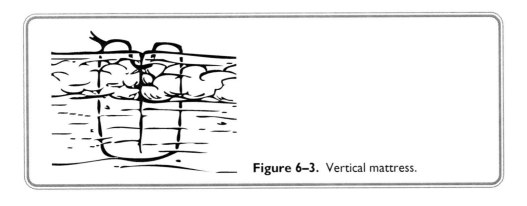

Figure 6–3. Vertical mattress.

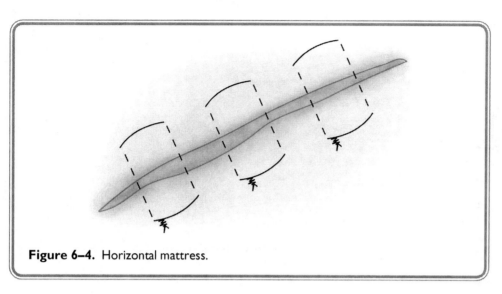

Figure 6–4. Horizontal mattress.

C. Wound Aftercare

1. Antibiotics. Topical antibiotic ointments provide a moist environment that assists epithelization and reduces the rate of infection. Prophylactic oral antibiotics are recommended for heavily contaminated wounds, significant animal or human bites, areas prone to infection (mouth, plantar aspect of the foot), open fractures, tendon or joint involvement, immunocompromised host, history of a heart valve replacement, or deep puncture wounds.

2. Tetanus. In patients with full childhood immunizations, tetanus toxoid, given with diphtheria toxoid (Td 0.5 cc IM), is administered after a minor, clean wound if the last booster was > 10 years ago. In all other wounds (contaminated, puncture, crush), tetanus toxoid is given if the last booster was > 5 years ago. Tetanus immune globulin (TIG) is administered to patients with a history of < 3 immunizations and a contaminated wound.

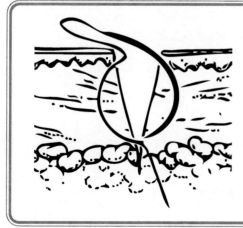

Figure 6–5. Deep dermal stitch. On the first pass, the needle enters at the depth of the wound so that the knot will end up at the bottom of the wound.

3. **Dressing.** Apply a topical ointment (eg, bacitracin) and then a sterile dressing. The dressing may be removed in 24 hours and the wound can be gently cleansed with soap and water, using caution to blot the sutures dry.
4. **Suture removal** in 3–5 days for face and neck; 7–10 days for upper extremity, chest, legs, and scalp; and 10–14 days for hand, back, buttocks, foot, and overlying joints.

V. Complications

A. **Infection.** Despite all efforts to reduce the risk of infection, this complication can still occur. The patient should be instructed to return upon the first signs of infection. Some patients with high-risk wounds should be asked to return to the ED within 24–48 hours to have the wound re-examined by a physician.

B. **Scarring.** Patients should be instructed that a scar will form with healing. Scarring is more significant after full-thickness wounds and when absorbable sutures are used.

CHAPTER 7
NEEDLE AND TUBE THORACOSTOMY

I. Indications

A. **Needle thoracostomy** for suspected tension pneumothorax.

B. **Tube thoracostomy** after needle thoracostomy for simple pneumothorax, traumatic hemothorax, or large pleural effusion with respiratory compromise.

II. Contraindications.

Always be sure that the suspected pneumothorax seen on CXR is not actually a pulmonary bullae or bleb. These are gas-filled spaces with thin walls in which lung parenchyma has been destroyed and alveolar size is greatly increased, sometimes mimicking a pneumothorax. Bullae tend to be localized in the upper lung fields, with normal lung markings to the periphery in the lower lung fields.

III. Equipment

A. **Needle thoracostomy.** 12- to 16-gauge angiocatheter (length 3 to 4 inches) and 5–10 ml syringe.

B. **Tube thoracostomy.** 36–40 French tube for hemothorax in adults (20–24 Fr in children); 18–28 French tube for simple pneumothorax in adults (14–16 Fr in children). (1 French = 0.33 mm). Povidone-iodine (Betadine), sterile field, sterile gloves, 20 mL of 1% lidocaine with epinephrine, scalpel with #10 blade, large curved and straight clamp, needle driver, and 2-0 silk suture.

IV. Procedure

A. **Needle thoracostomy.** Insert the catheter in the 2nd intercostal space (just over the rib) at the midclavicular line. If there is a sudden rush of air or improvement of patient vital signs, tension pneumothorax is confirmed. The procedure should be followed by chest tube placement.

B. **Tube Thoracostomy**

1. **Preparation.** Position the patient with the arm on the affected side placed above the head with a soft restraint. Prepare the chest wall with povidone-iodine and a sterile field in the area of the 5th intercostal space at the mid to anterior axillary line.

2. **Anesthesia.** Anesthetize the skin with lidocaine, then the deeper structures tunneling up over the 5th rib. Then, inject the intercostal muscles of the 4–5 interspace and through into the parietal pleura (3–4 mL). Procedural sedation or intercostal nerve block may also be used.

3. **Tube placement.** Make a 2–3 cm incision over the 5th rib between the mid and anterior axillary lines (Figure 7–1A). Using the large curved clamp, tunnel through the soft tissues up over the 5th rib to the 4–5 intercostal space. Puncture through the intercostal muscles with the curved clamp, being careful not to penetrate the pleural cavity too deeply (Figure 7–1B). Open the jaws of the clamp to widen the hole in the intercostals and slowly remove the clamp. Insert a gloved finger through the tract and into the pleural cavity, making sure there are no lung adhesions (Figure 7–1C). Using either a finger or the curved clamp, insert the chest tube into the thorax, directing it posterior and superior and making sure that all holes of the tube are within the thorax (Figure7–1D).
4. **Aftercare.** Attach the tube to a suction device (Figure 7–2). Secure the tube by placing a simple interrupted suture inferior to the tube. After tying a knot, use the remaining suture to wrap around the tube several times and tie a second knot. Close the skin above the tube with a simple interrupted suture. Cover with Vaseline gauze and a bandage. Order a CXR to check tube position and lung re-expansion (Figure 7–3).

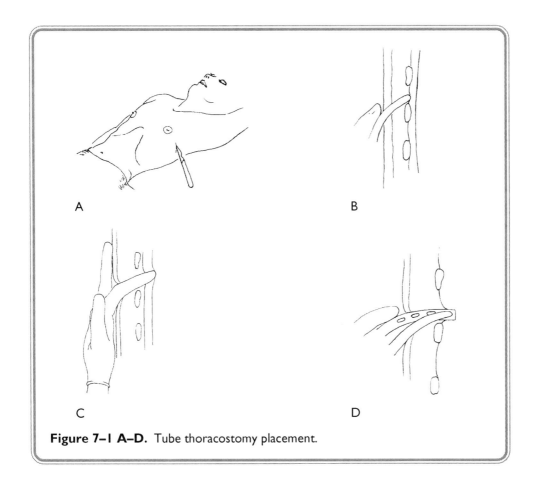

Figure 7–1 A–D. Tube thoracostomy placement.

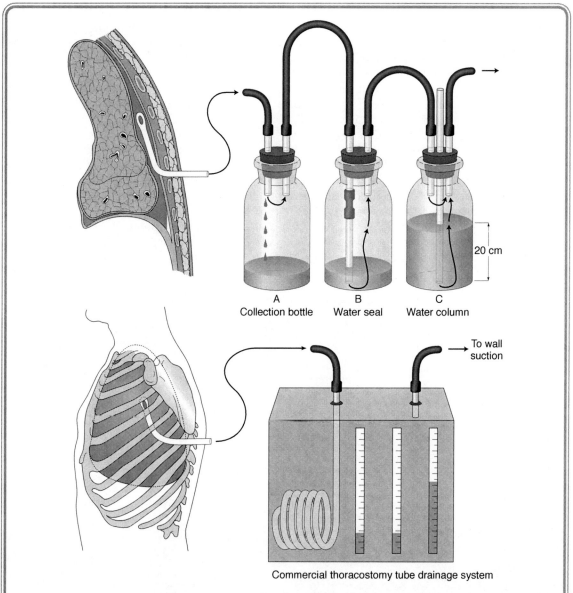

A
Collection bottle

B
Water seal

C
Water column

20 cm

To wall suction

Commercial thoracostomy tube drainage system

Figure 7–2. Diagram of tube thoracostomy and 3-bottle suction apparatus. **Bottle A** is connected to the thoracostomy tube and collects pleural drainage for inspection and measurement of volume. **Bottle B** acts as a simple valve to prevent collapse of the lung if tubing distal to this point is opened to atmospheric pressure. Pulmonary air leak can be detected by the escape of bubbles from the submerged tube. **Bottle C** is a system for regulating the negative pressure delivered to the pleural space. Wall suction should be regulated to maintain continuous vigorous bubbling from the middle open tube in bottle C. The resulting negative pressure (in cm H_2O) is equal to the difference in the height of the fluid levels in bottles B and C. The Pleur-evac system works in a similar manner. One end is attached to the chest tube and the other end is attached to suction. Each chamber of the Pleur-Evac id filled with sterile water to the level noted in the manufacturer's instructions.

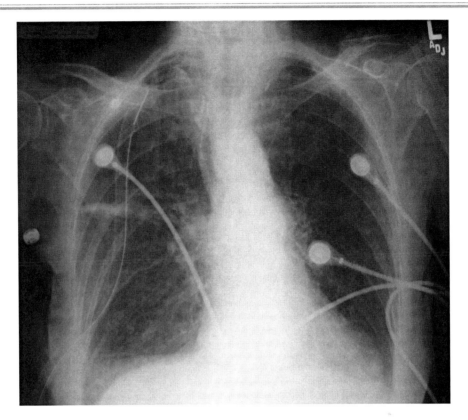

Figure 7–3. Chest x-ray showing the proper position of a chest tube.

Remember that the neurovascular bundle runs inferior to each rib. To avoid it, always enter over the 5th rib and never under.

V. Complications

    A. **Needle thoracostomy.** Unable to evacuate (use a catheter that is 3 to 4.5 inches long).

    B. **Tube Thoracostomy**

        1. **Infection.** Never advance or replace a tube if it has migrated out of the chest. Place a new tube.

        2. **Bleeding.**

        3. **Iatrogenic injury** to lung or abdominal organs.

        4. **Incorrect tube placement** (kinked tube, subcutaneous placement, drainage holes outside thorax, non-draining tube, or persistent air leak).

        5. **Re-expansion pulmonary edema,** a rare complication, is more common when the lung is completely collapsed for several days. Avoid by placing tube to water seal when lung is completely collapsed allowing gradual re-expansion.

CHAPTER 8
ULTRASONOGRAPHY

I. **Indications.** Emergency physicians perform and interpret "limited ED ultrasound" (US) examinations to answer specific clinical questions as part of the physical examination. Emergency US has the following applications

  A. **Abdominal and chest trauma.** The Focused Assessment with Sonography for Trauma (FAST) scan evaluates for blood in the pericardial, pleural, and peritoneal compartments.

  B. **Ectopic pregnancy.** US can assess pregnant patients in the first trimester who have pelvic pain, bleeding, or syncope. An intrauterine pregnancy rules out an ectopic pregnancy in the majority of patients.

  C. **Abdominal aortic aneurysm.** In the hypotensive patient with abdominal pain, US can quickly assess for the presence of an AAA. When present, rupture is the likely cause of hypotension. In addition, in patients with nonspecific abdominal or low back pain, a normal aorta on US rules out AAA without the need for a CT scan.

  D. **Acute cholecystitis.** Up to 20% of patients with RUQ pain in the absence of fever and elevated WBC count have evidence of acute cholecystitis on US, requiring admission for IV antibiotics and cholecystectomy.

  E. **Hydronephrosis.** In the uncomplicated patient with flank pain and hematuria, mild to moderate hydronephrosis supports the diagnosis of nephrolithiasis without the need for further imaging.

  F. **Procedural applications.** Placement of peripheral and central lines, abscess and foreign body localization, interspace visualization for LP, and US guidance of pericardiocentesis, thoracentesis, and paracentesis.

II. **Contraindications.** Relative contraindications include patient obesity and physician inexperience. If the specific clinical question is not answered or unexpected findings are encountered, then always proceed to the next test. Emergency medicine US is a diagnostic and procedural tool, not a replacement for definitive testing.

III. **Equipment**

  A. US is analogous to a submarine's sonar system. Sound waves are emitted by the US probe, travel through tissue, are reflected off structures, and then return to the probe. Travel time is translated by the computer into depth within the body.

Strength of returning echos is translated into brightness or intensity of the structure on the display.

B. **Sound** is a series of repeating pressure waves. Audible sound is in 16–20,000 cycle/sec or Hz range, while diagnostic US uses sound waves in the 2–12 MHz range (million cycles/sec).

C. **Probes** send out and receive information via the piezoelectric or the pressure-electricity effect. The probe relies on a complex, delicate, and expensive arrangement of crystals. When electricity is applied to these crystals, sound waves are emitted. Returning sound waves are translated back into electricity by the probe.

D. **Frequency.** The higher the frequency of sound waves emitted by the probe, the greater the tissue resolution, but the lower the depth of penetration. Different types of probes exist for different clinical questions. Low-frequency probes (2–5 MHz) are used in transabdominal imaging to visualize deeper structures in the abdomen. High-frequency probes (8–10 MHz) are used in procedural applications, such as central line placement, to visualize more superficial structures with more detailed resolution.

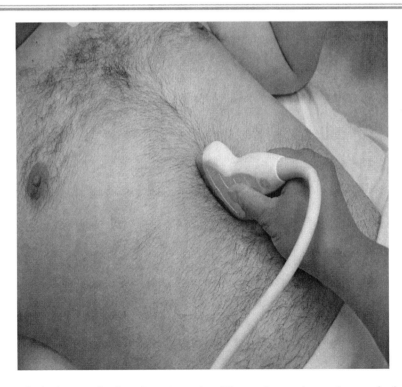

Figure 8–1. Longitudinal probe orientation. The probe marker points to the head of the patient.

E. **Echogenicity.** Images are described in terms of echogenicity. Dense bone is highly reflective, appearing bright or **hyperechogenic.** Less dense organ parenchyma appears grainy or echogenic. Fluid-filled structures or acute bleeding do not reflect, appearing black or **anechogenic.** Air has an irregular reflective surface and appears as scatter on the US monitor.

F. **Orientation.** A marker on the US probe corresponds to an indicator on the screen. By accepted standard in emergency medicine and radiology, the indicator is always on the left side of the screen. In the sagittal (longitudinal) anatomic plane, the probe marker is pointed at the patient's head, resulting in the head being displayed towards the left side of the screen and the feet towards the right (Figure 8–1). In the coronal (transverse) anatomic plane, the probe marker is pointed at the patient's right resulting in the patient's right side being displayed on the left side of the screen, similar to viewing a CT scan image (Figure 8–2).

G. **Modes.** The most commonly used mode is the brightness (B) mode on the US machine. Other modes include the motion (M) mode, often used to measure the fetal heartbeat, and the Doppler mode to measure blood flow.

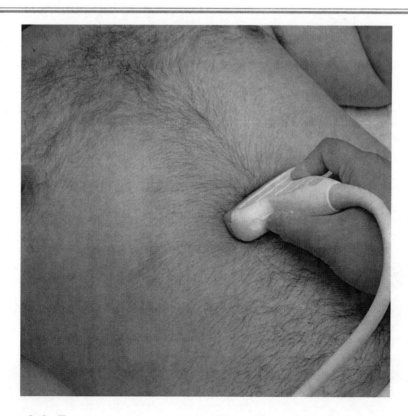

Figure 8–2. Transverse probe orientation. The probe marker points to the right of the patient.

IV. Procedure: FAST Scan

A. **Subxiphoid view.** The probe is placed in the transverse anatomic plane with the marker to the patient's right and is aimed at the patient's left shoulder. Blood between the visceral and pleural pericardial layers will appear anechogenic or black (Figure 8–3).

B. **RUQ view.** The probe is placed in the midaxillary line in the 10–12th interspace with the marker to the patient's head. Examine for blood in the right hemithorax, the hepatorenal fossae (Morison's pouch), and the inferior paracolic gutter. Morison's pouch is the most dependent portion of the abdominal cavity above the pelvis and the most common site to visualize free intraperitoneal fluid (ie, blood) (Figure 8–4).

C. **LUQ view.** The probe is placed in the posterior axillary line in the 9–10th interspace with the marker to the patient's head. Examine for blood in the left hemithorax, the subphrenic space, the splenorenal space, and the left inferior paracolic gutter.

D. **Pelvic view.** The probe is initially placed longitudinally in the midline just above the pubic symphysis. Examine for blood in the retrouterine pouch of Douglas in the female or in the retrovesicular space in the male.

V. Complications.

Complications may arise from inadequate visualization of structures or image misinterpretation, but usually do not occur because of the procedure itself.

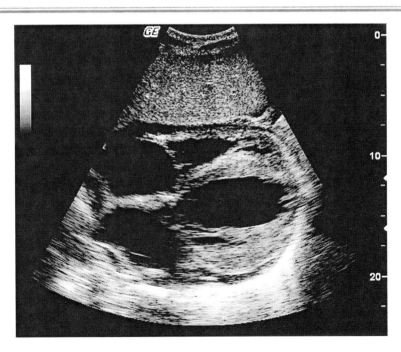

Figure 8–3. Subxiphoid view showing a pericardial effusion.

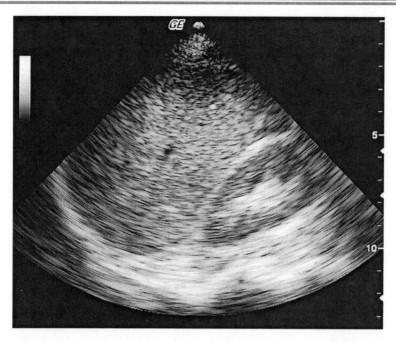

Figure 8–4. Right upper quadrant view showing Morison's pouch between the liver and kidney. No free fluid is present.

SECTION II
RESUSCITATION

CHAPTER 9
CARDIOPULMONARY ARREST

I. Defining Features

A. Cardiopulmonary arrest is defined by the triad of unconsciousness, apnea, and pulselessness.

B. **Sudden cardiac death** (SCD) is an unexpected natural death from a cardiac cause that occurs suddenly in a person without a prior condition that would appear to be fatal. SCD can occur as a result of ventricular fibrillation (VF), pulseless ventricular tachycardia (VT), pulseless electrical activity (PEA), or asystole.

C. **Asystole** is present when there is no discernible electrical activity on the cardiac monitor and there is no pulse. **PEA** is present when there is electrical activity on the cardiac monitor, but there is no discernible pulse.

II. Epidemiology

A. It is estimated that SCD accounts for about 15% of all deaths in the United States.

B. The risk of SCD is increased 6 to 10 times in the patient with known heart disease. The presence of coronary risk factors increases the risk of SCD 4-fold.

C. Although many advances have occurred in the field of cardiac resuscitation, the rate of survival of out-of-hospital SCD remains low, at 3–8%.

D. Survival to hospital discharge in out-of hospital cardiac arrest is predicted by the initial rhythm. Patients with an initial rhythm of VF are > 15 times more likely to survive than patients in asystole (34% vs. 0–2%).

III. Pathophysiology

A. **Atherosclerotic coronary artery disease** (CAD). CAD is present in 65–70% of all cases of SCD.

B. **Structural heart disease.** Patients with both acquired (heart failure, left ventricular hypertrophy, myocarditis) and hereditary (cardiomyopathy) structural heart disease account for approximately 10% of cases of SCD.

C. **No structural heart disease.** About 10% of cases of SCD are found in patients with no structural heart disease or CAD. These cases of SCD are thought to originate from several different pathologic etiologies, including Brugada syndrome, commotio cordis, prolonged QT syndrome, and familial VT.

IV. Risk Factors

A. Various risk factors are associated with an increased risk of SCD. Smoking, diabetes mellitus, hypertension, dyslipidemia, and a family history of cardiac disease increase risk for SCD.

B. Moderate alcohol intake of 1–2 drinks daily is protective for SCD, while heavy alcohol consumption of > 6 drinks daily increases the risk.

C. SCD, like MI, is more likely to occur within the first few hours after awakening, due to the body's sensitivity to sympathetic stimulation during this time period.

V. Clinical Presentation

A. **History**
   1. Obtain from paramedics or any available family members.
   2. Inquire about medications, past medical history, allergies, trauma, or events leading up to SCD.

B. **Physical Examination**
   1. Check ABCs.
   2. If the patient presents with an ET tube in place, ensure that it is positioned properly by listening to breath sounds.
   3. Continue CPR as outlined.

KEY COMPLAINTS

Obtain a thorough history from family members, paramedics, or other witnesses.

VI. Differential Diagnosis

A. **PEA** (5Hs and 5Ts)
   1. Hypovolemia, hypoxia, hydrogen ion (acidosis), hypothermia, and hyperkalemia.
   2. Tablets (drug overdose), tamponade (cardiac), tension pneumothorax, thrombosis (pulmonary embolism), and thrombosis (acute coronary syndrome).

B. Structural cardiac abnormalities (ie, cardiomyopathies, valvular disorders, myocarditis).

C. Electrophysiologic cardiac abnormalities (ie, prolonged QT syndrome, Wolff-Parkinson-White syndrome, Brugada's syndrome).

VII. Diagnostic Findings

A. **Laboratory Studies**
   1. **ABG** during a cardiac arrest is rarely helpful; however, an exception is if hyperkalemia is suspected.
   2. If pulse and BP can be detected in the patient, obtain CBC, electrolytes, renal function, and myocardial markers.

B. **Imaging studies.** If the patient regains a pulse and BP, obtain a **CXR** to check placement of the ET tube and an **ECG** to look for evidence of cardiac ischemia.

C. **Procedures**
   1. **Pericardiocentesis.** Indicated when there is suspicion of cardiac tamponade in the setting of PEA. Bedside ultrasound should be considered in these cases. The procedure requires a long spinal needle and a 60-mL syringe. The needle is inserted subxiphoid, aiming to the left shoulder. Pull back on the syringe plunger while advancing the needle until blood is obtained.

2. **Needle thoracostomy.** Indicated when there is suspicion of tension pneumothorax in the setting of PEA (see Chapter 7).

D. **Diagnostic Algorithm**

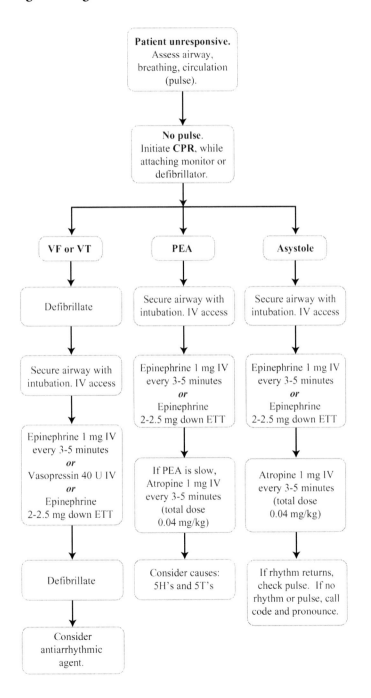

VIII. Treatment

A. The resuscitative team must orchestrate simultaneous assessment and management of patients in cardiopulmonary arrest.

B. **Defibrillation** is indicated for patients in VF or pulseless VT (Figure 9–1). A success rate of defibrillation within 1 minute of VF is > 90%, but this rate falls 10% with each passing minute.

C. **Airway.** In a hospital setting, the step after immediate defibrillation is airway control. The most common airway obstruction is due to the tongue falling back against the posterior pharynx. This can be managed immediately by using the jaw thrust or chin lift maneuver. Endotracheal intubation is the definitive airway management technique used for patients in cardiac arrest.

D. **Breathing.** After the airway is cleared, the rescuer looks, listens, and feels for an exchange of air. BVM ventilation is required prior to intubation if no spontaneous respirations are present.

E. **Circulation.** The carotid pulse is most reliable in low flow states. If no pulse is detected, CPR should be initiated. The cardiac output generated by CPR is < 10–30% of normal and drops precipitously with each passing minute. Recent studies clearly indicate that survival is *greatly increased* when **chest compressions** are performed properly (depth 1.5–2 inches and frequency > 100/min) and *greatly decreased* when there is significant **delay or interruption.**

F. **Pharmacologic Therapy**
   1. **Vasopressors.** The current recommended dose of **epinephrine** is 1 mg initially, with repeated doses every 3–5 minutes. "High-dose" epinephrine has

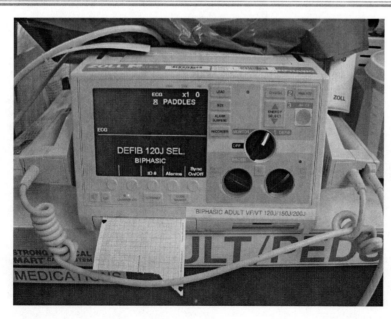

Figure 9–1. Defibrillator.

been shown to be of no benefit and potentially harmful. When IV access cannot be established, epinephrine can be given in the ET tube in a dose 2 to 2.5 times normal. **Vasopressin** (antidiuretic hormone) has been shown in clinical trials to improve return of spontaneous circulation (ROSC) in patients in cardiac arrest, but to be of no benefit over epinephrine in improving survival to hospital discharge. The dose of vasopressin is 40 units IV as a single bolus. The half-life is 10–20 minutes.

2. **Antiarrhythmic agents.** Suppress ectopic electrical activity of the heart and thus improve myocardial function in patients with VT or VF. **Amiodarone** 300 mg IV push in cardiopulmonary arrest. **Lidocaine** 1.5 mg/kg IV may be repeated once. **Procainamide** 17 mg/kg IV at a rate no faster than 50 mg/min. **Magnesium** 1–2 g IV over a 5-minute period in patients with torsades de pointes.

G. **Do Not Resuscitate** (DNR)
  1. If there is a clear advanced directive in writing, signed by the patient or medical power of attorney for the patient, stating that resuscitative efforts are not to be instituted.
  2. If resuscitation would be futile because the patient shows clear signs of irreversible death (decapitation, rigor).

IX. Disposition

A. Once the patient has ROSC, underlying conditions leading to the arrest must be managed for optimal outcome.

B. If ACS is the presumed diagnosis, all therapies and, especially PCI, should be considered.

C. All patients who survive a cardiopulmonary arrest should be admitted to an ICU.

CASE PRESENTATION

The paramedics call the ED to say that they are bringing in a 65-year-old man who was found unresponsive in a casino. Witnesses say that the patient collapsed without warning while playing the slot machines.

1. *The patient arrives at the ED. What should your initial approach to this patient include?*
  - *Assess ABCs. If no pulse, initiate and continue CPR while placing the defibrillator pads/paddles on the patient.*
2. *The defibrillator pads are secured to the patient. Describe your approach now.*
  - *Assess rhythm. If VF/pulseless VT, then attempt defibrillation. Continue CPR and secure the airway if defibrillation is unsuccessful.*

SUMMARY POINTS

- *SCD is the most common cause of nontraumatic death in the United States.*
- *It is usually due to underlying cardiac disease, in particular acute coronary ischemia.*
- *The survival rate is dependent on the length of time without a pulse, the underlying cardiac rhythm, and any co-morbid disease.*
- *VF has the highest rate of ROSC when compared to other rhythms.*
- *Early and uninterrupted chest compressions and early defibrillation are the keys to success in CPR.*

CHAPTER 10
AIRWAY MANAGEMENT

I. Defining Features

A. Airway management involves the recognition of an inadequate airway, the identification of risk factors that predict a difficult airway, and the techniques used to secure an airway.

B. Criteria for endotracheal intubation include failure to maintain a patent airway; failure to protect the airway from aspiration; failure to maintain adequate gas exchange (hypoxia, hypercarbia); the need to provide therapeutic hyperventilation (increased ICP) or decrease work of breathing (sepsis); or the need for sedation for diagnostic or therapeutic procedures in agitated patients.

C. Risk factors that predict a difficult airway should be assessed prior to attempts at orotracheal intubation, BVM ventilation, and the administration of paralytic agents.

D. Techniques to manage an airway include noninvasive procedures (eg, jaw-thrust and chin-lift maneuvers) and advanced procedures (eg, endotracheal intubation and cricothyrotomy). **Rapid sequence intubation (RSI)** involves the use of pretreatment, induction, and paralytic agents to create the most ideal circumstances to insert an ET tube.

II. Epidemiology.
The prevalence of a patient who cannot be intubated within 3 attempts is between 3% and 5%. The rate of surgical airway placement is approximately 0.6%.

III. Pathophysiology

A. The airway begins at the oral and nasal cavities and continues through the oropharynx. When the laryngoscope blade is properly positioned, the epiglottis, glottis, and vocal cords are seen (Figure 10–1).

B. In children and infants, the tongue is relatively larger in relation to the mandible. The glottis is higher and more anterior, and the epiglottis is larger and more floppy.

IV. Risk Factors

A. **Difficult orotracheal intubation.** Overbite or long upper incisors. Open mouth is < 3 finger breaths; distance from chin to hyoid bone is < 3 finger breaths; and the mandible to thyroid cartilage (thyromental) distance is < 2 finger breaths (3-3-2 rule). Only the soft palate or the hard palate is visible with

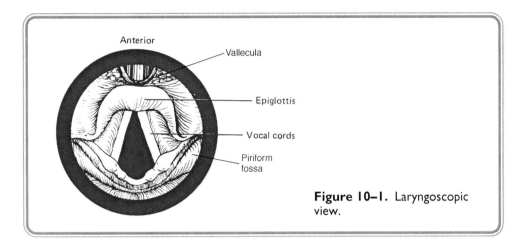

Figure 10–1. Laryngoscopic view.

mouth opening. Decreased cervical ROM or a short and/or thick neck. Airway distortion/obstruction (eg, angioedema).

B. **Difficult BVM ventilation.** The **seal** of the mask is difficult to achieve in patients with beards, no teeth, or facial trauma. Soft tissues obstruct the airway in **obese** patients. **Elderly,** secondary to loss of muscle tone. **High airway resistance,** such as occurs in an asthmatic patient.

V. Clinical Presentation

A. **History**
   1. In emergent situations, the need to perform immediate airway management supersedes the need to obtain a complete history and physical examination.
   2. Perform an airway assessment directed at detecting risk factors for a difficult airway whenever time allows.

B. **Physical Examination**
   1. Inspect the mouth (ie, dentures, size of teeth, view of soft palate). Determine the space available after the mouth is fully opened.
   2. Note the anatomical features of the neck (eg, thyromental distance). Cervical mobility should be tested in the absence of trauma.
   3. Stridor, hoarseness, or the inability to handle secretions is suggestive of airway obstruction.
   4. Gurgling, pooling of secretions, or sonorous respirations implies a lack of airway protection.

VI. Differential Diagnosis. Consider rapidly reversible causes of airway compromise (eg, hypoglycemia and opioid overdose).

VII. Diagnostic Findings

A. **Laboratory studies. ABG** and **pulse oximetry:** depending on the clinical scenario, the presence of normal values on these studies may have no impact on the need to perform an airway intervention. Increasing CO_2 levels in a patient who is clinically failing indicates a need for airway intervention.

B. **Imaging Studies**
   1. There is no imaging study that predicts the need for airway intervention.
   2. Patients with airway obstruction on imaging studies of the neck (plain soft tissue radiographs or CT scan) are likely to be difficult patients to intubate.
   3. **CXR** is indicated in patients with pulmonary conditions and after endotracheal intubation to ensure that the ET tube has not been advanced into the right mainstem bronchus. The end of the ET tube should be 2 cm above the carina.

CLINICAL SKILLS TIP

A patient with airway compromise should never be sent to radiology for imaging studies prior to securing the airway.

C. **Procedures**
   1. **BVM ventilation.** Proper BVM ventilation requires opening the airway and creating a seal with the patient's face (Figure 10–2). When used properly with high flow O_2, this method provides an FiO_2 of approximately 90%. BVM ventilation provides a much higher FiO_2 than the non-rebreather (NRB) mask (60%).
   2. **Oral and nasopharyngeal airways** are utilized to lift the tongue off the hypopharynx and facilitate BVM ventilation.
   3. **RSI** is the induction of anesthesia and paralysis in order to insert an ET tube.
   4. **"Awake" orotracheal intubation.** The suggestion of a difficult airway should prompt the physician to consider "awake" laryngoscopy, wherein the

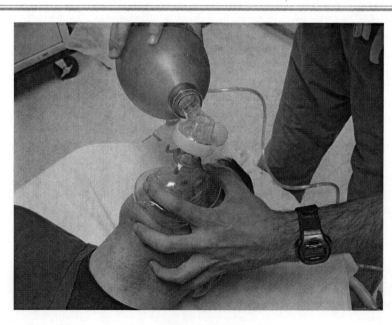

Figure 10–2. Proper method of BVM ventilation.

patient is sedated but not paralyzed. In this situation, the patient is still breathing and to some extent maintaining airway reflexes.

5. **Difficult airway devices** assist in getting the ET tube in the trachea. A **laryngeal mask airway (LMA)** conforms to the contours of the hypopharynx and allows blind insertion into the oropharynx. It is used to ventilate until a definitive airway is established. There is an aspiration risk with this device. **ET introducer (bougie)** is an airway adjunct used when the vocal cords are not well visualized. A bougie is a thin cylinder of plastic or rubber that allows blind placement of the ET tube when it is difficult to visualize the airway because it is anteriorly positioned. Placement in the airway is confirmed by feeling the bougie bump against the tracheal rings (Figure 10–3). The ET tube slides over the bougie, and the bougie is then removed. **Cricothyrotomy** is performed by making an incision in the cricothyroid membrane with insertion of a tracheostomy or small ET tube through the incision and into the airway (Figures 10–4A and 10–4B). It is indicated when other airway attempts have failed, or there is massive facial trauma or total upper airway obstruction. It is contraindicated when the larynx is crushed or there is an expanding neck hematoma. **Other airway techniques** include blind nasotracheal intubation, lighted stylet, Combitube, fiberoptic intubation, retrograde tracheal intubation, and percutaneous translaryngeal ventilation.

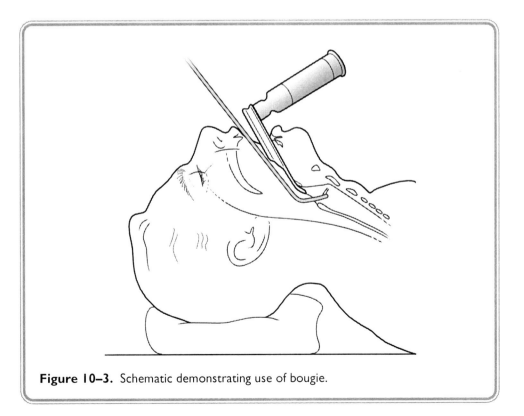

Figure 10–3. Schematic demonstrating use of bougie.

D. **Diagnostic Algorithm**

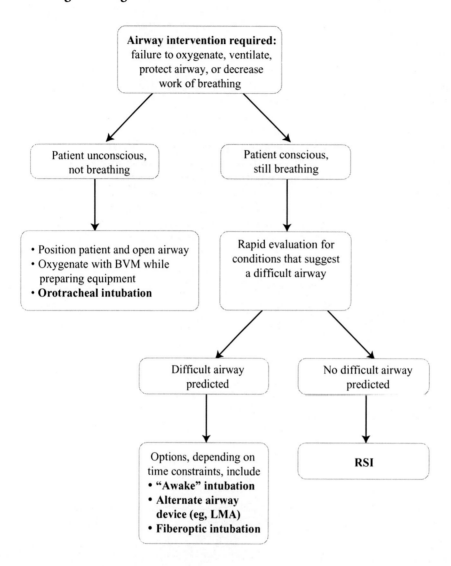

VIII. Treatment

A. **RSI** is performed with the administration of an induction and neuromuscular blocking agent to facilitate endotracheal intubation. Steps to perform RSI include preparation, preoxygenation, pretreatment, induction, paralysis, protection, tube placement, and confirmation.

B. **Preparation** (Figure 10–5). Check the laryngoscope blade light; place a stylet in the ET tube; check the ET tube balloon with a 10-mL syringe; and hook up

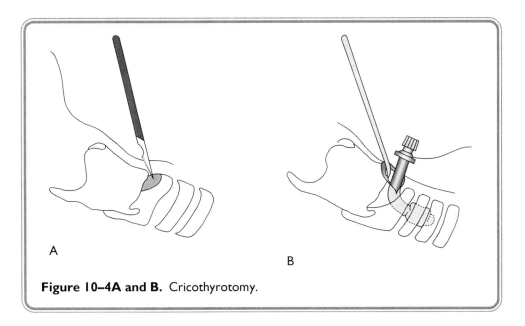

Figure 10–4A and B. Cricothyrotomy.

suction. Different blades are available for laryngoscopy, with most adults requiring a Macintosh 3 or 4 blade. The straight blade (Miller) is useful when the airway is particularly anterior. ET tubes range in diameter from 2.5 mm to 9 mm. In most adult females, a 7.5-mm tube is appropriate, and in adult males, an 8.0 mm tube is used. Smaller, uncuffed tubes are available for children (up to age 8), since the subglottic ring/cricoid cartilage is the narrowest part of the airway. In adult patients, sheets are placed under the head to provide the best position for visualization of the cords. Dentures are removed along with any debris in the mouth or oropharynx.

C. **Preoxygenation.** The patient should be preoxygenated with a BVM. Preoxygenation prevents desaturation during intubation, increasing the time available to insert the ET tube. The ability to preoxygenate depends on the time available and the patient's condition. Positive pressure (ie, squeezing the bag) is not recommended if the patient has adequate spontaneous respirations.

D. **Pretreatment.** Medications are used to attenuate the adverse responses to laryngoscopy and intubation (ie, increase in HR, BP, and ICP). The most common indication for pretreatment is suspected increased ICP. In these patients, a nondepolarizing neuromuscular blocker (eg, pancuronium 0.01mg/kg) and lidocaine (1.5 mg/kg) should be given prior to induction.

E. **Induction** is the process of achieving sedation so that intubation can be accomplished. A variety of induction agents are available, including etomidate (0.3–0.5 mg/kg), thiopental (3–5 mg/kg), ketamine (2 mg/kg), and propofol (1 mg/kg). The preferred agent depends on the clinical scenario. In patients with hypotension or increased ICP, etomidate is the agent of choice. In the setting of reactive airway disease, ketamine should be considered because it causes bronchodilation.

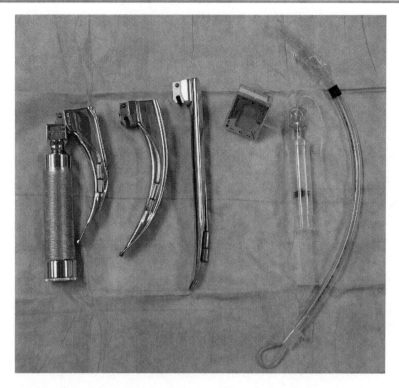

Figure 10–5. Equipment needed for orotracheal intubation in an adult. From left to right, laryngoscope handle attached to Macintosh 3 blade, Macintosh 4 blade, Miller 4 blade, end-tidal CO_2 detector, 10 cc syringe, and endotracheal tube with stylet.

F. **Paralysis** is performed to facilitate orotracheal intubation in patients without risk factors for a difficult airway. It is achieved with neuromuscular blocking agents. Succinylcholine (1–2 mg/kg) is the primary depolarizing agent, commonly used because of its short duration of action. Complete relaxation occurs at 1 minute, with maximal paralysis at 2–3 minutes and loss of effect at approximately 10 minutes. Succinylcholine may increase intraocular pressure and may cause a transient increase in ICP. Succinylcholine is not used in patients with suspected hyperkalemia or denervated musculature (ie, Guillain-Barré syndrome or spinal cord injury). Nondepolarizing paralytic agents (vecuronium, rocuronium, atracurium) produce a longer duration of paralysis (at least 25 min), which may not be desirable, particularly when securing a difficult airway.

G. **Protection.** When the patient is sedated and paralyzed, gentle pressure is applied to the cricoid cartilage (Sellick maneuver) to prevent aspiration and gastric distension. This pressure should be maintained during the entire procedure unless the patient vomits.

H. **Tube placement.** The laryngoscope handle is grasped with the left hand, and the blade is positioned in the oropharynx. The blade is lifted upward and toward the patient's feet until the vocal cords can be seen. The tube is advanced through the cords to a depth (at the teeth) that is 3 times the size of the tube.

I. **Confirmation.** ET tube placement is confirmed by direct visualization of the tube passing through the cords, auscultation, and confirmatory capnometry. Once tube placement is confirmed, secure it firmly to the lips.

IX. **Disposition.** Any patient requiring airway management should be admitted to an ICU setting.

CASE PRESENTATION

A 42-year-old man is brought to the ED after a gunshot wound to the head. The patient does not open his eyes spontaneously and is nonverbal when stimulated. There is pooling of secretions and sonorous respirations. The patient's vital signs are BP 170/90 mm Hg, HR 110 beats/min, RR 8 breaths/min, and pulse oximeter is 98% on an NRB mask. You can find no factors predictive of a difficult airway.

1. What steps are necessary to secure the airway?

  · *Open the airway with jaw thrust. Prepare equipment, preoxygenate with 100% O_2 via BVM, and premedicate with lidocaine and a defasiculating dose of a nondepolarizing paralytic. Administer induction and short-acting paralytic agent. Intubate with ET tube and inflate cuff. Confirm placement with direct visualization, auscultation, and capnometry.*

SUMMARY POINTS

· *The decision to intubate is usually a clinical one.*

· *Time permitting, the patient should be evaluated for risk factors suggestive of a difficult airway.*

· *When an airway intervention has failed and the patient cannot be ventilated, an alternate technique (eg, cricothyrotomy) is indicated.*

CHAPTER 11
SHOCK

I. Defining Features

A. Shock is the inability of the circulatory system to deliver sufficient O_2 and other vital nutrients to meet the metabolic demands of the patient. Although the effects of inadequate tissue perfusion are initially reversible, prolonged O_2 deprivation leads to cellular hypoxia and derangement of critical biochemical processes.

B. **Hypovolemic shock** is due to an inadequate blood volume, most commonly following hemorrhage. Severe dehydration may also result in hypovolemic shock. **Distributive shock** is secondary to a loss of vascular tone (eg, sepsis, adrenal crisis, anaphylaxis, neurogenic shock). **Obstructive shock** results from a blockage of blood flow to the heart (eg, massive pulmonary emboli, pericardial tamponade). **Cardiogenic shock** refers to a state in which the heart is unable to produce forward flow of blood to the tissues. MI is the largest contributor to cardiogenic shock. About 40% of the myocardium must be dysfunctional before cardiogenic shock is evident.

II. Epidemiology

A. In the United States, it is estimated that over 1 million patients a year are brought to the ED to be treated for shock.

B. The most common cause of shock in patients < age 40 is hypovolemia due to traumatic causes. After age 40, septic shock and cardiogenic shock are more prevalent.

C. The mortality rate for cardiogenic shock remains high despite advances in cardiac care.

III. Pathophysiology

A. Shock pathophysiology is divided into 3 basic categories: autonomic response, cellular hypoxia, and inflammatory mediators.

B. **Autonomic response.** The initial insult to tissue is a reduction of O_2 delivery. Cardiac output increases in an attempt to compensate. As O_2 delivery continues to decrease, blood is shunted away from skin, kidneys, muscles, and splanchnic beds. The kidneys activate the renin-angiotensin axis, and the body releases vasoactive substances such as dopamine, cortisol, glucagon, growth hormone, and antidiuretic hormone (ADH). The net effect is to preserve O_2 and nutrient delivery to the most critical organs—the brain and the heart.

C. **Cellular hypoxia.** When O_2 extraction is maximal, cells switch from aerobic to anaerobic metabolism. Anaerobic metabolism does not produce enough ATP to continue regular cellular function. Lactate accumulates, resulting in an acidosis. Eventually, the breakdown in cellular metabolism produces cell death.

D. **Inflammatory mediators.** Hypoxic cells in the vascular endothelium lead to the production of harmful inflammatory mediators. This results in the development of fever, elevated HR, increased RR, and an elevated WBC count.

IV. **Risk Factors.** Elderly, debilitated, immunocompromised (sepsis); CNS trauma (neurogenic); MI (cardiogenic); serious blunt or penetrating trauma (hypovolemic); history of allergic reactions, bee sting (anaphylaxis).

V. **Clinical Presentation**

A. **History**
  1. Vague complaints, such as fatigue and malaise, may be the only presenting symptoms.
  2. AMS due to the high metabolic demands of the brain is not uncommon. History should be obtained from friends, family, or paramedics.
  3. Medications provide information about immunosuppression (eg, steroids, HIV medications), potential allergic reactions, and any underlying medical conditions.

B. **Physical Examination**
  1. **Vital signs.** The body has many means of compensating for shock, so a large percentage of shock patients will present with a normal BP and HR.
  2. **Neurologic examination.** The patient may have AMS.
  3. Other essential components of the physical examination include skin (urticaria, purpura, mottling, increased capillary refill), cardiovascular (jugular venous distention, murmurs, rales), and abdominal examination (peritonitis, pulsating mass). The patient may have decreased urine output.

CLINICAL SKILLS TIP

Abnormalities in vital signs (hypotension, fever, tachycardia, tachypnea) are frequently absent in subtle cases of shock.

VI. **Differential Diagnosis (Table 11–1)**

A. **Hypovolemic shock.** Anemia (severe), aortic aneurysm (ruptured), burns, DKA and hyperglycemic hyperosmolar syndrome, ectopic pregnancy, GI bleed, postpartum hemorrhage, and trauma.

B. **Cardiogenic shock.** Cardiomyopathy, conduction abnormalities or dysrhythmia, MI, myocardial contusion, myocarditis, pericardial tamponade, tension pneumothorax, and valvular dysfunction.

C. **Septic shock.** Abscess and cellulitis, cholangitis and cholecystitis, endocarditis, infected indwelling catheter, meningitis, peritonitis, pneumonia, and UTI.

Table 11–1. SHOCK: differential diagnosis.

Shock Mnemonic
S Septic, spinal (neurogenic)
H Hypovolemic, hemorrhagic
O Obstructive (pulmonary embolism, tamponade)
C Cardiogenic
K Kortisol (adrenal crisis), anaphyla K tic

      D. **Anaphylactic shock.** Drug reaction, food allergy, insect sting, and radiographic contrast material.

      E. **Neurogenic shock.** Spinal cord injury.

VII. **Diagnostic Findings**

    A. **Laboratory Studies**

      1. No single laboratory test is diagnostic of shock.

      2. **CBC** may reveal an elevated, normal, or low WBC count. A differential with a band count >10% (even if the WBC count is normal) suggests an infectious process.

      3. **Electrolytes and renal function.** This will assess kidney function as well as acid-base status. Elevation of the anion gap may be due to lactic acidosis, uremia, or toxic ingestions.

      4. **Lactate.** This test is a sensitive marker of tissue hypoperfusion. In septic shock, a high lactate level predicts mortality. Lactate levels > 4 mmol/L signify continued cellular hypoxia.

      5. **Other tests** useful in the correct clinical scenario include myocardial markers, blood gas analysis, urinalysis, coagulation profile, toxicologic screens, hepatic enzymes, and a pregnancy test. Blood and urine cultures (and possibly CSF) if sepsis is a concern.

    B. **Imaging Studies**

      1. No single radiological test is diagnostic of shock.

      2. **CXR.** Evidence of an infiltrate (sepsis), enlarged cardiac silhouette (cardiac tamponade), free air under the diaphragm (sepsis), heart failure, or pneumothorax may be noted.

      3. **Bedside ultrasound** has been shown to be a simple, effective, and safe tool for assistance in the work-up, treatment, and disposition of the shock patient in the following situations: abdominal trauma, pregnancy, AAA, and pericardial tamponade.

      4. **CT scan** has become the modality of choice for assessing PE, aortic dissection, or intra-abdominal pathology.

C. **Diagnostic Algorithm**

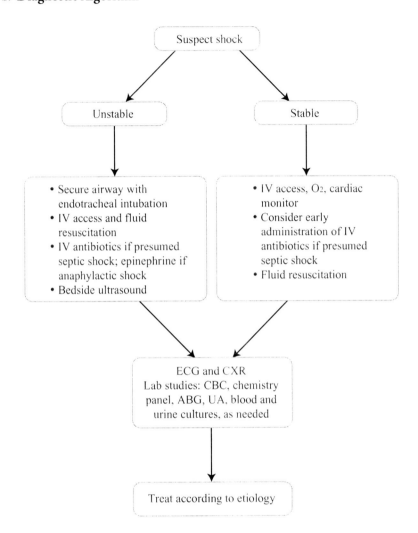

VIII. Treatment

A. The goal of treatment is to restore normal aerobic metabolism.

B. **Airway and breathing.** Supplemental O_2 is provided to all patients. Respiratory muscles can reduce cerebral blood flow by 50% due to shunting of blood to the muscles of respiration. Mechanical ventilation leads to a reduction in the O_2 consumption of the muscles of respiration.

C. **Circulation.** IV access, usually with 2 large bore peripheral lines is initiated. If peripheral lines cannot be placed, central access is established. IV fluids (crystalloid) are administered to replenish an absolute or relative vascular depletion. Blood may be required to improve O_2-carrying capacity. Vasopressors may also be required to assist or maintain the body's inherent hemodynamic parameters. A Foley catheter is used to measure urine output.

D. **Hypovolemic shock.** Administer 2 L bolus of crystalloid, followed by the addition of packed RBCs if the patient remains unstable.

E. **Distributive Shock**
1. **Septic shock.** The goal of treatment is to eradicate infection through early administration of IV antibiotics and/or surgical drainage. IV fluid is the starting point in the resuscitation of the septic patient. If there is no improvement of the shock state with crystalloid resuscitation, pressor therapy is initiated. Norepinephrine is more reliable, rapid, and effective in BP control than dopamine. Many patients in septic shock have a relative adrenal insufficiency. Consider low dose corticosteroid supplementation.
2. **Neurogenic shock.** Atropine is given to counter the unopposed vagal tone, but if ineffective, pressor support is required. Dopamine is recommended.
3. **Anaphylactic shock.** Epinephrine is the drug of choice to treat anaphylaxis. If the patient is in profound shock, 0.1–0.3 mg epinephrine should be administered *IV SLOWLY* over 2–3 minutes to avoid dysrhythmias. Steroids, antihistamines, and IV fluids are administered.

F. **Obstructive Shock**
1. **Pericardial tamponade.** In penetrating thoracic trauma, thoracotomy in the ED is life saving. In the medical setting (eg, renal failure), pericardiocentesis (performed with a long spinal needle and 60 mL syringe) may relieve enough pressure to stabilize the patient for more definitive treatment (ie, pericardial window).
2. **Massive pulmonary embolism.** In contrast to other forms of shock, IV fluid is administered cautiously and may exacerbate symptoms. Norepinephrine is the vasopressor of choice. Thrombolytic therapy is indicated in the hypotensive patients with PE.

G. **Cardiogenic shock.** Initial management consists of judicious fluid administration. Nitrates, β blockers, ACE inhibitors, and antidysrhythmic medications have adverse effects on the myocardium, and their use is contraindicated. Patients who remain hypotensive despite fluid resuscitation require the addition of pressor therapy. If BP is > 80 mm Hg, dobutamine is the agent of choice because it increases contractility and cardiac output; it may exacerbate hypotension, however. For BP in the range of 70–80 mm Hg, dopamine is the recommended vasopressor. When BP is < 70 mm Hg, norepinephrine is recommended. The definitive management of cardiogenic shock is to re-establish perfusion to the myocardium (ie, thrombolytics or PCI) to improve pump function.

IX. **Disposition.** Patients with the diagnosis of shock should be admitted to ICU settings where appropriate clinical and laboratory parameters can be monitored.

CASE PRESENTATION

A 75-year-old woman presents with AMS. At the nursing home where she resides, she was noted to have had a progressive decline in the preceding 12 hours. She has a history of CAD and lymphoma. Her vital signs reveal a HR of 130 beats/min and a systolic BP of 60 mm Hg. She is afebrile, and her RR is 24

breaths/min. She has dry mucous membranes. Cardiovascular examination reveals no murmurs or extra heart sounds. Abdominal examination is normal. Stool sample is brown and positive for blood. No rashes are seen.

1. What are the potential causes of shock in this patient?
   - Septic, hypovolemic (hemorrhagic), cardiogenic.
2. What would be your definitive management if
   - ST elevation on ECG. The definitive management of cardiogenic shock is reperfusion of the myocardium.
   - Urinalysis revealing clumps of WBCs. The management of septic shock is the initiation of antibiotics, fluids, and pressors, if necessary.
   - The patient's hemoglobin is 5 g/dL. The presumptive diagnosis of hemorrhagic shock includes rapid re-establishment of circulating blood volume with crystalloid solutions as well as return of O_2-carrying capacity with blood transfusion.

SUMMARY POINTS

- Do not wait for hypotension to diagnose shock.
- Survival from shock can be improved by early identification and initiation of aggressive therapy.

SECTION III
CARDIOVASCULAR EMERGENCIES

CHAPTER 12
CHEST PAIN

I. Defining Features
   A. Chest pain is one of the most common complaints of patients presenting to the ED.
   B. Diagnosing the etiology of chest pain requires a thorough evaluation in the form of a history and physical examination, ECG, laboratory studies, and radiographic imaging.
   C. Many of the diagnoses in the differential are life-threatening conditions that require rapid diagnosis and treatment.

II. Epidemiology. Acute coronary syndrome (ACS) is the most significant cause of chest pain and is responsible for over 50% of all non-traumatic deaths in the United States.

III. Pathophysiology
   A. **Somatic nerve fibers** innervate the dermis and parietal pleura. Stimulation of these fibers results in pain that is precisely localized and is experienced as a sharp sensation.
   B. **Visceral nerve fibers** are found in internal organs. Because the fibers enter the spinal cord at many levels, pain is imprecisely localized and described as vague, heavy, or aching. Many visceral nerve fibers synapse at the same dorsal root ganglia, leading to radiation of pain to other areas of the body.

IV. Risk Factors
   A. **ACS.** Previous CAD, diabetes mellitus, smoking, hypertension, hypercholesterolemia, family history of heart disease, cocaine use, male gender, and elderly.
   B. **Pulmonary disease.** Previous asthma, COPD, pneumonia, or pneumothorax. Previous pulmonary embolus, DVT, or hypercoagulable state.
   C. **GI disease.** Prior diseases of the gallbladder, pancreas, or esophagus.

V. Clinical Presentation
   A. **Initial Approach**
      1. Ensure adequate ABCs.
      2. Vital signs, in conjunction with general appearance, are the first steps in patient assessment. Alteration of vital signs requires immediate intervention.
      3. The patient should have vascular access, pulse oximetry, supplemental O_2, and cardiac monitoring (Figure 12–1).

61

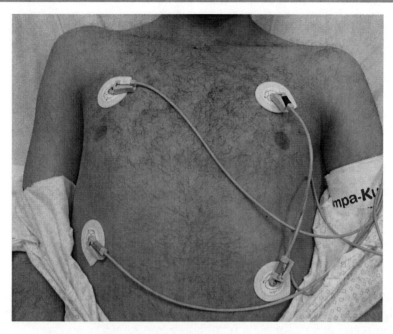

Figure 12–1. Proper placement of cardiac monitor leads. Remember "salt, pepper, ketchup" or "white is right, smoke over fire." Right arm = white; left arm = black; left leg = red; right leg = green. The "leg" leads are commonly placed on the abdomen.

    4. A diagnosis that must not be missed is **tension pneumothorax.** Patients present with chest pain, dyspnea, shock, and unilateral loss of breath sounds. ***Immediate needle decompression followed by tube thoracostomy is required.***

    5. Once immediate life threats are excluded, a more extensive evaluation is performed.

B. **History**

    1. **Character.** Some descriptive terms pertaining to pain include squeezing, crushing, burning, or pressure. Sharp pains are less likely due to cardiac ischemia; however, myocardial sources of chest pain can present with any quality due to its visceral innervation.

    2. **Location.** Substernal or left-sided chest pain is most characteristic of ACS, but pain in other locations does not exclude the diagnosis.

    3. **Radiation.** Radiation of pain to the arms, neck, or jaw is suspicious for myocardial disease. Aortic dissection frequently presents with severe chest pain radiating between the shoulder blades. Myocardial and GI diseases may also cause chest pain that radiates to the back.

    4. **Duration.** Pain that lasts a few minutes with exertion suggests angina. Pain that is constant and lasts several days is less likely to be due to cardiac ischemia.

5. **Exacerbating and alleviating factors.** Exertion increases myocardial O_2 demand and may trigger chest pain in individuals with significant coronary atherosclerosis. Pain that occurs with meals is often related to GI pathology. Pain that is exacerbated by lying down and is alleviated by sitting up and leaning forward suggests pericardial disease. Pleuritic pain may be of pulmonary, cardiac, or musculoskeletal origin.

6. **Associated symptoms** such as diaphoresis, nausea and vomiting, shortness of breath, or syncope should alert the physician to stimulation of visceral nerve fibers. These symptoms are associated with myocardial disease, PE, and aortic dissection.

C. **Physical Examination**

1. **General appearance.** The patient's appearance can give an overall impression of the severity of disease and subsequently the speed at which to pursue the work-up.

2. **Vital signs.** Hypotension suggests the possibility of tension pneumothorax, cardiogenic shock, pericardial tamponade, or a large PE.

3. **Cardiovascular examination.** A significant BP differential (> 20 mm Hg) or pulse discrepancy in the arms or lower extremities is suggestive of aortic dissection. Careful auscultation for new murmurs suggests ACS or aortic dissection. Pericardial friction rub may be auscultated in pericarditis. Elevation of jugular venous pressure is found in tension pneumothorax, pericardial tamponade, ACS, PE, and heart failure.

4. **Lung examination.** Unilateral loss of breath sounds is indicative of a pneumothorax or pleural effusion. Pleural rubs may be appreciated in PE. Subcutaneous emphysema may be present in tension pneumothorax, pneumothorax, or esophageal rupture. Crackles in the lung fields may be due to CHF or a primary pulmonary focus of infection or MI.

5. **Abdominal examination.** Examination of the abdominal area is often neglected in the patient with chest pain. GI pathology may present primarily as chest pain due to visceral innervation.

6. **Extremity examination.** Examine the extremities for redness, warmth, or swelling. Findings may suggest a diagnosis of PE (eg, DVT) or CHF.

7. **Neurologic examination.** Focal neurologic deficits may be found if aortic dissection involves spinal and/or cerebral vessels.

VI. **Differential Diagnosis**

A. **Cardiovascular.** ACS, aortic dissection, pericarditis, myocarditis, or cardiac tamponade.

B. **Pulmonary.** PE, tension pneumothorax, pneumothorax, mediastinitis, or pneumonia.

C. **GI.** Esophageal rupture, cholecystitis, pancreatitis, or GERD.

D. **Musculoskeletal.** Muscle strain, rib fracture, costochondritis, or fibromyalgia.

E. **Neurologic.** Thoracic outlet syndrome, herpes zoster, or postherpetic neuralgia.

VII. **Diagnostic Findings**

A. **ECG**

1. **Myocardial ischemia.** ECG should be obtained immediately to identify ST-segment elevation MI. Other ECG findings indicative of ischemia include

ST depression, T wave inversion, and Q waves. Many patients with ACS have non-diagnostic or normal ECGs.

2. **PE.** An S-wave in lead I, a Q-wave in lead III, and a T-wave inversion in lead III (S1Q3T3) are present in only 12% of patients. More commonly, sinus tachycardia, right-axis deviation, or T-wave inversions in the precordial leads (ie, right-sided heart strain) are present.

3. **Pericarditis.** The ECG will show diffuse ST-segment elevations and PR-segment depressions.

B. **Laboratory Studies**

1. **Cardiac markers.** Cardiac markers should be used serially for maximum sensitivity (see Chapter 13).

2. **ABG** studies have limited use.

3. **D-dimer.** Depending on the type of D-dimer available, a normal D-dimer will safely rule out the presence of a PE in patients with a low risk for PE.

C. **Imaging Studies**

1. **CXR.** A widened mediastinum (> 8 cm) causes concern for an aortic dissection. Pneumothorax is visualized directly. Subcutaneous air, pneumomediastinum, or pleural effusion is seen in esophageal rupture.

2. **CT angiography of chest** may be indicated in patients who are suspected of having a PE or aortic dissection.

D. **Diagnostic Algorithm**

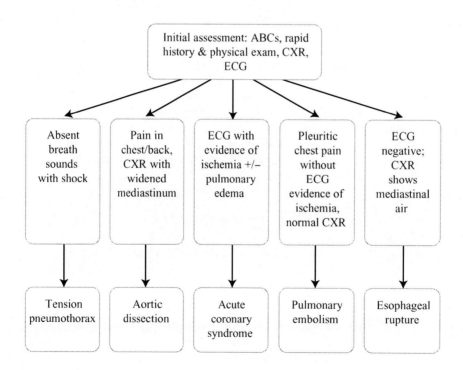

VIII. Treatment

A. **ACS** should be considered in any patient who presents with chest pain when no other clear etiology is present. Patients should be given aspirin, nitroglycerin, O_2, and morphine as needed for pain.

B. **Aortic dissection** requires immediate control of BP and HR with a β blocker (eg, esmolol) and nitroprusside. An alternative single agent is labetalol.

C. **Tension pneumothorax** requires needle thoracostomy followed by chest tube placement.

D. **PE** will require anticoagulation. Thrombolytics are indicated in patients with hemodynamic compromise.

E. **Esophageal tear and mediastinitis** require immediate surgical intervention. Patients with this diagnosis should be given broad-spectrum antibiotics and appropriate fluid resuscitation.

F. **Pericardial tamponade** requires emergent pericardiocentesis to remove enough fluid to improve cardiac output and reverse hypotension.

IX. Disposition

A. **Admission.** Most patients with chest pain will require hospital admission.

B. **Discharge.** Discharge is appropriate only for patients with clear-cut, non-emergent causes of chest pain (eg, muscle strain, herpes zoster). When doubt exists, admission is prudent.

CASE PRESENTATION

A 57-year-old woman is brought to the ED by her husband. She awakened from sleep 1 hour ago complaining of retrosternal chest pain radiating to the back. The pain has remained constant and is currently 9/10 in severity. She denies any previous pain episodes. She has associated nausea but no vomiting or diaphoresis. The pain is described as aching. There is no associated cough, sputum, fever, or chills. She has a history of hypertension. Physical examination reveals an anxious woman with a BP of 160/90 mm Hg and an HR of 110 beats/min. O_2 saturation is 98% on room air. She is afebrile. She has an intact airway and is speaking in complete sentences. The chest is clear, and the cardiovascular examination is normal. There is no swelling of her ankles, and the remainder of her physical examination is normal.

1. *What other historical facts do you want to know?*
   - *Exacerbating or alleviating factors? Numbness/tingling or weakness? Syncope?*
2. *What testing will you need to perform to assess the etiology of the chest pain?*
   - *ECG to determine if there is ischemia. CXR for possible widened mediastinum or other active process. Myocardial markers in serial fashion to maximize sensitivity of MI. CT angiography of chest to diagnose aortic dissection, depending on above findings.*

SUMMARY POINTS

- *Chest pain is a very common complaint of patients presenting to the ED.*
- *Physicians must be able to rapidly assimilate data from history and physical examination, ECG, and laboratory and imaging studies to determine accurate diagnoses.*
- *Exclude the life-threatening causes of chest pain first.*

CHAPTER 18
ACUTE CORONARY SYNDROME

I. Defining Features

   A. ACS is a spectrum of disease that includes unstable angina and acute myocardial infarction (AMI).

   B. AMI is categorized as ST elevation MI (STEMI) and non-ST elevation MI (NSTEMI). This distinction has important prognostic and treatment implications.

   C. The diagnosis of ACS is based on the characteristics of chest pain and associated symptoms, ECG abnormalities, and serum markers of cardiac injury.

II. Epidemiology

   A. ACS is the leading cause of death in the United States, accounting for approximately 1 million deaths a year.

   B. Chest pain is the chief complaint in over 5 million visits to the ED annually. Of these visits, 10% of patients will have a diagnosis of AMI.

   C. About 2–4% of patients with AMI are incorrectly discharged from EDs in the United States. About 20% of monetary settlements from malpractice lawsuits are spent on patients with ACS.

III. Pathophysiology

   A. Atherosclerosis is responsible for almost all cases of ACS. This insidious process begins with fatty streaks that are first seen in patients in adolescence, progressing into plaques by early adulthood, and culminating in thrombotic occlusions in middle age and later life.

   B. Fixed atherosclerotic lesions are the initial predisposing factor for ACS. Secondary reduction of coronary flow is due to coronary artery spasm and disruption of plaques, followed by platelet aggregation and thrombus formation.

IV. Risk Factors

   A. **Age**

   B. **Male.** Incidence of ACS is 3-fold higher and the mortality rate is 5-fold higher in men.

   C. **History of CAD** is the largest single risk factor for subsequent myocardial ischemia.

   D. **Hypertension.**

   E. **Elevated cholesterol.**

F. **Smoking.** The risk of AMI increases 6-fold in men and 3-fold in women who smoke > 20 cigarettes a day. Upon smoking cessation, the risk of AMI is reduced by over 50% at 1 year and normalizes to that of nonsmokers by 2 years.

G. **Diabetes mellitus** carries a 2- to 3-fold increase in the incidence of ACS.

H. **Family history** of significant cardiac disease carries a 2-fold increased risk.

I. *Approximately one half of all patients with ACS have no established risk factors other than age and gender.*

V. Clinical Presentation

A. **History**

1. History is the most sensitive tool for the detection of ACS, and is a more powerful predictor for cardiac ischemia than a normal or non-diagnostic ECG.

2. **Pain character.** The character of the pain can be described as pressure, squeezing, or fullness. Burning and pleuritic pain may also be consistent with ACS (Table 13–1).

3. **Pain radiation.** Pain may radiate to the shoulder, arm, neck, jaw, abdomen, or back, depending on the anatomic region of the heart affected. Radiation to the left arm is 55% sensitive and 76% specific for ACS, whereas radiation to the right arm is 41% sensitive and 94% specific for ACS.

4. **Associated symptoms** include dyspnea, diaphoresis, nausea, or vomiting.

5. *A significant number of patients present with atypical pain or no pain.* Atypical presentations of ACS are more common in patients with advanced age, diabetes mellitus, co-morbid disease, or substance abuse. Elderly patients may present with mental status changes. Diabetic patients account for up to 40% of unrecognized AMI. Patients presenting with atypical symptoms of ACS have a 3-fold increase in mortality rate.

B. **Physical Examination**

1. **Vital signs.** Hypotension suggests cardiogenic shock.

2. **Heart failure** is present in patients with an elevated jugular venous pressure, crackles, an S3, lower extremity swelling, or hepatojugular reflux.

3. **Neurologic and rectal examinations** are useful for patients who may receive antiplatelet and/or thrombolytic therapy.

VI. Differential Diagnosis. Aortic dissection, aortic stenosis, asthma, biliary tract disease, cardiomyopathy, esophagitis/esophageal spasm, gastritis and PUD,

Table 13–1. Terms used to describe chest pain in patients with ACS.

Crushing, heaviness	24% of AMI; 30% of unstable angina
Burning pain	23% of AMI; 21% of unstable angina
Pleuritic pain	19% of AMI
Reproducible pain	8–15% of AMI

myocarditis, pericarditis, pneumonia, pneumothorax, pneumomediastinum, and PE.

VII. **Diagnostic Findings**

A. **ECG**

1. A normal ECG does not preclude the diagnosis of ACS. The ECG provides only a snapshot of time. Serial assessments improve sensitivity and specificity for detecting ACS.

2. ECG leads represent various areas of the heart. Based on the affected area, the most likely coronary artery involved can be predicted. Reciprocal changes reflect electrical alterations identified on the opposite wall of the myocardium during an AMI (Table 13–2). The presence of reciprocal changes is not only further evidence that ST elevation is due to an AMI, but it is also predictive of a larger infarct and a higher mortality rate.

3. Changes on the ECG in 2 or more contiguous leads that are suspicious for ACS include Q waves, ST segment elevation, ST segment depression, or T wave changes. Q waves are the only diagnostic waveform of AMI. However, these present late, indicate myocardial necrosis, and are not useful in the acute decision making process.

4. **ST elevation** is not sensitive or specific for an AMI. STEMI is found in approximately 50% of AMI (Figures 13–1 and 13–2). Other causes of ST elevation include LVH, left ventricular aneurysm, bundle branch blocks, paced rhythms, benign early repolarization, pericarditis, and hyperkalemia. The morphology of the ST elevation in patients with an AMI is straight or convex ("tombstone" shape), while concave ST segments (upward slope) suggest a more benign etiology.

5. **Hyperacute T waves** occur in the first few moments after the occlusion of a coronary vessel. These T waves are prominent and generally asymmetric with a wide base. They are usually transient and progress to ST elevation within minutes to hours.

6. **T wave inversion** (TWI) is a common finding in patients with myocardial ischemia. TWI is usually symmetric and narrow. Isolated TWI is found in

Table 13–2. Portions of the heart represented by ECG leads.

Anatomic Location	Occluded Artery	Leads	Reciprocal Leads
Anterior wall	LAD	V2, V3, V4	II, III, aVF
Lateral wall	LCX	I, aVL, V5, V6	V1, V2
Inferior wall	RCA (90%). LCX	II, III, aVF	Variable
Posterior	LCX	V8, V9	V1, V2
Right ventricle	RCA	V1, V4R	Variable

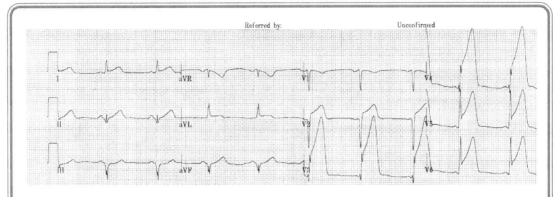

Figure 13–1. Anterior wall MI. This patient had a 100% occlusion of the left anterior descending artery.

10% of patients with an AMI. Other causes of TWI include LVH, myocarditis, PE, stroke, and Wolfe-Parkinson-White syndrome.

7. **Posterior wall** and the **right ventricle** are areas of the heart that are not seen well on the standard 12-lead ECG. They may be more appropriately assessed using a 15-lead ECG (12 lead ECG + V4R, V8, and V9 leads). Leads V8 and V9 are placed on the posterior thorax at the level of the anterior 5th intercostal space, with V8 at the mid-scapular line and V9 along the left paraspinal border. V4R is attached to the right side of the chest, mirroring the position of V4. Right ventricular involvement is seen in 30% of inferior wall infarctions.

8. **Heart block.** High-degree (2nd or 3rd degree) AV block is present in 6% of patients with AMI. In inferior MI, the incidence is higher (15%), and is sec-

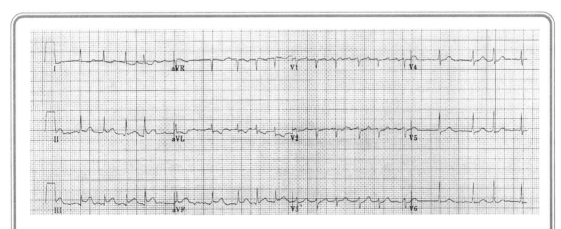

Figure 13–2. Inferior wall MI. Note the ST segment elevation in leads II, III, and aVF. This patient also has atrial fibrillation.

ondary to increased vagal tone or ischemia of the AV node. Anterior wall infarctions result in heart block due to ischemia of the bundle of His or both bundle branches, resulting in a wide QRS complex.

B. **Laboratory Studies**
  1. When myocardial tissue is damaged, enzymes (eg, creatine kinase, myoglobin, troponin) leak into the vascular space and are measured in the serum.
  2. No single marker measurement has sufficient accuracy to reliably identify or exclude AMI within 6 hours of symptom onset. Serial measurements offer increased sensitivity and are obtained every 2–4 hours for a period of 8–12 hours.
  3. **Troponin (Tn)** is the most specific marker for myocardial necrosis and thus has become the "gold standard" for detection of AMI. Elevated levels of troponin are detected in the serum within 4–6 hours of injury, peak at 12 hours, and remain elevated for 3–10 days. The prolonged period of elevation allows the physician to diagnose myocardial damage during the preceding week. The amount of myocardial damage and mortality correlate with the degree of Tn elevation. Tn elevation may also be seen in unstable angina, myocarditis, CHF, cardiac surgery, PE, or after defibrillation.
  4. **Creatine kinase (CK)** is found in skeletal and cardiac muscle. The CK-MB portion is a subunit of CK and is more specific for myocardial tissue. CK-MB typically begins to increase 4–6 hours after the onset of infarction, but is not elevated in all patients until after about 12 hours. Levels return to normal within 24–36 hours after the ischemic event.
  5. **Myoglobin (Mb)** has the most rapid increase in serum concentrations after AMI, but its poor specificity limits its utility. It is released from damaged myocardial cells starting at 3 hours.

C. **Imaging Studies**
  1. **CXR** should be performed to look for evidence of heart failure as well as alternative diagnoses (eg, widened mediastinum in aortic dissection).
  2. **Transthoracic echocardiogram** has been demonstrated to be an effective tool for detecting regional wall motion abnormalities associated with ACS. Lack of availability in the acute setting limits its usefulness.

D. **Diagnostic Algorithm (see page 71)**

VIII. **Treatment**

  A. Initial attention to ABCs.

  B. Cardiac monitor, O_2, and IV access.

  C. **Nitrates.** Nitroglycerin decreases myocardial O_2 demand by decreasing ventricular preload and improves myocardial perfusion by dilating the coronary vascular bed. The usual starting dose of nitroglycerin is 0.4 mg sublingually with tablet or spray. This can be repeated every 5 minutes as long as systolic BP remains > 100 mm Hg. If chest pain persists after 3–5 sublingual doses, then IV nitroglycerin should be initiated. The usual starting dose of IV nitroglycerin is 10–20 µg/min, which can be titrated upward in 10–20 µg/min increments every 5 minutes according to clinical parameters (pain and blood pressure). If nitroglycerin induces hypotension, stop the agent and administer fluid. Right ventricular infarctions are particularly sensitive to nitroglycerin due to their dependence on preload.

Diagnostic Algorithm

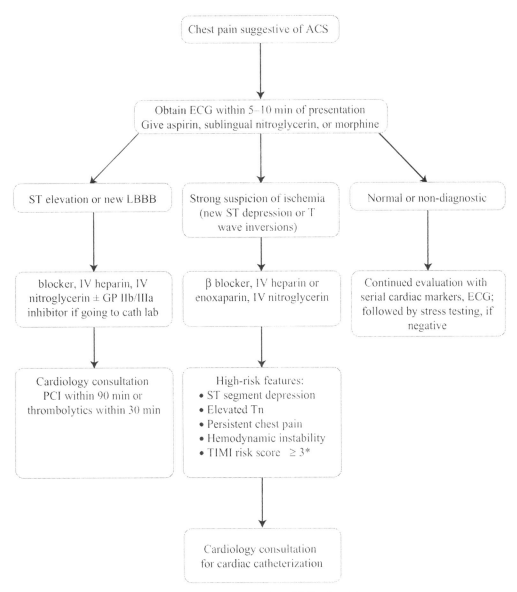

*TIMI risk score for NSTEMI/unstable angina = number of following 7 items present: age ≥ 65, > 3 CAD risk factors, known CAD, have taken aspirin in past 7 days, recent angina, elevated cardiac markers, ST deviation > 0.5 mm. Score of 3 carries a 13% risk of adverse cardiac event (AMI, death, revascularization) within 14 days.

D. **Morphine.** IV morphine should be administered to patients who continue to experience pain after taking nitroglycerin. Morphine decreases venous tone (preload) and sympathetic catecholamine surge.

E. **Antiplatelet Agents**
   1. **Aspirin.** The usual dose is 163–325 mg of a nonenteric-coated formula. This simple intervention has been shown to have a relative reduction in mortality rates by 23% without reperfusion therapy and 42% if given with thrombolytics.
   2. **Clopidogrel (Plavix)** 300 mg results in a significant reduction in subsequent cardiovascular events in patients with NSTEMI. However, major bleeding is increased in patients who undergo coronary artery bypass grafting (CABG); therefore, it is appropriate to withhold clopidogrel in patients who will undergo cardiac catheterization until it is known if they will require subsequent CABG.
   3. **Glycoprotein IIb/IIIa receptor antagonists.** Glycoprotein IIb/IIIa antagonists prevent platelet aggregation and improve short and long-term outcome. The absolute mortality reduction of these agents is 1%. They are useful in high-risk patients (elevated Tn levels, ischemic ECG findings, history of ACS), especially if cardiac catheterization will be performed within 24 hours.

F. **Heparin** should be given to patients with ST depression or T wave inversion and ischemic-type chest pain. It interferes with thrombus formation and inhibits clot propagation. Low molecular weight heparin (LMWH) is as effective as unfractionated heparin (UFH). LMWH has the advantage of ease of administration, no need to monitor blood levels, uniform bioavailability, and less heparin-induced thrombocytopenia than UFH. LMWH has less ability for reversal than UFH, so if clinical situations exist where rapid reversal may be required, administer UFH.

G. **β Blockers** reduce O_2 demand by decreasing heart rate, afterload, and ventricular contractility. β blockers should be administered to patients who have ACS, providing there are no contraindications. Contraindications include reactive airway disease, heart block, hypotension, acute CHF, or allergy. A standard regimen is metoprolol given in 5 mg increments every 5 minutes to a total of 15 mg, followed by 100 mg PO.

H. **Reperfusion Therapy**
   1. **Thrombolytics** are recommended for patients with > 1 mm ST elevation in 2 or more contiguous leads or new LBBB in the clinical setting of AMI. *The goal of thrombolysis is to begin administration within 30 minutes of patient presentation to the ED.* The best outcomes are achieved when reperfusion is administered within 4 hours. Thrombolytics administered after 12 hours have minimal effect and are not recommended. Thrombolytics have no use in unstable angina or NSTEMI due to the elevated risk of bleeding and increased mortality rate with administration. If thrombolytics are to be given, patient consent must be obtained and the risks explained to the patient. Absolute contraindications for thrombolytic therapy include previous history of hemorrhagic stroke, known intracranial neoplasm, active internal bleeding (not menses), and suspected aortic dissection or pericarditis. Relative contraindications are uncontrolled hypertension (> 180/110 mm Hg), significant trauma in the preceding month, history of ischemic CVA, pregnancy, known bleeding disorder, active PUD, current use of oral anticoagulants in therapeutic doses, or non-compressible vascular punctures.

2. Percutaneous coronary intervention (PCI) is preferred to thrombolytics due to lower mortality rates and reduced re-infarction rates. PCI should be performed as soon as possible for maximal myocardial salvage. ***The goal is to have the balloon blown up in the "culprit artery" within 90 minutes after patient presentation to the ED.*** PCI may also be useful in patients with unstable angina as well as those with NSTEMI, which is not the case for thrombolytics. Combination therapy with both thrombolytics and PCI has not been shown to be beneficial for AMI patients.

IX. Disposition

   A. **Admission.** Patients with suspected ACS should be admitted to the hospital. High-risk patients (elevation of myocardial markers or ischemia on ECG) should be monitored in a CCU setting and undergo early PCI.

   B. **Discharge.** Patients at low risk of ACS (atypical history, normal ECG, and normal myocardial markers) who remain pain free and have negative serial myocardial markers are candidates for early stress testing as an outpatient.

CASE PRESENTATION

A 55-year-old man presents to the ED complaining of chest pain. He describes the pain as heavy and retrosternal.

1. *Describe your initial treatment of this patient if the ECG is normal.*
   - *Assess ABCs. IV, O_2, and monitor. Portable chest radiograph. Administer aspirin, morphine, and nitroglycerin.*
2. *The patient's myocardial markers return with an elevated Tn level. What further treatments would be indicated for this patient?*
   - *β blocker, heparin. Cardiology consultation for PCI. If the patient were going to the catheterization laboratory, GP IIb/IIIa administration would be indicated. If the hospital is without PCI capabilities, clopidogrel should be initiated. Admit to the CCU.*

SUMMARY POINTS

- *ACS should be considered in the assessment of all patients with chest pain.*
- *Atypical presentations of ACS are common, especially in the elderly and in diabetics.*
- *An ECG should be obtained rapidly in patients presenting with chest pain to ensure timely treatment.*
- *For patients with STEMI, reperfusion therapy with thrombolytics should occur within 30 minutes or PCI within 90 minutes of presentation.*

CHAPTER 14
CONGESTIVE HEART FAILURE

I. Defining Features

A. CHF is due to the inability of the heart to meet the metabolic demands of the body.

B. In patients with CHF exacerbations, it is important to consider the underlying etiology of this disease process as well as the explanation for the acute exacerbation.

C. Pulmonary edema occurs when the pulmonary capillary pressure is elevated and fluid leaks into the alveoli. When this process is sudden and severe, respiratory distress ensues.

II. Epidemiology

A. About 1–2% of the population has CHF. In persons > age 75, 10% have CHF.

B. The annual cost of treating CHF is $60 billion. About 2% of yearly hospital admissions are due to acute exacerbations of CHF.

C. The mortality rate of patients with CHF is 50% at 5 years.

III. Pathophysiology

A. CHF is due to one or a combination of disorders, including diminished contractility of the myocardium (ischemic heart disease), mechanical inhibition (valvular heart disease), and increased systemic afterload (hypertension). Other less common causes include pericardial disease and high output states (thyrotoxicosis).

B. Precipitating causes of acute exacerbations of CHF include myocardial ischemia or MI, infection, noncompliance with medications, arrhythmias, increased metabolic demands (fever, trauma, pregnancy), anemia, thyroid disorders, sodium-retaining medications, dietary noncompliance, pulmonary embolus, or progressive hypertension.

IV. Risk Factors. CAD, cigarette smoking, hypertension, obesity, diabetes mellitus, valvular heart disease, cardiomyopathy, and cocaine use.

V. Clinical Presentation

A. **History**

1. **Dyspnea** is the most common presenting complaint of CHF patients. Activity level, associated symptoms, and duration of symptoms should be evaluated.

2. **Orthopnea** is dyspnea that occurs rapidly in the supine position (within 1–2 min) and is relieved by sitting up. It is often quantified based on the number of pillows a patient sleeps on at night. Orthopnea is a result of an increased venous return to the heart when the lower extremities are elevated. Pulmonary congestion results because the heart is unable to pump out the extra volume.

3. **Paroxysmal nocturnal dyspnea** (PND) is the occurrence of sudden dyspnea that awakens the patient from sleep. Usually the patient feels the need to sit upright or to go to an open window. The mechanism is similar to orthopnea. Symptoms are usually relieved after sitting upright for 5–20 minutes.

4. **Cough** that is worse when lying down may also herald pulmonary congestion from CHF.

5. **Review of systems** should cover precipitating symptoms of a heart failure exacerbation. Chest pain (myocardial ischemia or PE); palpitations (dysrhythmia); fever, chills, cough, sputum, urinary tract symptoms (UTIs); dietary indiscretion; noncompliance with medications; or initiation of new medications.

B. **Physical Examination**

1. **General appearance.** Patients in severe respiratory distress may only be able to speak in short sentences, words, or gasps.

2. **Vital signs.** Tachycardia occurs as a compensatory mechanism to maintain cardiac output in the face of decreased stroke volume. Patients with low or normal BP with signs of hypoperfusion (cyanosis, chest pain, or AMS) are in cardiogenic shock.

3. **Cardiovascular examination.** An S3 gallop is associated with increased left atrial and ventricular pressures. An S4 may also be present due to a noncompliant left ventricle.

4. **Lung examination.** Crackles (rales) are heard in the bilateral lung fields in most moderate to severe CHF exacerbations. The absence of crackles does not exclude the diagnosis. Wheezing may also occur and should not be confused with COPD or asthma.

5. **Jugular venous distention** (JVD). The neck veins reflect right atrial pressure. When the right ventricle fails, there is an increase in right ventricular volume and pressure, which is referred back to the right atrium and jugular veins.

6. **Hepatojugular reflux.** Manual compression of the RUQ elevates the central venous pressure via increased venous return due to compression of the inferior vena cava.

7. **Peripheral edema** manifests as swelling of the legs, scrotum, sacral region, and abdominal wall.

VI. **Differential Diagnosis.** ARDS, anaphylaxis, anemia, bronchitis, COPD, pericarditis with cardiac tamponade, pneumonia, PE, MI, shock, tension pneumothorax, or venous air embolism.

RULE OUT

Myocardial ischemia is the cause of an acute exacerbation of CHF in approximately 50% of patients. Unless another cause is readily apparent, ischemia should be excluded, even in patients who do not present with chest pain.

VII. Diagnostic Findings

A. **Laboratory Studies**

1. **CBC.** Anemia exacerbates CHF.

2. **Serum chemistry.** Hypokalemia may give rise to cardiac irritability and dysrhythmias. Diuretic therapy frequently causes abnormalities of electrolytes and renal function (BUN/creatinine).

3. **Myocardial enzymes** are sent to determine the presence of cardiac injury.

4. **Brain natriuretic peptide** (BNP). A ventricle with high filling pressures releases BNP. Rapid bedside measurement of plasma BNP is useful for distinguishing between heart failure and a pulmonary cause of dyspnea (eg, COPD). Serum levels of BNP < 100 pg/mL are unlikely to be caused by CHF, while levels of > 500 pg/mL are consistent with CHF. Levels between 100–500 pg/mL may be CHF, but other conditions that elevate right ventricular filling pressures (pulmonary embolus, cor pulmonale, renal failure, or cirrhosis) may cause an elevated BNP.

5. **Thyroid-stimulating hormone** (TSH) **and free thyroxine** (T4) are indicated if other signs and symptoms of hyperthyroidism or hypothyroidism exist.

B. **Imaging Studies and ECG**

1. **CXR.** Findings suggestive of CHF include cardiomegaly (cardiac-to-thoracic width > 50%) and cephalization of pulmonary vessels. High hydrostatic pressures cause fluid to accumulate in the alveoli, represented by diffuse fluffy alveolar infiltrates (Figure 14–1).

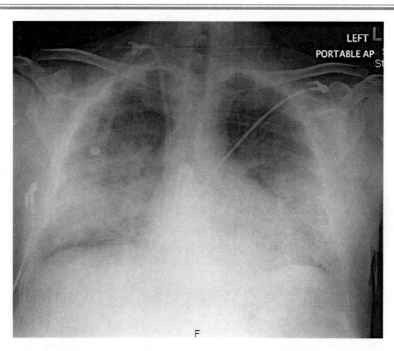

Figure 14–1. Bilateral fluffy infiltrates in a patient with pulmonary edema.

2. **ECG** may show evidence of ischemia and can also detect arrhythmias, which may cause or exacerbate CHF.
3. **Echocardiography** (ECHO) should be performed on an inpatient basis in patients with new-onset CHF and can provide important information about ventricular size and function. The sensitivity and specificity of ECHO for the diagnosis of CHF is 80–100%.

C. **Diagnostic Algorithm**

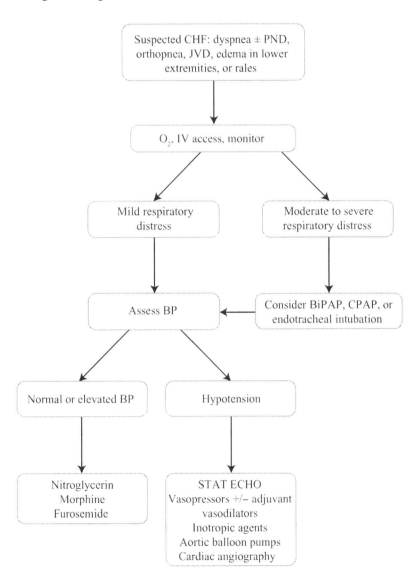

VIII. Treatment

A. The goals of therapy for CHF are to optimize oxygenation and reverse decompensation. This is accomplished by decreasing afterload (improves ejection fraction, tissue perfusion, and minimizes the work of the heart) and preload (lower end-diastolic volumes and pressures).

B. **Supplemental O$_2$** should be administered immediately via high-flow face mask in spontaneously breathing patients to maintain O$_2$ saturation at > 90%. Continuous positive airway pressure (CPAP) and biphasic positive airway pressure (BiPAP) are noninvasive respiratory techniques that can be used in patients with severe respiratory distress due to pulmonary edema. These techniques result in decreased left ventricular preload and afterload, which result in more rapid restoration of normal vital signs and oxygenation. Patients with agonal respirations or AMS are not candidates.

C. **Nitrates** are first-line therapy for patients with an exacerbation of CHF. Nitroglycerin is primarily a venodilator, but at higher doses, arterial vasodilation also occurs. Myocardial function is improved by reduction of preload and afterload. Nitroglycerin may be of further benefit due to direct coronary vasodilation. Initiate nitroglycerin 0.4 mg sublingually every 5 minutes. In severe exacerbations, therapy should proceed quickly to the IV form. Initial dosages depend on the desired clinical responses. Doses of 10–20 µg/min will result primarily in venodilation and preload reduction, while doses > 50 µg/min cause arterial vasodilation that decreases afterload and has the most rapid effect in alleviating the patient's pulmonary congestion. Titrate the dosages up quickly, every 3–5 minutes, according to the patient's BP and clinical status.

D. **Morphine** (2–4 mg IV initially) reduces patient anxiety and work of breathing. This leads to a reduction in sympathetic outflow and results in improved cardiac filling pressures.

E. **Loop diuretics** (furosemide 40–120 mg IV) are used to increase salt and water excretion. This leads to a reduction in plasma volume, which decreases preload and pulmonary congestion. Peak effect of diuresis occurs at 30 minutes to 1 hour.

F. **Cardiogenic shock.** If the patient has severe CHF with hypotension, inotropic vasopressor therapy, aortic balloon pumps, and endotracheal intubation with mechanical ventilation may be indicated. Cardiology consultation and ECHO should be obtained in the ED.

G. **Chronic heart failure.** ACE inhibitors (improve survival and prevent acute exacerbations), diuretics, and β blockade (reduction of death or hospitalization by up to 35%). *It should be stressed that β blockers are administered ONLY in the face of CHRONIC heart failure. Patients with acute presentations should NOT receive β blockers because these drugs reduce myocardial contractility.*

IX. Disposition

A. **Admission.** Patients with exacerbations of CHF generally require admission to a monitored setting.

B. **Discharge.** Patients may be discharged if they have a defined etiology for heart failure and the precipitating cause has been identified and appropriately treated.

The patient should receive clear discharge plans and have appropriate followup and medications.

CASE PRESENTATION

A 65-year-old man presents to the ED in respiratory distress. The patient awoke at 5 AM with acute onset shortness of breath and chest pain. He has never had an episode like this before. He has a history of hypertension and diabetes mellitus. The patient is speaking in single words before stopping to take another breath. His BP is 170/110 mm Hg, and his pulse oximetry is 92% on room air. Auscultation of the chest reveals crackles in both lung fields. Massive jugular venous distension is also noted.

1. *What are the initial steps in the management of this patient?*
   - *High-flow O_2. Consider noninvasive techniques such as BiPAP or CPAP. IV access. Cardiac monitor and ECG.*
1. *What medications are indicated acutely in this patient?*
   - *Nitroglycerin. Morphine. Furosemide.*

SUMMARY POINTS

- *Always think of ACS as a primary precipitant for heart failure.*
- *Nitroglycerin is the first-line therapy because it reduces both preload and afterload.*
- *Do not administer a β blocker to a patient with an acute exacerbation of CHF.*
- *Cardiogenic shock and heart failure have a very high mortality rate despite appropriate medical management. A cardiologist should be involved early in the care of these patients.*

CHAPTER 15
ARRHYTHMIAS

I. Defining Features

A. Arrhythmias are defined as either bradyarrhythmias or tachyarrhythmias, based on HR < 60 beats/min or > 100 beats/min, respectively.

B. Clinically, arrhythmias are further classified as stable or unstable, based on the presence or absence of end-organ hypoperfusion (ie, hypotension, cardiac ischemia, pulmonary edema, or mental status changes).

II. Epidemiology

A. In 75% of patients with cardiac arrest, VF is the initial rhythm. Almost all of the remaining 25% have a bradyarrhythmia or asystole.

B. Atrial fibrillation (AF) is very common and affects 5% of the population > age 70.

C. Third-degree heart block occurs within the AV node in 20% of cases, within the bundle of His in 20% of cases, and below the bundle of His in 60% of cases.

III. Pathophysiology

A. Normal cardiac conduction originates in the SA node and conducts to the AV node. Impulses then travel via the His bundle to the right and left bundle branches, which produce ventricular depolarization via the Purkinje fibers.

B. The normal ECG waveform contains a P wave, QRS complex, and T wave. The P wave corresponds to atrial depolarization. It is followed by the PR interval, which is normally < 0.2 sec. The QRS complex represents ventricular depolarization. It is normally < 0.1 sec. Any delay in intraventricular conduction results in a widened QRS complex. The ST segment is due to the plateau of ventricular depolarization. This segment is normally isoelectric. Finally, the T wave is caused by ventricular repolarization.

C. Bradyarrhythmias occur because of depressed sinus node activity or blocks in the conduction system. This commonly occurs with structural heart damage or increased vagal tone.

D. Tachyarrhythmias occur because of enhanced automaticity from a normal or an ectopic focus. They also occur with re-entry loops in normal or accessory pathways.

E. Wide complex rhythms occur when the ventricles are not depolarized by the normal conduction system.

IV. Risk Factors

A. **Bradyarrhythmia.** Sinus bradycardia is a common finding in healthy adults. Risk factors for pathologic causes of bradyarrhythmia include elderly patients, CAD, electrolyte imbalances (eg, hyperkalemia), or medications (eg, β blockers, calcium channel blockers, digoxin).

B. **Tachyarrhythmia.** Elderly, CAD, valvular heart disease, pulmonary disease, increased sympathetic tone (eg, fever, caffeine, thyroid disease, cocaine) and medications (eg, tricyclic antidepressants or anticholinergic overdose).

C. **Wide complex rhythm.** Structural or ischemic heart disease (eg, Wolfe-Parkinson-White, VT, bundle branch block), drug ingestions (eg, tricyclic antidepressant overdose), hyperkalemia, or pacemaker.

V. Clinical Presentation

A. **History**

1. **Start with ABCs.** Patients are frequently unstable and will require immediate intervention before a detailed history and physical examination can be completed. Make sure the patient is connected to a cardiac monitor for continuous rhythm and BP monitoring.

2. Inquire about symptoms that would classify the patient as unstable, including chest pain, dizziness, lightheadedness, shortness of breath, or syncope.

3. **Onset of symptoms.** Supraventricular tachycardias (SVTs) usually start abruptly, whereas onset of sinus tachycardia is more gradual.

B. **Physical Examination**

1. Always note the triage vital signs and repeat them frequently.

2. Palpate pulses to see if they correspond with the arrhythmia on the monitor.

3. Assess for signs of end-organ hypoperfusion, including a detailed cardiac (murmurs, rhythm), pulmonary (rales), neurologic (AMS), and vascular (diminished pulses, delayed capillary refill) examinations.

VI. Differential Diagnosis

A. **Bradyarrhythmias**

1. **Sinus bradycardia.** P wave before each QRS complex. Usually a normal variant (Figure 15–1A).

2. **Junctional bradycardia.** No P waves in front of a narrow (< 0.1 sec) QRS. Usually occurs secondary to medications (eg, β blockers) (Figure 15–1B).

3. **Idioventricular rhythm.** Wide complex QRS (> 0.1 sec) without preceding P waves at a rate of approximately 40 beats/minute. Usually associated with myocardial ischemia or infarct.

B. **Tachyarrhythmias**

1. **Sinus tachycardia.** P wave before each QRS complex. Regular R-R interval. Secondary to pain, fever, anxiety, PE, drug use (cocaine), alcohol withdrawal, thyrotoxicosis, volume depletion, or anemia (Figure 15–2A).

2. **SVT.** No P wave in front of QRS. Regular R-R intervals (Figure 15–2B). QRS complex usually < 0.1 sec, unless it is associated with a bundle branch block. SVT with a bundle branch block (SVT with aberrancy) or conduction through an accessory pathway is often difficult to distinguish from VT. Always assume VT until proven otherwise, especially in elderly patients with heart disease.

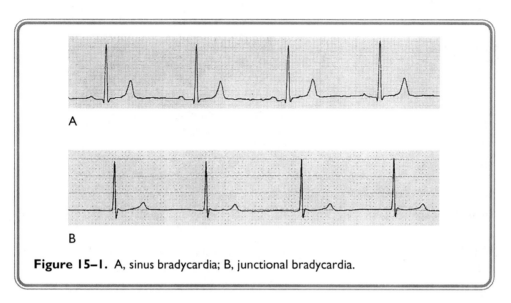

Figure 15–1. A, sinus bradycardia; B, junctional bradycardia.

3. **Atrial flutter.** More P waves than QRS complexes. Frequently a "saw toothed" appearance (Figure 15–2C). Regular R-R intervals unless there is variable blocking of the atrial impulses. The most common presentation is atrial rate of 300 with 2:1 block and a consistent ventricular rate of 150 beats/minute.

4. **AF.** Irregular R-R intervals. No discernible P waves. Frequently with a rapid ventricular rate (Figure 15–2D). One third of patients are without structural heart disease (Table 15–1). This rhythm may be confused with multifocal atrial tachycardia (MAT).

5. **MAT.** The R-R and P-R intervals are irregular, but multiple different P wave morphologies are related to and precede each QRS complex. This rhythm is common in patients with pulmonary disease (Figure 15–2E).

6. **VT.** Rate > 120 beats/minute and QRS interval > 0.12 sec. No discernible P waves. Requires antiarrhythmic agent or defibrillation if unstable (Figure 15–2F).

7. **VF.** No discernible P waves or QRS complexes. Requires immediate defibrillation (Figure 15–2G).

C. **Atrioventricular Blocks**
   1. **Second-degree A-V block Mobitz type I (Wenckebach).** Progressive increase in P-R interval with intermittent dropped beat (non-conducted QRS). Usually benign (Figure 15–3A).
   2. **Second-degree A-V block Mobitz type II.** P-R interval is constant, and a beat is dropped without warning (non-conducted QRS). May degenerate into third-degree block (Figure 15–3B).
   3. **Third-degree A-V block.** No relationship between P wave and QRS complex (Figure 15–3C).

VII. Diagnostic Findings
   A. **ECG.** Initial work-up on all patients with suspected arrhythmia should include an immediate 12-lead ECG unless the patient is unstable and requires immediate

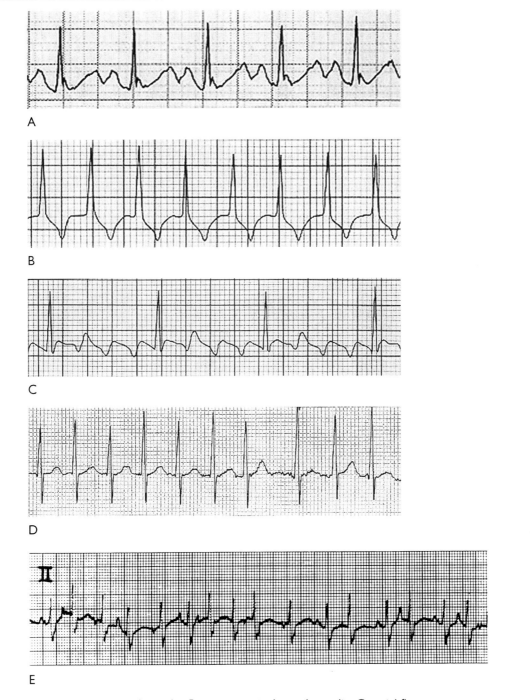

Figure 15–2. A, sinus tachycardia; B, supraventricular tachycardia; C, atrial flutter; D, atrial fibrillation; E, multifocal atrial tachycardia;

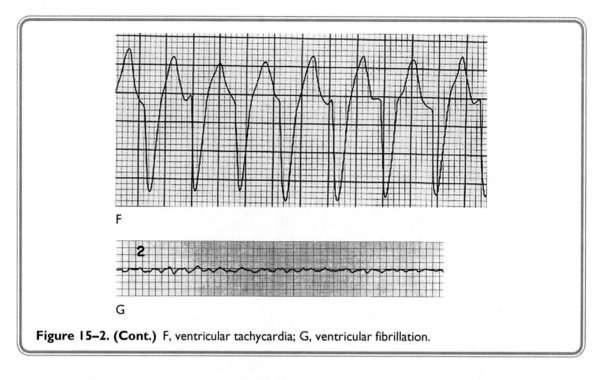

Figure 15–2. (Cont.) F, ventricular tachycardia; G, ventricular fibrillation.

cardioversion or pacing. Determine the rate. Determine if the rhythm is regular or irregular (may need additional rhythm strip). Determine QRS complex width: narrow (< 0.1 sec) or wide (> 0.1 sec).

CLINICAL SKILLS TIP

A rhythm that is fast, narrow, and regular has 1 of 3 diagnostic possibilities: **sinus tachycardia, atrial flutter,** *or* **SVT.** *When uncertain which is present, administer adenosine to transiently slow the rate and make the diagnosis clear.*

Table 15–1. PIRATES: causes of atrial fibrillation.

P	PE, pneumonia, pericarditis
I	Ischemia (CAD and MI)
R	Rheumatic heart disease, respiratory failure
A	Alcohol ("holiday heart")
T	Thyrotoxicosis
E	Endocrine (Ca), enlarged atria (mitral valve disease, cardiomyopathy)
S	Sepsis, stress (fever)

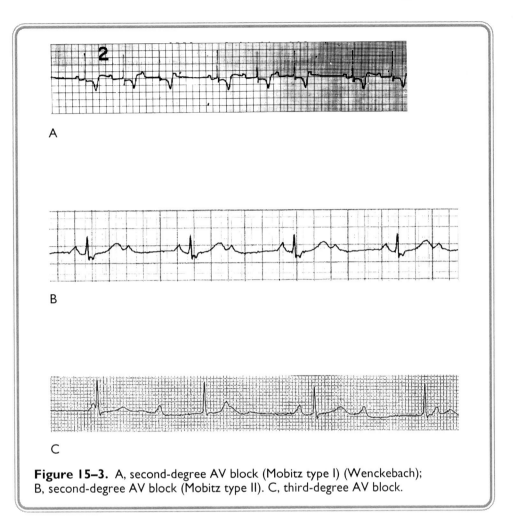

Figure 15–3. A, second-degree AV block (Mobitz type I) (Wenckebach); B, second-degree AV block (Mobitz type II). C, third-degree AV block.

B. **Laboratory Studies**
   1. **CBC** to exclude anemia.
   2. **Serum chemistry** to diagnose electrolyte abnormalities such as hyperkalemia.
   3. **Cardiac enzymes** when cardiac ischemia is suspected.
   4. **Digoxin level** in any patient taking digoxin.
   5. **D-dimer** and **thyroid function tests** in select patients with tachycardia at risk for PE or thyroid disease.
C. **Imaging studies. CXR** to aid in the diagnosis of heart failure.

D. **Diagnostic Algorithm**

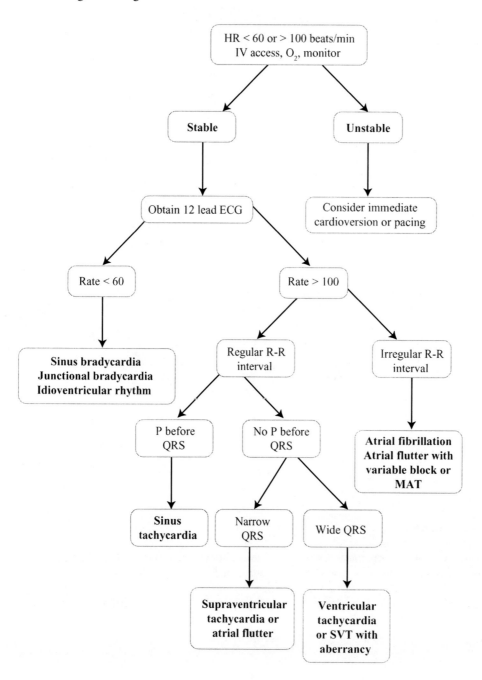

VIII. Treatment

A. Bradyarrhythmia

1. Asymptomatic bradycardia

a. *Sinus bradycardia or first-degree AV block.* No intervention if asymptomatic. Treat underlying conditions.

b. *Second-degree AV block (Mobitz type II) or third-degree block (asymptomatic).* Transcutaneous pacemaker pads placed on the patient for possible use if clinical condition changes. Cardiology consultation for pacemaker placement.

2. Symptomatic bradycardia

a. Patients require emergent treatment, especially if bradycardia is the most likely cause of the symptoms.

b. *Atropine.* First-line treatment for symptomatic bradycardia. Give dose of 0.5 to 1.0 mg IVP.

c. *Transcutaneous pacemaker.* Used for patients refractory to atropine. Place pads on the patient's chest and back and connect to the defibrillator/pacer. Turn the dial to PACE. Set the rate to 80/minute and dial up the energy level until capture is obtained. Use the lowest energy level that will maintain capture. Patients will require IV sedation and analgesia.

d. *Transvenous pacemaker.* Placed through a central venous catheter. Is needed emergently if unable to capture or pace transcutaneously.

B. Tachyarrhythmia

1. Unstable. *Immediate cardioversion:* To cardiovert a patient, turn on the defibrillator, place the pads or paddles on the patient, and turn the dial to DEFIBRILLATE. *Push the SYNC button so the electricity is delivered outside of the refractory period of the cardiac cycle.* Select an energy level and deliver the shock after signaling the rest of the team. Afterward, the defibrillator automatically reverts to defibrillation mode so that another shock can be delivered rapidly if the resulting rhythm has deteriorated (ie, VF). To cardiovert a second time, push the SYNC button again.

2. Stable

a. *Sinus tachycardia.* Treat the underlying cause.

b. *SVT.* Vagal maneuvers can be attempted. If unsuccessful, give adenosine IV in doses of 6 mg, followed by 12 mg if preceeding dose unsuccessful. Adenosine must be administered rapidly and followed by saline flush. The onset and duration are short. Record a rhythm strip while giving the medication.

c. *Atrial flutter or AF.* Control rate with diltiazem 0.25 mg/kg bolus. A second bolus (0.35 mg/kg) 15 minutes later is administered if the first dose is unsuccessful. Monitor for hypotension. An infusion of 5–15 mg/hr can be administered after the bolus.

d. *Wide complex tachycardia* of uncertain etiology (VT vs. SVT with aberrancy). In elderly patients with underlying heart disease, the etiology is VT until proven otherwise. Start with amiodarone 150 mg IV over a 10-minute period. If there are no signs of heart failure, an alternative agent is procainamide.

CLINICAL SKILLS TIP

Vagal maneuvers include carotid artery massage for 5 seconds, immersion of the face in ice water, or having the patient "bear down" (Valsalva maneuver).

CASE PRESENTATION

A 58-year-old man presents to the ED with palpitations and is noted in triage to have a pulse of 160 beats/min.

1. *What else do you want to know?*
   - *Does the patient have any other symptoms, including fevers, dizziness, chest pain, shortness of breath, or syncope? Any signs of hypoperfusion, including hypotension, AMS, or anginal chest pain?*
2. *Once you have made the clinical diagnosis of arrhythmia, what is your next step?*
   - *Determine if the patient is stable or unstable based on the above information. If unstable, prepare for cardioversion. If stable, obtain 12-lead ECG and treat accordingly.*

SUMMARY POINTS

- *When an arrhythmia is discovered, provide O$_2$, IV access, and continuous cardiac monitoring.*
- *A 12-lead ECG should be obtained on all patients with arrhythmias unless they are unstable and require immediate intervention.*
- *Evaluate the patient for signs of end-organ hypoperfusion, including hypotension, AMS, pulmonary edema, or chest pain.*
- *If the patient is stable, investigate for the possible underlying cause, including medications, heart disease, or potential ingestions.*

CHAPTER 16
AORTIC DISSECTION

I. Defining Features

    A. Aortic dissection is initiated with an intimal tear in the aorta. Blood travels into the media and "dissects" toward the adventitia.

    B. **Stanford classification system** divides aortic dissection into type A (dissection with any involvement of the ascending aorta) and type B (dissection restricted to the descending aorta).

    C. Left untreated, death occurs in one-third of patients within 24 hours and in half within 2 days.

II. Epidemiology

    A. Peak incidence is in patients aged 50–70 years.

    B. The incidence is higher in males (3:1).

    C. Aortic dissection is uncommon in persons < age 40, except in cases of congenital heart disease, connective tissue disease, or pregnancy.

III. Pathophysiology

    A. The aortic wall has 3 layers (intima, media, and adventitia). In aortic dissection, blood enters via an intimal tear and travels along the media, creating a false lumen. Blood may re-enter the intima or dissect through the adventitia.

    B. The most common site of dissection is the ascending aorta. About 90% of cases occur within 10 cm of the aortic valve.

    C. An aortic dissection may propagate anterograde, retrograde, or both. Anterograde propagation can result in stroke, MI, mesenteric ischemia, renal failure, paralysis, or limb ischemia. Retrograde dissection causes aortic valve insufficiency or pericardial tamponade.

IV. Risk Factors

    A. **Hypertension** in 70–90% of patients.

    B. Rare in patients < age 40 unless connective tissue disorders (eg, Marfan's syndrome), congenital heart disease (eg, bicuspid aortic valve), aortic stenosis, stimulant use (eg, cocaine), pregnancy, or trauma.

V. Clinical Presentation

A. History

1. **Pain** is reported in 96% of cases. The pain is most common in the chest (73%), but also occurs in the back, neck, and abdomen. Pain is usually abrupt (84%) and severe (90%), and is commonly described as sharp (64%), tearing, or ripping (50%).

2. **Location.** Anterior chest pain correlates with dissection of the ascending aorta. Neck or jaw pain is associated with the aortic arch. Back or intrascapular pain correlates with the descending arch.

3. ***Dissections can obstruct any branch of the aorta, resulting in complaints attributed to several organ systems.*** Presentations consistent with aortic dissection include syncope, weakness, stroke, paraplegia, hematemesis, dyspnea, hemoptysis, abdominal pain, and flank pain.

B. Physical Examination

1. **General appearance.** The patient will usually appear anxious, and may be diaphoretic.

2. **Vital signs.** The presenting BP is frequently elevated, but may be normal or low.

3. **Cardiovascular examination.** A murmur of aortic regurgitation is present in 30% of cases. There is evidence of pericardial tamponade if the dissection extends proximally into the pericardium. Examine distal pulses. Unequal pulses are present in only 15% of cases. A BP differential of > 20 mm Hg in the arms is also supportive evidence of an aortic dissection.

4. **Neurologic examination.** Focal neurologic deficits may be present if the dissection obstructs spinal arteries or involves the cerebral circulation.

VI. Differential Diagnosis. MI or ischemia, pneumothorax, pulmonary embolism (PE), pericarditis, esophageal rupture, pneumonia, or musculoskeletal chest pain.

VII. Diagnostic Findings

A. Laboratory Studies

1. Laboratory studies are of little value in patients with aortic dissection, but may be used to exclude other diagnoses.

2. **Renal function (BUN/creatinine)** is tested before giving IV contrast. New onset renal insufficiency suggests involvement of the renal arteries.

3. **Myocardial markers** are obtained when ECG changes suggest ischemia from involvement of the coronary arteries.

4. **D-dimer** is usually elevated in aortic dissection.

B. ECG

1. Useful to exclude acute MI.

2. Proximal dissections can extend into coronary arteries and cause changes in the ECG consistent with acute MI. The most common location of associated infarction is inferior.

C. Imaging Studies

1. **CXR** is abnormal in 80–90% of cases and should be taken in the upright position. Findings suggestive of dissection include mediastinal widening > 8 cm (60%); obliteration or abnormal contour of aortic knob (50%); left pleural ef-

fusion (20%); or intimal calcification of the aorta that is separated by > 5 mm from the outer aortic border (15%).

   2. CT angiogram of chest is the diagnostic test of choice (Figure 16–1). CT scan may reveal an alternative diagnosis if dissection is not apparent. The patient must be clinically stable before being taken to radiology for the examination.

   3. Transesophageal echocardiography (TEE) is the diagnostic test of choice in the unstable patient. It is highly sensitive, requires minimal sedation, and is performed at the bedside by the cardiologist.

  D. **Diagnostic Algorithm (See page 92)**

VIII. Treatment

  A. **Medical Management**

   1. Pulse and BP reduction to diminish the forces that propagate the dissection should be initiated in patients where there is high clinical suspicion of aortic dissection, especially when diagnostic testing is delayed for any reason.

   2. Pulse is initially controlled to a rate of 60–80 beats/minute using IV β blockers. Esmolol (500 mcg/kg over 1-minute period, followed by an infusion of 50–200 mcg/kg/min) is an excellent choice due to the drug's short half life.

   3. Systolic BP is then reduced to 100–120 mm Hg using IV nitroprusside (0.3 mcg/kg/min and titrate up slowly). If nitroprusside is given first, a reflex tachycardia may cause dissection propagation.

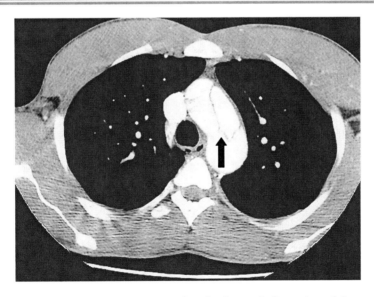

Figure 16–1. CT scan demonstrating a Stanford type A dissection of the aortic arch (*arrow*).

Diagnostic Algorithm

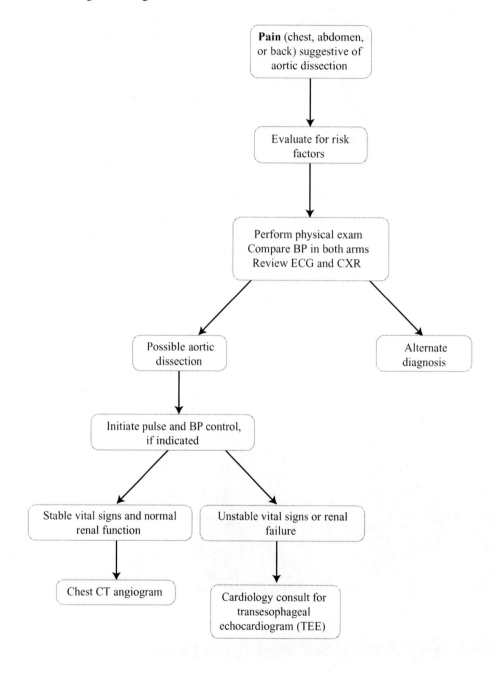

4. Alternatively, labetalol (10–20 mg IV boluses) can be used as a single agent because it blocks both α-1 and β-1 receptors, controlling both BP and pulse.
   B. **Surgical Management**
      1. Stanford type A dissections require surgical management in addition to pulse and BP control, as indicated.
      2. When proximal dissection is discovered, immediate cardiothoracic surgery consult is obtained.

IX. Disposition

   A. **Admission.** All patients with a new diagnosis of aortic dissection should be admitted to an ICU setting.
   B. **Discharge** is indicated only in patients with previously diagnosed Stanford type B dissections who maintain good BP control and symptoms are unrelated to the aortic dissection.

CASE PRESENTATION

A 62-year-old man presents to the ED complaining of chest pain radiating to the back. The pain is described as sharp in character. The patient states that the pain occurred "all of the sudden" and has been unrelenting for the past hour. The patient appears anxious and diaphoretic.

1. What information do you want to know?
   · *Risk factors for aortic dissection? BP differential in the arms? Aortic insufficiency murmur or signs of cardiac tamponade? Absent or unequal pulses?*
2. CT scan reveals a dissection of the ascending aorta. What is the next step?
   · *Pulse and BP control with a β blocker and nitroprusside. Consult cardiothoracic surgery.*

SUMMARY POINTS

· *Consider aortic dissection in patients with a history of hypertension who present with pain of sudden onset in the chest, neck, abdomen, or back.*
· *If the index of suspicion for dissection is high, medical management of pulse and BP should begin before diagnostic testing (CT or TEE).*
· *Treatment of Stanford type A aortic dissection is pulse and BP control and surgical management, while treatment of a Stanford type B dissection is pulse and BP control only.*

CHAPTER 17
HYPERTENSIVE EMERGENCIES

I. Defining Features

A. Hypertension is among the most misunderstood and mismanaged of "acute" medical problems seen in clinical practice. Emergent lowering of the BP based on numbers alone, without considering the clinical context, can be deleterious.

B. **Hypertension** is classified according to the degree of BP elevation.
   1. **Mild hypertension** is defined as systolic BP 140–159 mm Hg or a diastolic BP 90–99 mm Hg.
   2. **Moderate hypertension** is defined as systolic BP 160–179 mm Hg or diastolic BP 100–109 mm Hg.
   3. **Severe hypertension** is defined as systolic BP ≥ 180 mm Hg or diastolic BP ≥ 110 mm Hg.

C. **Hypertensive emergency** (crisis) is defined as a sudden increase in systolic and diastolic BP associated with acute end-organ damage (ie, CNS, heart, eyes, or kidneys). The term malignant hypertension has been used interchangeably with hypertensive emergency. Examples of end-organ injury include
   1. Hypertensive encephalopathy
   2. Acute aortic dissection
   3. Acute pulmonary edema with respiratory failure
   4. Acute MI or unstable angina
   5. Preeclampsia or eclampsia
   6. Acute renal failure

D. **Hypertensive urgency** refers to patients with severely elevated BP and chronic end-organ damage (eg, history of a stroke, MI, renal insufficiency) but without acute end-organ damage.

II. Epidemiology

A. About 25% of the United States population suffers from hypertension, with the vast majority having essential hypertension.

B. About 75% of these patients have poorly controlled hypertension.

C. Less than 1% of hypertensive patients will develop a hypertensive emergency.

III. Pathophysiology

A. Severe elevations of BP lead to endothelial injury and fibrinoid necrosis of the arteriole. This injury results in platelet and fibrin deposition and a breakdown of autoregulatory function. The subsequent ischemia gives rise to release of vasoactive substances, initiating a vicious cycle.

B. Chronic hypertension leads to a rightward shift of cerebral and renal autoregulation that allows patients to tolerate high BP without end-organ damage. Rapid lowering of BP in this setting may be associated with significant morbidity and mortality due to hypoperfusion of end-organ vascular beds and subsequent ischemia.

IV. **Risk Factors.** Obesity, diabetes mellitus, elderly, African American, family history, sedentary lifestyle, alcoholism, emotional stress, medications (eg, steroids, NSAIDs), or pain. Many patients with hypertension are without any risk factors.

V. **Clinical Presentation**

A. **History**
1. **Hypertensive encephalopathy.** Headache and AMS are classic findings. The mental status changes may include drowsiness, confusion, or coma. Patients may have seizures, blindness, or focal neurologic deficits.
2. **Pulmonary edema.** Patients present with acute shortness of breath and chest pain and/or pressure. They may also have slowly progressive symptoms of paroxysmal nocturnal dyspnea or orthopnea.
3. **Myocardial ischemia.** Patients usually present with chest pain; however, subtle signs of CHF may be the only presenting symptom.
4. **Aortic dissection.** Patients present with severe chest or back pain. Associated symptoms include neurologic deficits, syncope, and abdominal pain as well as constitutional symptoms such as nausea, vomiting, or diaphoresis.
5. **Renal failure** may manifest as urinary tract complaints such as hematuria, oliguria, or anuria. Patients may also present with swelling of the extremities or shortness of breath due to fluid retention.

KEY COMPLAINTS

A patient with elevated BP should be assessed for end-organ damage, beginning with historic factors. Review of systems should address chest pain, back pain, shortness of breath, numbness, tingling, weakness, headache, visual disturbances, abdominal pain, and urinary tract complaints.

B. **Physical Examination**
1. **Vital signs.** Begin by verifying that the elevated BP reading was obtained with a cuff of the appropriate size for the patient. Cuffs that are too small will lead to spuriously high BP readings. The width of the cuff bladder (inflatable portion of the cuff) should be approximately 40% of the circumference of the arm. The length of the cuff bladder should be 80% of the circumference of the arm.
2. **Neurologic examination.** Encephalopathic patients may have mental status changes or focal findings. These findings may not be in a normal vascular distribution, as seen in a stroke syndrome, due to the global diffuse breakdown of the entire cerebral autoregulatory system. Careful funduscopic examination may show retinal hemorrhages and papilledema.
3. **Cardiovascular examination** should note murmurs, bruits, or pericardial rubs. S3 heart sound is indicative of ventricular failure, while an S4 may be indicative of reduced compliance of the left ventricle. BP should be checked

in both arms and a comparison made to readings in the lower extremities. A differential > 20 mm Hg suggests the presence of aortic dissection or coarctation.

4. **Pulmonary examination.** Crackles in patients with pulmonary edema.
5. **Abdominal examination.** Assess for pulsatile masses, tenderness, or evidence of a gravid uterus.

CLINICAL SKILLS TIP

Calculate the MAP from the BP. The formula for determining MAP can be easily remembered by knowing that systole occurs one third of the time and diastole the other two thirds. Therefore,

$$MAP = 1/3(SBP) + 2/3(DBP)$$

VI. **Differential Diagnosis (elevated BP).** Essential hypertension, fever, pain, anxiety, thyrotoxicosis, glomerulonephritis, polycystic renal disease, renovascular stenosis, hyperaldosteronism, pheochromocytoma, or preeclampsia.

VII. **Diagnostic Findings**
   A. **Laboratory Studies**
      1. **Urinalysis** and **BUN/creatinine.** The renal system is evaluated by assessing the presence of protein, blood, or glucose in the urine as well as measuring serum BUN and creatinine.
      2. **Urine pregnancy test** should be considered in all females of reproductive age.
      3. **Cardiac enzymes** for patients complaining of chest pain, back pain, or shortness of breath.
   B. **Imaging**
      1. **ECG** should be performed when there is suspicion of cardiac ischemia, arrhythmias, or conduction defects.
      2. **CXR** can be performed to determine the presence of pulmonary edema or to assess the width of the mediastinum in patients with suspected aortic dissection.
      3. **Head CT scan** is indicated in patients presenting with AMS, papilledema, or focal neurologic deficits.
      4. **Chest and abdominal CT scan** in patients with suspicion of aortic dissection.
      5. **Ultrasound** may be used as an initial screening tool to assess the kidneys and abdominal aorta.
   C. **Diagnostic Algorithm (See page 97)**

VIII. **Treatment**
   A. **Hypertensive emergency.** Requires immediate control of the BP to terminate ongoing end-organ damage. ***The goal is not to return BP to normal limits, but to reduce MAP by 20% in the first ½ hour.*** This is accomplished with IV medications (Tables 17–1 and 17–2). The exception to this rule is aortic dissection, in which the systolic BP should be reduced to 100–120 mm Hg.
   B. **Hypertensive urgency.** BP is gradually reduced over a period of 24 to 48 hours with oral medications.

Diagnostic Algorithm

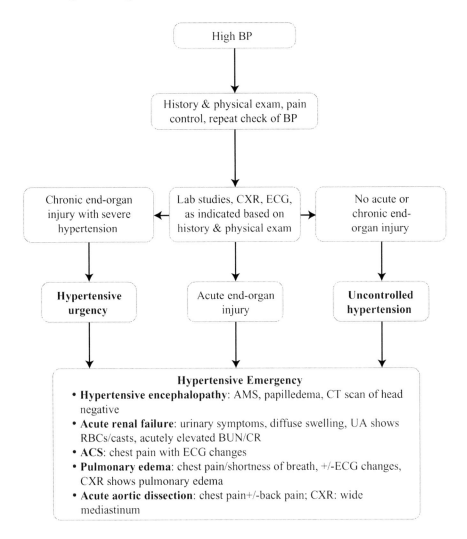

C. **Hemorrhagic stroke.** The value of emergently reducing BP has not been proven. However, with radiologic evidence of a major intracerebral bleed, cautious reduction of systolic BP < 200 mm Hg or diastolic BP < 120 mm Hg is recommended with the use of parenteral agents.

D. **Ischemic stroke.** There is no evidence that hypertension has a deleterious effect on the outcome of ischemic strokes in the acute phase. On the contrary, reducing BP in patients with cerebral ischemia may result in further injury. Therapy is usually only recommended if diastolic BP is >130 mm Hg, with the therapeutic goal to reduce MAP by only 20% in the first 24 hours using parenteral agents.

Table 17–1. Recommended agents for specific hypertensive emergencies.

Emergency	First-line	Alternative
Hypertensive encephalopathy	Nitroprusside	Labetalol or nicardipine
Acute pulmonary edema	Nitroglycerin and loop diuretic	Nitroprusside or ACE inhibitor
Acute coronary syndrome	Nitroglycerin and β blocker	Labetalol or nitroprusside
Aortic dissection	Nitroprusside and β blocker	Labetalol
Acute renal failure	Nitroprusside	Nicardipine
Preeclampsia/eclampsia	Labetalol	Hydralazine or nicardipine

Table 17–2. IV antihypertensive medications used in the treatment of hypertensive emergency.

Agent	Mechanism	Onset	Duration	Contraindications	Adverse Effects
Nitroprusside (0.3–2 mcg/kg/min)	Vascular smooth muscle dilator	Seconds	3–5 min	Hepatic or renal dysfunction	Prolonged use (> 48 hr) gives cyanide toxicity
Labetalol (20–40 mg every 10 min up to 300 mg)	α and β blockers	5 min	4–8 hr	Asthma, COPD, bradycardia, heart blocks	Bradycardia, bronchoconstriction
Nitroglycerin (10–100 mcg/min)	Vascular smooth muscle dilator	2–5 min	5–10 min	Right ventricular infarction	Headache
Hydralazine (10–20 mg)	Arteriolar dilator	10 min	4–6 hr	Aortic dissection, coronary syndromes	Tachycardia, increases catecholamines
Enalaprilat (0.625–1.25 mg)	ACE inhibitor	15 min	6 hr	Renal artery stenosis	Acute renal failure, angioedema
Nicardipine (5–15 mg/hr)	Calcium channel blocker	15–30 min	40 min	Aortic stenosis	Headache, tachycardia

IX. Disposition

A. **Admission.** Patients with hypertensive emergency require admission to an ICU. Patients with hypertensive urgency are admitted for BP control over the following 24–36 hours.

B. **Discharge.** Patients with uncontrolled severe hypertension without acute or chronic end-organ injury can be discharged with close follow-up.

CASE PRESENTATION

A 42-year-old man presents with AMS. Family members have noted progressive confusion over the past several hours. The patient was diagnosed with hypertension, but has been noncompliant with his medications. His BP is 250/150 mm Hg. There are no meningeal findings or focal neurologic deficits. Retinal hemorrhages are present on funduscopic examination.

1. *What other testing is required for this patient?*

   • *Blood glucose, pulse oximetry, O_2 saturation. Urinalysis, CBC, and blood chemistry. ECG (myocardial ischemia), CXR (widened mediastinum or pulmonary edema), and CT scan of head.*

2. *Your work-up is negative. What will your working diagnosis be, and how will you initiate treatment?*

   • *Hypertensive encephalopathy. Initiate treatment with nitroprusside or labetalol to reduce the MAP 20%.*

SUMMARY POINTS

• *Hypertension is very common in patients presenting to the ED.*

• *Evidence of end-organ dysfunction in the setting of hypertension is rare, but requires emergent diagnosis and treatment.*

• *Asymptomatic hypertension without evidence of end-organ dysfunction does not require emergent BP control.*

CHAPTER 18
SYNCOPE

I. Defining Features

A. Syncope is a sudden transient loss of consciousness associated with an inability to maintain postural tone.

B. The etiology of syncope covers a wide variety of disorders ranging from benign to life threatening.

C. In the ED, the cause often remains elusive, but identifying a high-risk group who require admission can be achieved through a careful history and physical examination.

II. Epidemiology

A. Between 12% and 48% of the United States population will experience syncope at some time in their lives.

B. Syncope is the presenting complaint in 1–3% of visits to the ED.

C. About 3–5% of all ED hospital admissions are for treatment of syncope.

III. Pathophysiology

A. Syncope occurs via impaired blood flow to the reticular activating system or both cerebral hemispheres.

B. Transient impaired blood flow to the brain may be due to systemic hypotension or to a rapid increase in ICP (eg, subarachnoid hemorrhage).

C. Reduced cerebral blood flow results in loss of postural tone and unconsciousness.

IV. Risk Factors.
Elderly, cardiovascular disease, medications (eg, diuretics, β blockers, α blockers), dehydration, anemia, and pregnancy (inferior vena cava compression by the uterus).

V. Clinical Presentation

A. **History**

1. History is crucial in determining the cause of syncope. Ask about the events prior, during, and after the episode. Interview any witnesses, if possible.

2. Concerns for immediate life-threatening syncope include associated chest pain (ie, aortic dissection), headache (ie, SAH), or back or abdominal pain (ie, ruptured AAA, ectopic pregnancy).

3. *Arrhythmia should be suspected if the patient had a sudden syncopal event without a prodrome.* In a young patient, lightheadedness when moving from a

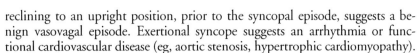

reclining to an upright position, prior to the syncopal episode, suggests a benign vasovagal episode. Exertional syncope suggests an arrhythmia or functional cardiovascular disease (eg, aortic stenosis, hypertrophic cardiomyopathy).
   4. **Past medical history** and **medication profile.** Patients with significant cardiac history are at a higher risk of arrhythmia as the cause of syncope.
B. **Physical Examination**
   1. **Vital signs.** Always examine triage vital signs and repeat them when abnormal. Obtain BP measurements in both arms, looking for unequal pressures that might suggest aortic dissection. Orthostatic vital signs suggest volume depletion, anemia, or side effects due to medications.
   2. **Cardiovascular examination** auscultating for murmurs (eg, aortic stenosis) and irregular heart rhythms.
   3. **Rectal examination** for occult or gross blood.
   4. **Neurologic examination** for focal neurologic deficits.

VI. **Differential Diagnosis**
A. **Syncope.** Cardiac (23%) (arrhythmia, acute MI, PE, valvular heart disease); orthostatic hypotension (hypovolemia, anemia); reflex mediated (58%) (vasovagal episode, micturition syncope); neurologic (SAH); or medications (β blockers, diuretics, vasodilators).
B. **Syncope mimickers.** Psychogenic, hypoglycemia, hypoxia, or seizures.

RULE OUT

Cardiac syncope due to an arrhythmia must be differentiated from other, more benign causes. Patients with any risk factors for cardiac syncope should be admitted to a monitored setting. Risk factors include > age 45, abnormal ECG, symptoms compatible with ACS, history of ventricular arrhythmia, or CHF.

VII. **Diagnostic Findings**
A. **Laboratory Studies**
   1. Useful only when indicated by history and physical examination.
   2. **Bedside glucose** in patients with altered sensorium.
   3. **CBC** in patients with GI bleeding or evidence of anemia.
   4. **Urine pregnancy test** in females of childbearing age.
   5. **Myocardial enzymes** are indicated when the event was preceded or followed by chest pain or other cardiovascular symptoms.
B. **ECG**
   1. Obtain on all patients with syncope.
   2. An abnormal ECG is a significant risk factor for cardiac syncope. Significant abnormalities include evidence of ischemia, arrhythmia, bundle branch block, or prolonged QT interval.
   3. Brugada syndrome (RBBB with ST segment elevation in leads V1-V3) carries a high mortality rate (10% per year) due to the development of VT and should prompt admission to a monitored setting with cardiology consultation.
C. **Imaging Studies**
   1. **CXR.** Indicated when history and physical examination suggests heart failure or aortic dissection.
   2. **Head CT scan.** Studies fail to show any indication for routine CT scan of the head unless headache or focal neurologic deficits are present.

D. **Diagnostic Algorithm**

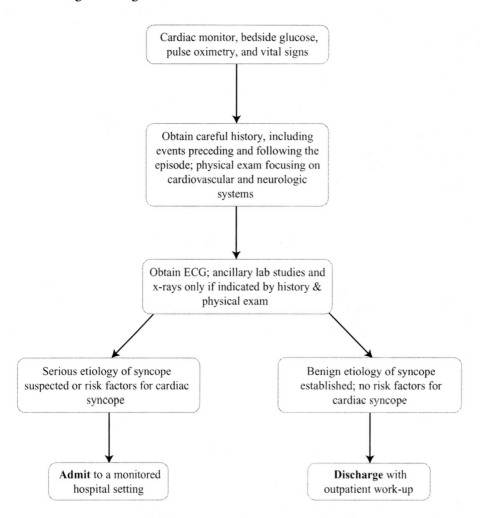

VIII. Treatment

A. Treatment in the ED is usually supportive.

B. Continuous cardiac monitoring, especially if an arrhythmia is suspected.

C. Supplemental O_2 if the patient is hypoxic.

D. IV fluids if the patient is dehydrated. Blood transfusion is indicated in patients with anemia or significant GI bleeding.

IX. Disposition

A. **Admission** to a monitored setting if risk factors for a cardiac etiology are present. Also, admit all patients with ECG evidence of *Brugada syndrome.* Admit all patients with life-threatening non-cardiac causes for their syncope (eg, GI bleeding, SAH).

B. **Discharge** if low risk for cardiac etiology (normal physical examination, no CHF, normal ECG, < age 45) and no life-threatening non-cardiac cause is suspected.

CASE PRESENTATION

A 55-year-old woman presents to the ED complaining of "passing out" while walking to the grocery store earlier this morning. The patient states that she never had this happen before and feels fine now.

1. What other information do you want to know?

  • *What events preceded the episode? What occurred after the episode? Did anyone witness the event? Any associated chest pain, headache, abdominal or back pain? Abnormal vital signs? Abnormalities in the cardiovascular or neurologic examinations?*

2. If you have failed to find an explanation for the syncopal event based on the history and physical examination, what is your next step?

  • *ECG. Admit the patient to a telemetry bed because her age puts her at an increased risk for a cardiac cause of syncope.*

SUMMARY POINTS

• *Place all patients with syncope on a cardiac monitor and obtain a bedside glucose level and pulse oximetry reading.*

• *Take a detailed history of events surrounding the episode; interview witnesses, if possible.*

• *All patients with a syncopal episode require an ECG.*

• *Admit patients with risk factors for a cardiac etiology or another acute life-threatening condition.*

SECTION IV
PULMONARY
EMERGENCIES

CHAPTER 19
DYSPNEA

I. **Defining Features**

    A. **Dyspnea,** or shortness of breath, is the sensation of breathlessness or "air hunger," and is manifested by signs of difficult or labored breathing.

    B. **Tachypnea** is rapid breathing and is usually defined by RR > 20 breaths/minute in adults.

    C. **Hyperventilation** is tachypnea due to nonphysiologic causes. Hyperventilation may cause symptoms of lightheadedness or even syncope by reducing the CO_2 concentration in blood.

    D. **Hyperpnea** is an increase in the rate of breathing that is proportional to an increase in metabolism.

    E. **Upper airway obstruction** is defined by blockage of airflow in the larynx or trachea. It is characterized by **stridor,** an inspiratory sound caused by airflow through a partially obstructed upper airway. The onset may be abrupt or gradual, and if not recognized and treated promptly, death may result.

II. **Epidemiology**

    A. Dyspnea is the presenting complaint in over 2.5 million physician visits a year.

    B. Most patients with chronic dyspnea have 1 of 4 conditions: asthma, COPD, CHF, or interstitial lung disease.

III. **Pathophysiology**

    A. Dyspnea is a symptom of many disorders that involve alterations or abnormalities in gas exchange, pulmonary circulation, respiratory mechanics, O_2-carrying capacity, and cardiovascular function.

    B. A mismatch between supply and demand of O_2 and failure of CO_2 elimination is the basis for dyspnea.

    C. Hypoxemia occurs secondary to several potential mechanisms: decreased alveolar pO_2 (eg, high altitude), hypoventilation (eg, neuromuscular disorder), V/Q mismatch (eg, PE), shunting of blood (eg, cardiac defect), and decreased O_2-carrying capacity (eg, anemia, CO).

IV. **Risk Factors.** Elderly, history of COPD, asthma, interstitial lung disease, CHF, immunocompromise (eg, pneumonia), hypercoagulability (eg, pulmonary embolus), and trauma (eg, pneumothorax, pulmonary contusion).

V. Clinical Presentation

A. History

1. A thorough history is extremely important in developing an appropriate differential diagnosis.
2. **Onset.** Sudden onset suggests a pneumothorax, MI, or airway obstruction, while a slow progression is more consistent with an infectious process such as pneumonia.
3. **Duration.** Long-standing symptoms that have changed little suggest a more chronic or benign disease process.
4. **Associated symptoms.** Chest pain is frequently present and suggests ACS, especially when it is exertional. Pleuritic chest pain supports the diagnosis of PE, but is also present in patients with a pneumothorax, pneumonia, and occasionally ACS. Cough and fever suggest pneumonia, but are also seen in patients with a URI or an exacerbation due to asthma. Swelling in the lower extremities suggests CHF if it is bilateral and venous thromboembolism if it is unilateral.
5. **Prior medical history.** The patient's prior history will provide clues to the diagnosis. It is helpful to ask the patient whether the current episode is similar to previous attacks.

B. Physical Examination

1. **Vital signs with pulse oximetry** are the most important portion of the initial assessment.
2. **General appearance.** Level of distress is ascertained by noting patient position (eg, "tripoding"), presence of retractions, and the patient's ability to speak.
3. **Neck examination.** A deviated trachea suggests a tension pneumothorax. Stridor is present in patients with upper airway obstruction. JVD is evidence of increased right-sided heart pressures seen in pericardial tamponade or CHF.
4. **Lung examination.** Wheezes suggest an exacerbation due to asthma or COPD, but may also be present in heart failure or anaphylaxis. The presence of rales suggests CHF, pneumonia, or in the setting of trauma, a pulmonary contusion. Decreased breath sounds on one side of the chest are consistent with a pneumothorax.
5. **Cardiac examination.** Muffled heart sounds are present in a patient with a pericardial effusion. The presence of a murmur should be noted.
6. **Extremity examination.** Unilateral edema and calf tenderness may be present in patients with DVT. Bilateral pitting edema is present with right-sided heart failure.
7. **Skin examination.** Wheals suggest an anaphylactic reaction with edema of the airway as the cause of dyspnea.
8. **Neurologic examination.** An ascending paralysis is present in Guillain-Barré syndrome and may cause respiratory depression due to diaphragmatic muscle weakness.

VI. Differential Diagnosis

A. **Pulmonary.** Foreign body airway obstruction, epiglottitis, croup, pleural effusion, neoplasm, COPD, asthma, pulmonary embolus, anaphylaxis, pneumothorax, pneumonia, or non-cardiogenic edema.

B. **Cardiovascular.** Pulmonary edema/CHF, MI, pericarditis, or cardiac tamponade.

C. **Traumatic.** Tension or simple pneumothorax, flail chest segment, cardiac tamponade, inhalation injury, or pulmonary contusion.

D. **Hematologic.** Anemia or CO poisoning.

E. **Neuromuscular.** Guillain-Barré syndrome, ALS, botulism, or myasthenia gravis.

F. **Metabolic/endocrine/toxicologic.** Toxic ingestion, electrolyte abnormalities, metabolic acidosis, or organophosphate poisoning.

VII. **Diagnostic Findings**

A. **Laboratory Studies**

1. **Pulse oximetry.** This is a rapid, non-invasive test that is useful to screen for hypoxia. An $SaO_2 > 98\%$ predicts a $PaO_2 > 80$ mm Hg with 100% sensitivity and an $SaO_2 \geq 90\%$ predicts a $PaO_2 > 60$ mm Hg.

2. **ABG.** This test is the most accurate method for determining oxygenation and ventilation. The PaO_2 (oxygenation) and pCO_2 (ventilation) is directly measured. The pCO_2 is useful in the management of patients with COPD, asthma, or sleep apnea.

3. **CBC.** Anemia is a common cause of dyspnea.

4. **Electrolytes and renal function.** These tests will detect metabolic abnormalities and uremia.

5. **Blood cultures.** Two blood cultures should be obtained in febrile patients when there is suspicion of pneumonia.

CLINICAL SKILLS TIP

A-a gradient is the pO_2 difference between the alveolar gas and arterial blood. It is used to detect abnormalities of ventilation or perfusion of the lung. The normal A-a gradient increases with patient age (age/4 + 4). If the calculated A-a gradient is greater than the age-based estimation, then a ventilation-perfusion abnormality exists.

The most common formula for the A-a gradient (assuming the patient is breathing room air at sea level) is

$$A\text{--}a \ gradient = 150 - [pO_2 + (pCO_2/0.8)]$$

B. **Imaging Studies**

1. **ECG.** To assess for cardiac ischemia and arrhythmias.

2. **CXR.** Useful to evaluate bony structures, soft tissue, mediastinum, heart silhouette, and lung parenchyma.

3. **Echocardiogram.** The most common use in the ED is to exclude pericardial fluid. In the setting of suspected cardiac disease, valvular disorders or wall motion abnormalities may also be detected.

4. **Chest CT angiogram.** This test is used to further assess mass lesions, adenopathy, or trauma. CT angiogram is helpful to rule out pulmonary emboli.

5. **Soft tissue lateral neck radiograph** is used in stable patients to determine the presence of epiglottitis, foreign body, or retropharyngeal abscesses in patients with upper airway obstruction.

C. **Procedures. Pulse oximetry** uses a microprocessor to continuously measure oxyhemoglobin saturation. The technique takes advantage of the difference in the wavelength of oxygenated and deoxygenated hemoglobin. The probe is placed on the index finger, but may also be attached to the earlobe. Colored nail polish, COHb, hypothermia, or an inflated BP cuff on the same arm will result in inaccurate readings.

D. **Diagnostic Algorithm**

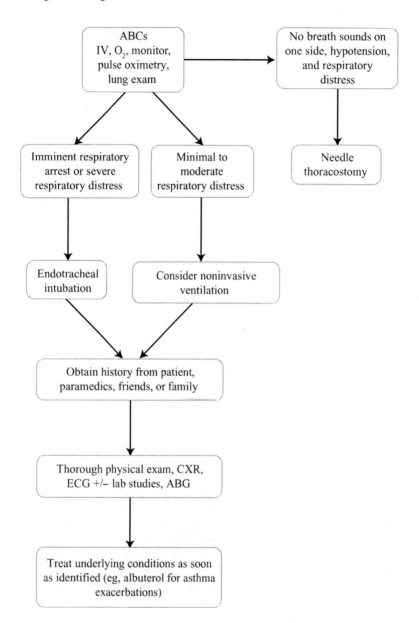

VIII. Treatment

A. Emergent interventions are frequently necessary before proceeding to a complete diagnostic work-up and definitive treatment. (Treatment of specific causes of dyspnea is discussed in Chapters 20–23.)

B. **ABCs.**

C. **IV access, cardiac monitor,** and a **pulse oximeter.**

D. **Supplemental O_2** is provided. A nasal cannula with 2–6 L/min of O_2 is used for patients with mild symptoms (room air has an FiO_2 of 21%; each L/min adds an additional 2–4% to the FiO_2). For patients in severe distress, a nonrebreather (NRB) mask with 15 L/min flow of O_2 will provide a FiO_2 of approximately 60–70% (Figure 19–1). BVM-assisted ventilation provides 90–100% FiO_2 with 15 L/min of O_2. If respiratory arrest is imminent, immediate endotracheal intubation is performed.

E. In general, allow the patient to assume the position that is most comfortable for them. For patients with acute pulmonary edema or asthma, forcing them to lie down will only exacerbate their symptoms.

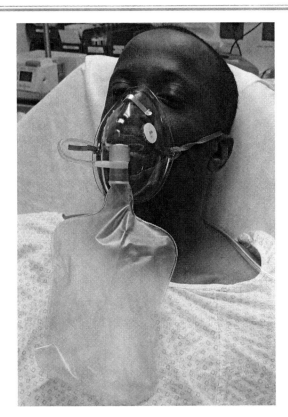

Figure 19–1. Patient with non-rebreather mask.

IX. Disposition

A. **Admission.** Patients who are unstable or have the potential to become unstable should be admitted to an ICU. Patients who were initially unstable but improved after treatment may be observed on a telemetry unit.

B. **Discharge.** Patients who are stable with improvement in symptoms, an identified non-emergent condition, and good medical follow-up may be discharged.

CASE PRESENTATION

A 20-year-old man presents to the ED acutely short of breath and in severe distress. His examination reveals decreased breath sounds on the right side.

1. *What should be done initially?*

 • *ABCs. Needle decompression. IV, O_2, cardiac monitor.*

2. *The dyspnea improves after needle decompression. What is the next step?*

 • *Complete physical examination. Tube thoracostomy (chest tube). CXR. Admission.*

SUMMARY POINTS

• *Emergent conditions must be identified and treated before proceeding to a complete diagnostic work-up.*

• *After patient stabilization, obtaining a thorough history and performing a physical examination are necessary to determine an appropriate differential diagnosis.*

• *Reassess the patient frequently and note any changes in condition or response to therapy.*

CHAPTER 20
ASTHMA

I. Defining Features

   A. Asthma is a chronic inflammatory disorder of the airways that results in recurrent wheezing and breathlessness. It is associated with variable airflow obstruction that is **reversible with treatment.**

   B. Controlling an acute asthma exacerbation is dependent on suppressing the inflammatory process and alleviating the obstruction to airflow.

II. Epidemiology

   A. In the United States, 5% of the population has asthma.

   B. Asthma exacerbations account for up to 10% of all ED visits.

   C. Asthma can occur at any age, but is more common in children and adolescents. About 50% of patients develop asthma before age 10.

   D. Asthma-related morbidity and mortality rates have been increasing over the past 20 years, despite advances in treatment.

III. Pathophysiology

   A. The inflammatory process is responsible for both acute and chronic asthma.

   B. Bronchial hyperactivity results from multiple potential triggers that cause a release of cytokines and recruitment of inflammatory cells to the airway.

   C. Inflammatory mediators produce bronchoconstriction, mucus hypersecretion, and airway edema.

   D. Increases in airway resistance and the subsequent decrease in expiratory flow rates result in air trapping and barotrauma.

IV. Risk Factors.

Features that increase mortality from asthma include history of sudden severe exacerbations, prior intubations, prior ICU admissions, overuse of medications leading to delays in seeking treatment, illicit drug use (eg, inhaled cocaine and heroin), ≥ 2 hospitalizations a year, ≥ 3 ED visits a year, and low socioeconomic status.

V. Clinical Presentation

   A. **History**

     1. In the acutely dyspneic patient, a brief assessment is made and treatment is initiated.

2. Most patients with acute asthma have a constellation of symptoms consisting of cough, dyspnea, chest tightness, and wheezing. Fever may indicate the presence of a URI or pneumonia.

3. Patients should be questioned about recent steroid or inhaler use, history of intubations, and the number of ED visits and hospitalizations within the past 12 months. This information will allow the physician to gauge the severity of the patient's disease.

4. Identifying triggers for asthma may help avoid future exacerbations. Potential triggers include weather changes, cigarette smoke, intranasal heroin or cocaine use, URI, and pets.

5. Patients with severe asthma, especially those with recurrent exacerbation, have a blunted perception of dyspnea. These patients are at risk for bad outcomes because they may underestimate the severity of an attack.

6. Alternate diagnoses must be explored in the history, even in patients who report a history of "asthma." Be especially careful in the elderly population. Unless a thorough history is obtained, the true diagnosis can be missed.

B. **Physical Examination**
1. Wheezing depends on the air velocity and turbulence. The intensity of the wheezing varies with the radius of the airway. *Therefore,* **in a severe exacerbation, there may be little or no wheezing with minimal air movement on examination.**

2. Severe asthma exacerbations present with the patient in an upright position, tachycardia, tachypnea, poor air movement, inability to speak in complete sentences, accessory muscle use (retractions), and alterations in mentation or consciousness.

CLINICAL SKILLS TIP

With severe bronchoconstriction, increased use of accessory muscles (intercostals, sternocleidomastoid) occurs.

VI. **Differential Diagnosis.** COPD exacerbation, CHF, pneumonia, pulmonary embolus, upper airway obstruction, or aspirated foreign body.

VII. **Diagnostic Findings**
A. **Laboratory Studies**
1. **ABG.** An increasing pCO_2 level indicates ventilatory failure and is an indication for admission to the ICU. The patient's clinical condition is more important than an ABG to predict outcome or the need for intubation.

2. **CBC, electrolytes, and renal function.** These studies may be helpful if the patient has co-morbidities that make metabolic derangements more likely. An elevated WBC may aid in the diagnosis of concomitant pulmonary infection.

B. **Imaging Studies**
1. **CXR.** Hyperinflation of the lungs is seen in moderate to severe exacerbations. CXR should be considered in patients not responding to treatment and those requiring hospitalization. About 15% of these patients have unsuspected pneumonia, CHF, pneumothorax, or pneumomediastinum.

2. **ECG.** In severe asthma exacerbations, the ECG may demonstrate a right ventricular strain pattern that normalizes with improvement of airflow. Dysrhythmias and ischemia may occur in older patients with coexistent heart disease.

C. **Procedures**
1. **Peak expiratory flow rate** (PEFR). PEFR is an objective measurement of the degree of airway obstruction, which aids the physician in monitoring the progress of treatment and in determining patient disposition. Predicted values are based on patient's age, gender, and height. PEFR can be used as a screen for hypercarbia. PEFR < 25% of predicted is a sensitive marker for hypercarbia. Use the percent of personal best peak flow to further individualize the value.
2. **Nebulizer.** The components of a nebulizer treatment include the mouthpiece, medication reservoir, O_2 tubing, and "accordion" extension tube. The albuterol is placed within the reservoir, and the components are fastened together. The extension tube provides a reservoir of "trapped" O_2 and nebulized albuterol that can be inhaled with each breath. The O_2 tubing is hooked up to the green wall O_2 port and turned to 6 L/min. The yellow wall port delivers air (21% FiO_2) only. The patient holds the nebulizer during the treatment (Figure 20–1). If the patient is unable to hold the treatment, a similar set-up with a facemask is used instead.

CLINICAL SKILLS TIP

A PEFR or "peak flow" is obtained by having the patient stand (or sit up) and take a deep inspiratory breath. Then, with the lips tightly wrapped around the peak flow meter mouthpiece, the patient blows as hard as possible.

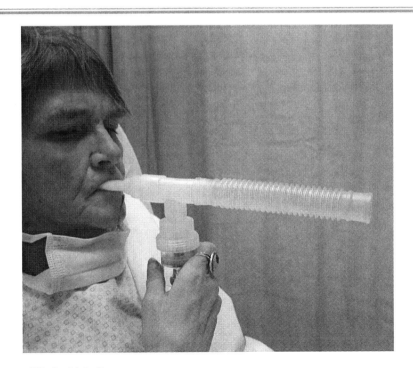

Figure 20–1. Nebulizer treatment.

D. **Diagnostic Algorithm**

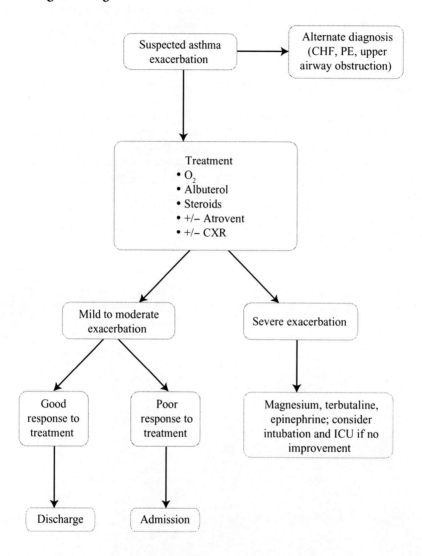

VIII. Treatment

A. **O$_2$** via nasal canula or facemask.

B. **Cardiac monitor** and **IV** in moderate to severe asthmatics.

C. **β Agonists**

1. **Albuterol** is the most commonly used agent and is considered first-line therapy. It bronchodilates by increasing cyclic AMP and relaxing airway smooth muscles. Onset of action is < 5 minutes.

2. **Nebulized form or metered dose inhaler** (MDI). Albuterol 2.5 mg in 3 cc of saline q 20 minutes x 3, or albuterol 10 mg continuous nebulizer over a period of 1 hour, or albuterol MDI 8 puffs with a spacer q 20–30 minutes.
3. **Spacer.** Delivery of β agonist using an MDI with a spacer can achieve bronchodilation equivalent to that achieved by nebulization. MDI requires more patient effort; therefore, it should be reserved for mild or moderate exacerbations only.
4. **Parenteral β agonists.** Terbutaline 0.25 mg or epinephrine 0.2 mg SQ. Useful in a life-threatening exacerbation. Avoid in patients with a history of ischemic heart disease.

D. Corticosteroids
   1. *First line treatment for ALL but the mildest attacks.*
   2. **Mechanism.** Suppresses the inflammatory component. Increases the responsiveness of β adrenergic receptors in the airway smooth muscle. Decreases the recruitment and activation of inflammatory cells.
   3. **Indications.** < 10% improvement in PEFR after first nebulizer treatment, current attack while taking steroids, or PEFR < 70% of predicted after 1st hour of treatment.
   4. **Onset of action.** Gradual, with a peak effect within 6–12 hours.
   5. **Route of administration.** PO and IV routes are equally effective. Prednisone 80 mg PO or methylprednisolone (Solu-Medrol) 125 mg IV. Continue steroids for 5–14 days, depending on the severity of the exacerbation and the prior experience of the patient. Aerosolized corticosteroids are important in chronic treatment and prevention of relapse in asthmatic patients. They play no role in the treatment of acute exacerbations but should be prescribed upon discharge from the ED.

E. **Anticholinergic agents.** Ipratropium bromide (Atrovent) 0.5 mg via nebulizer. Used in conjunction with β agonist therapy for moderate to severe asthma exacerbations. Competitively antagonizes acetylcholine and subsequently decreases cyclic GMP, causing bronchodilation. Onset of action is 20 minutes, with peak effect within 1–6 hours.

F. **Magnesium sulfate** 2 g IV. Given for severe asthma exacerbations. Causes relaxation of smooth muscle.

G. **Antibiotics** if evidence of pneumonia.

H. **Mechanical ventilation.** Use the largest ET tube possible to decrease airway resistance. Ketamine (2 mg/kg) is the best induction agent because it causes bronchodilation. Beware of high airway pressures causing barotrauma. Increase the expiration time to prevent air trapping. Low tidal volume (5–7 mL/kg) and low respiratory rate (permissive hypercarbia).

I. **Pregnancy.** All of the above drugs are safe to use during pregnancy except epinephrine, which is associated with congenital malformations and premature labor.

IX. Disposition
   A. **Admission.** Disposition is based on the combination of patient symptoms, physical examination findings, responses to treatment, O_2 saturation, peak flow measurements, and the patient's social limitations to medical care. ICU admission should be considered in patients with severe exacerbations and poor

response to treatment judged by AMS or continued respiratory distress. Floor admission is considered for patients with continued symptoms and a PEFR that remains < 70% of predicted despite treatment.

B. **Discharge** is acceptable for patients without respiratory distress or hypoxia, good aeration and diminished wheezing, and a sustained response after the final treatment. All discharged patients should be instructed on the proper use of the inhaler, spacer, and peak flow meter. Proper technique for use of the MDI is to remove the cap and shake; exhale completely; activate the canister and start inspiration; continue slow, deep inspiration; hold breath 5–10 seconds; and wait 20 seconds between each puff. In addition, patients should be given instructions to avoid asthma triggers (eg, smoking) and be provided with appropriate follow-up information.

CASE PRESENTATION

A 28-year-old woman with a history of asthma presents to the ED with an exacerbation. She has never been intubated nor been to the ICU before.

1. What historical questions do you want to ask?

   • *How severe is this attack compared to previous exacerbations? Triggers? What inhalers or medications does she use and how frequently is she using them?*

2. She appears comfortable and has expiratory wheezes on examination. Her PEFR is 60% of predicted. She is given a dose of prednisone and responds well to albuterol. What medications will you prescribe at discharge?

   • *Albuterol. Inhaled and oral corticosteroids.*

SUMMARY POINTS

• *Patients with severe asthma exacerbations may have such severe restriction of airflow that they do not exhibit wheezing on examination.*

• *β Agonists (albuterol) and corticosteroids are the mainstay of treatment for acute asthma exacerbations.*

• *The peak flow meter is used as objective evidence of the severity of a patient's asthma exacerbation and should be followed serially to measure improvement.*

• *There is no one factor or finding that reliably determines whether a patient is safe to be discharged home.*

CHAPTER 21
PNEUMONIA

I. Defining Features

  A. Pneumonia is an infection in the pulmonary alveoli.

  B. **Community-acquired pneumonia** (CAP) occurs in patients who neither have been recently hospitalized nor have been in a nursing home.

  C. **Nosocomial pneumonia** occurs in patients with recent hospitalizations. The distinction is important when considering the causative agents and the appropriate therapy.

  D. **Aspiration pneumonia** occurs in patients with diminished mental status when a foreign substance (eg, gastric contents) enters the lungs. A pneumonitis results due to both chemical and bacterial injury. The pathogens causing infection are typically polymicrobial.

II. Epidemiology

  A. In the United States, pneumonia is the 6th leading cause of death and the leading cause of death from an infectious disease.

  B. The annual incidence of CAP in the United States is 2–4 million cases and results in about 500,000 hospital admissions.

  C. Most deaths occur in the elderly or immunocompromised.

III. Etiology

  A. It is difficult to determine the specific organism responsible. In about half of cases, the etiologic agent will not be determined.

  B. **"Typical" pathogens (25%).** *Streptococcus pneumoniae, Haemophilus influenzae,* and *Klebsiella pneumoniae.* The most common pathogen that requires admission in adults is *S. pneumoniae.*

  C. **"Atypical" pathogens (15%).** Legionella species, *Mycoplasma pneumoniae* and *Chlamydia pneumoniae.*

  D. **Viral pathogens (17%).** The most commonly implicated viral agents are influenza, parainfluenza, and adenovirus.

  E. **Nosocomial pneumonia.** May be due to any of the above agents, as well as *Pseudomonas aeruginosa, Staphylococcus aureus,* and Enterobacter species.

  F. **Acquired immunodeficiency syndrome (AIDS).** Patients frequently have infection due to unusual pathogens, such as TB and *Pneumocystis carinii* pneumonia (PCP).

IV. Risk Factors

A. **Aspiration.** Decreased LOC, intoxication, seizure, stroke, or anesthesia.

B. **Damage to mucociliary function.** Cigarette smoking, underlying pulmonary disorder (eg, COPD, asthma), or elderly (decline in mucociliary clearance, elastic recoil of lungs, humoral and cellular immunity).

C. **Immunosuppression.** HIV/AIDS or post-transplantation.

V. Clinical Presentation

A. **History**

1. In most adolescents and adults, diagnosis can be made by history and physical examination alone.

2. **General symptoms.** Cough productive of purulent sputum, shortness of breath, pleuritic chest pain, and fever.

3. Infants, young children, elderly, debilitated, or immunocompromised patients with pneumonia often present with nonspecific complaints and may not demonstrate classic symptoms. In many cases, they present with mental status changes or deterioration of baseline function.

B. **Physical Examination**

1. **Vital signs.** Tachycardia, hypotension (sepsis), increased respiratory rate, or decreased pulse oximetry.

2. **Lung examination.** Evidence of consolidation (egophony, tactile fremitus, or dullness to percussion). Coarse rales or rhonchi.

CLINICAL SKILLS TIP

Tactile fremitus refers to an increase in the palpable vibration transmitted through the bronchopulmonary system to the chest wall when a patient speaks. Ask the patient to repeat the words "ninety-nine" or "one-to-one." Increased tactile fremitus suggests an underlying consolidation.
Egophony is tested by asking the patient to say "ee" while you are auscultating with the stethoscope. Normally, you would hear a muffled long E sound. When "ee" is heard as "ay," egophony is present, indicating an underlying consolidation.

VI. Differential Diagnosis (see Chapter 19)

RULE OUT

TB. Any patient suspected of having pulmonary TB (history of TB, history of exposure to TB, persistent weight loss, night sweats, hemoptysis, incarceration, HIV/AIDS, homelessness, alcohol abuse, immigrant from a high-risk area) should be masked and moved to a negative pressure isolation room.

VII. Diagnostic Findings

A. **Laboratory Studies**

1. **CBC.** There is often an elevated WBC count in patients with bacterial pneumonia.

2. **Chemistry.** Obtain in ill patients to rule out metabolic derangement.

3. **Blood cultures.** Obtain in hospitalized patients prior to initiating antibiotics. More than 25% of hospitalized patients with pneumonia have bacteremia.

4. **Sputum Gram stain and culture.** Recommended as a means to determine the bacterial pathogen, allowing more specific antimicrobial therapy. Rarely obtained in the ED.

B. **Imaging Studies. CXR.** Evidence of lobar consolidation, segmental or subsegmental infiltrate, or interstitial pattern (Figure 21–1). Cavitation is seen with anaerobic, aerobic gram-negative bacilli, *S. aureus,* mycobacterial, or fungal infections (Figure 21–2). Radiographic findings are nonspecific for predicting a particular infectious etiology and may lag behind clinical findings. Also, radiographic signs of pneumonia persist well after clinical resolution. A normal CXR cannot be relied on to completely exclude pneumonia, especially in patients with immunosuppression (HIV/AIDS).

C. **Diagnostic Algorithm**

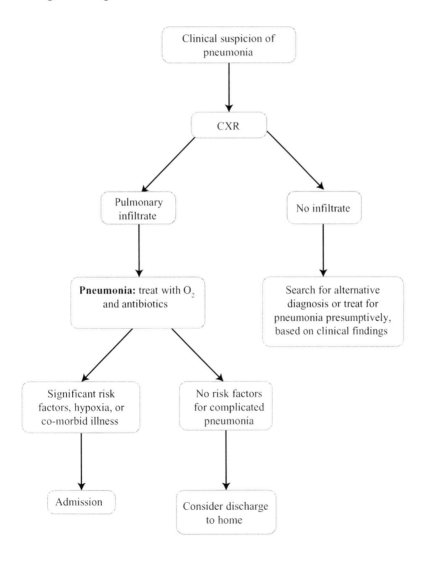

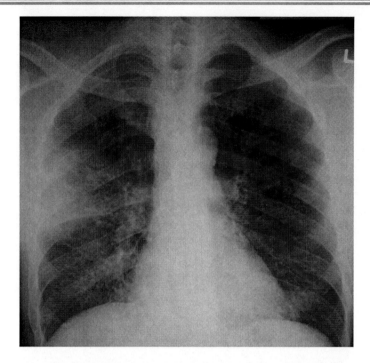

Figure 21–1. Chest radiograph showing pneumonia in the right middle lobe.

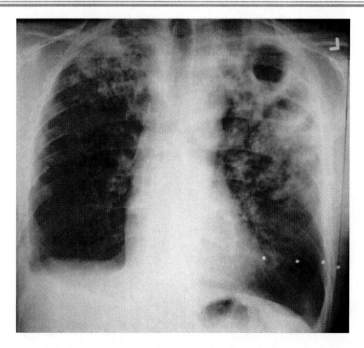

Figure 21–2. Chest radiograph of a patient with tuberculosis. Note the bilateral apical infiltrates and the cavitary lesion in the left upper lobe.

VIII. Treatment

A. **ABCs.**

B. **O₂** via nasal cannula or face mask. **IV fluids.**

C. **Endotracheal intubation.** For patients in severe respiratory distress or shock, mechanical ventilation will decrease the work of breathing and can be lifesaving.

D. **Isolation** of patients suspected of having TB.

E. **Antibiotics**

1. Empiric antibiotics are started based on the spectrum of likely pathogens and the overall clinical picture. *Timely administration of antibiotics (< 8 hr from presentation) is associated with improved outcomes for patients requiring hospital admission.*

2. **Outpatient < age 60 and otherwise healthy.** Doxycycline 100 mg PO BID × 14 days *or* azithromycin 500 mg PO × 1 day, then 250 mg PO × 4 days *or* levofloxacin 500 mg PO QID × 14 days.

3. **Outpatient > age 60 or co-morbidities.** Amoxicillin-clavulanate (Augmentin) 500 mg PO BID × 14 days *or* levofloxacin 500 mg PO QID × 14 days.

4. **Inpatient community-acquired pneumonia.** Third-generation cephalosporin *and* a macrolide. Ceftriaxone 1 g IV q 24 hours and azithromycin 500 mg IV q 24 hours.

5. **Aspiration pneumonia.** Cefoxitin 2 g IV q 8 hours *or* clindamycin 900 mg IV q 8 hours +/– aminoglycoside.

6. **Neutropenia or nosocomial.** Anti-pseudomonal β lactam (eg, Zosyn) and levofloxacin.

7. **Suspected PCP in HIV/AIDS patient.** Prednisone 40 mg PO 30 minutes before antibiotic when pO₂ is < 70 mm Hg. Trimethoprim/sulfamethoxazole 5 mg/kg IV q 8 hours.

IX. Disposition

A. **Admission.** There are a number of well-recognized risk factors associated with an increased risk of death or a complicated clinical course. They include elderly or nursing home resident, co-morbid illness (neoplastic disease, CHF, liver disease, CVA, chronic renal disease), AMS, RR > 30 breaths/min, systolic BP < 90 mm Hg, temperature < 35°C (95°F) or > 40°C (104°F), pulse >125 beats/min, pH < 7.35, BUN > 30 mg/dL, Na < 130 mEq/L, glucose > 250 mg/dL, Hct < 30%, arterial pO2 < 60 mm Hg, and pleural effusion. Patients with risk factors should be considered for admission to an observation unit, medical floor, or ICU, based on the number of factors present and overall clinical presentation.

B. **Discharge.** Patients without risk factors for death or a complicated course and who have a good social situation may be discharged home with appropriate follow-up.

CASE PRESENTATION

A 65-year-old man presents to the ED with complaints of a cough productive of green sputum. He is in moderate respiratory distress and has an O₂ saturation of 92% on room air.

1. *What interventions should occur immediately?*

   · *ABCs, IV, O₂, monitor.*

2. *CXR reveals an infiltrate. What historic features should you consider when choosing an antibiotic?*

- *Does he live at home or in a nursing home? Any co-morbid history (neutropenia, COPD, asthma, HIV, transplantation)? Recent hospitalizations?*

SUMMARY POINTS

- *ED evaluation should concentrate on making the diagnosis of pneumonia and determining the presence of risk factors that influence decisions regarding the need for hospitalization.*
- *Empiric antibiotic therapy should be started in the ED for patients admitted with pneumonia.*
- *TB should be considered for patients with HIV or other significant risk factors.*

CHAPTER 22
PNEUMOTHORAX

I. Defining Features

A. Pneumothorax is an accumulation of air in the pleural space.

B. **Spontaneous pneumothorax** is acquired in the absence of trauma. A **primary** spontaneous pneumothorax is found in healthy persons without underlying pulmonary pathology. A **secondary** spontaneous pneumothorax is found in persons with underlying lung pathology and damage to the alveolar-pleural barrier.

C. **Traumatic pneumothorax** is secondary to a penetrating (eg, knife) or blunt (eg, rib fracture) mechanism.

D. **Tension pneumothorax** is a life-threatening complication caused by progressive accumulation of air in the pleural cavity and resulting in impairment of venous return and shock.

II. Epidemiology

A. Spontaneous primary pneumothoraces have the greatest incidence of occurrence in young adults. They are more common in males than in females (5:1), and occur more often in tall, thin males who smoke. Recurrence rates are 20–50% within the following 2–5 years.

B. Spontaneous secondary pneumothoraces are most common in patients > age 40 with COPD.

III. Pathophysiology

A. Secondary spontaneous pneumothoraces are the result of a damaged alveolar-pleural barrier or underlying lung problems that cause an increase in intrabronchial pressures.

B. Tension pneumothoraces occur when air enters the pleural space on inspiration but cannot escape on expiration (ball-valve effect). There is progressive accumulation of air in the pleural space, resulting in collapse of the affected lung. Subsequently, there is a shift of the mediastinal structures to the opposite side, causing compression of the contralateral lung, impairment of venous return, decreased cardiac output, and signs of cardiovascular collapse.

IV. Risk Factors

A. **Primary spontaneous pneumothorax.** Atmospheric pressure changes (eg, scuba diving, fighter pilots), Valsalva maneuvers in association with drug abuse, Marfan's syndrome, or cigarette smoking.

125

B. **Secondary spontaneous pneumothorax.** Chronic airway disease (eg, COPD, chronic bronchitis, asthma, cystic fibrosis), acute airway disease (eg, pneumonia, tuberculosis), interstitial lung disease, neoplasm, pneumonitis, pulmonary infarction, or endometriosis.

V. **Clinical Presentation**

A. **History**
1. Patients present with a sudden onset of ipsilateral pleuritic chest pain (95%) and/or dyspnea (80%).
2. Patients may also present with agitation, restlessness, and/or with AMS if severe respiratory compromise is present.

B. **Physical Examination**
1. **Vital signs.** Mild tachycardia and mild tachypnea (> 24 breaths/min in only 5% of patients).
2. **Lung examination.** Findings may be subtle if there is a small pneumothorax. Decreased breath sounds (85%) or hyperresonance to percussion (< 33%).
3. **Tension pneumothorax.** Hypotension, cyanosis, severe respiratory distress, and trachea deviated to the contralateral side.

VI. **Differential Diagnosis (see Chapter 19)**

RULE OUT

Tension pneumothorax. Any patient presenting with hemodynamic instability requires rapid assessment. If the patient has decreased or absent breath sounds on one side, a tension pneumothorax is present and immediate needle decompression is performed before obtaining a CXR.

VII. **Diagnostic Findings**

A. **Laboratory studies** generally are not indicated unless other co-morbidities are present.

B. **Imaging Studies**
1. **CXR** (Figure 22–1). An inspiratory PA CXR is obtained initially. The edge of the collapsed lung runs parallel to the chest wall. Beyond this line, there are no lung markings. The size of the pneumothorax is estimated as a percentage (eg, 2 cm is approximately 20%). If a pneumothorax is not seen on the inspiratory film, but still suspected, an expiratory film should be taken. The intrapulmonary pressure is decreased during expiration, causing decreased lung volume and a relative increase in the size of the pneumothorax.
2. **Chest CT scan.** CT scan has higher sensitivity for the detection of pneumothoraces, especially in the supine patient. Patients with pneumothoraces identified solely on a CT scan, however, uncommonly require tube thoracostomy.

C. **Procedures**
1. **Needle decompression.** Needle thoracostomy is performed if a tension pneumothorax is suspected. Using a long 14- or 16-gauge angiocatheter, puncture the 2nd intercostal space at the mid-clavicular line on the affected side. A gush of air will be heard, and the hemodynamics should improve. Ultimately, a tube thoracostomy (chest tube) must be placed in the patient.
2. **Tube thoracostomy** (see Chapter 7).

D. **Diagnostic Algorithm**

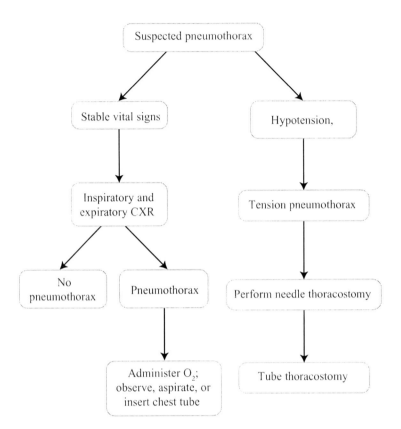

VIII. Treatment
  A. **O$_2$.** Reabsorption, which normally occurs at a rate of 1% per day, is hastened with O$_2$; 3–4 L/min of O$_2$ increases the rate of resorption 4-fold.
  B. **Observation.** Small (< 20%) pneumothoraces can be observed, and the patient can be discharged if there is no progression seen on a CXR repeated after 6 hours. Failure rates, defined by the eventual need for tube thoracostomy, with observation alone are as high as 40%.
  C. **Catheter aspiration.** Reduces a large/moderate pneumothorax to a small one that will resolve on its own. A CXR is needed immediately after aspiration and again 6 hours later to verify successful aspiration and to ensure that there is no re-accumulation of air.
  D. **Tube Thoracostomy (chest tube)**
     1. Indications. Underlying pulmonary pathology (secondary spontaneous pneumothorax), expanding pneumothorax, pneumothorax > 20%, bilateral

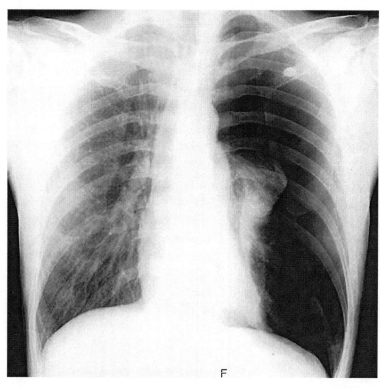

Figure 22–1. Complete pneumothorax of the left lung.

or tension pneumothoraces (after needle decompression), significant symptoms, positive pressure ventilation, and need for future air transport.

2. **Size.** In adults, tube size depends on the etiology. In a spontaneous pneumothorax, an 18–26 French tube is usually sufficient. In the setting of trauma, a larger 36–40 French tube is preferred. In children, the chest tube size can be estimated by multiplying the estimated size of an ET tube (4 + age/4) × 3.

IX. **Disposition**

A. **Admission.** If a chest tube is inserted, patients are admitted to the hospital. The chest tube must be attached to a water seal and vacuum device (Pleur-Evac). Patients with small (< 20%) traumatic pneumothoraces that are managed conservatively are usually admitted for observation.

B. **Discharge.** If the pneumothorax is small (< 20%) and patients are healthy, reliable, and minimally symptomatic, they may be observed. A second CXR 6 hours later should be performed to ensure that there has been no change in the size of the pneumothorax before discharge. Close follow up with a thoracic surgeon should be arranged.

CASE PRESENTATION

A 32-year-old man presents to the ED with sudden onset of shortness of breath after smoking crack. He is noted to be in mild respiratory distress. His O_2 saturation is 93% on room air.

1. *What other information do you want to know?*
   - *Other vital signs. Decreased breath sounds, deviated trachea, or hypotension.*
2. *The patient has decreased breath sounds on the left lung field, normal vital signs, no tracheal deviation, and no JVD. What are your next steps?*
   - *O_2 and monitor. CXR. Tube thoracostomy or catheter aspiration.*

SUMMARY POINTS

- *Always consider the diagnosis of tension pneumothorax in any patient with shock and respiratory distress. This is a clinical diagnosis; do not wait for confirmation with CXR.*
- *Appropriate treatment of a tension pneumothorax is needle thoracostomy, followed by tube thoracostomy.*
- *Unless a pneumothorax is spontaneous, small (< 20%), minimally symptomatic, and primary (no underlying lung pathology), definitive treatment is tube thoracostomy. Small traumatic and iatrogenic pneumothoraces may also be observed.*

CHAPTER 23
PULMONARY EMBOLISM

I. Defining Features

- A. Pulmonary embolism (PE) is a complication of DVT. An embolism from a peripheral vein migrates via the right side of the heart and lodges in the pulmonary artery circulation.
- B. PE often presents with nonspecific findings that mimic other disease processes.

II. Epidemiology

- A. Approximately 650,000 cases of PE occur each year.
- B. PE is the 3rd most common cause of death in hospitalized patients in the United States.
- C. Asymptomatic PE occurs in 50% of patients with DVT.
- D. Massive PE accounts for only 5% of cases, but has an associated mortality rate of 40%.
- E. About 90% of emboli originate from venous thrombi in the lower extremities and pelvis.

III. Pathophysiology

- A. A thrombus becomes lodged in the pulmonary vasculature, blocking normal blood flow to the lung.
- B. Obstruction increases pulmonary vasculature resistance. This, in turn, increases pulmonary artery pressure and right ventricular pressure. When > 50% of the vasculature is occluded, patients experience significant pulmonary hypertension and acute cor pulmonale. Undetected, this leads to long-term morbidity and death.

IV. Risk Factors. **Virchow's triad:** venous stasis (eg, bed rest > 48 hours, long-distance auto or air travel, recent hospitalization), hypercoagulable (eg, malignancy, previous PE/DVT, pregnancy, or protein C deficiency), and intimal damage (eg, trauma, recent surgery, central lines, IV drug use).

V. Clinical Presentation

- A. **History**
  1. **Shortness of breath** is the most common symptom. Sudden onset of shortness of breath is more specific for PE. Dyspnea may be intermittent or exertional.
  2. **Chest pain** is the 2nd most common symptom. It is usually pleuritic, and is more common with a peripheral PE.
  3. Other findings include cough, hemoptysis, diaphoresis, and syncope.

B. **Physical Examination**
1. **Vital signs.** Tachypnea (RR > 16) is present in 92% of patients. Tachycardia is present in 44%, while an elevated temperature (> 37.8°C) is seen in 43% of patients. Hypotension may be present in a patient with a massive PE.
2. **Lung examination** may be clear or reveal rales.
3. **Extremity examination** for swelling suggestive of a DVT.
4. **Rectal examination** for gross or occult blood if the patient requires anticoagulation therapy.
C. **Pretest probability of PE (Well's criteria).** Calculated based on the findings of the history and physical examination (Table 23–1). The results risk-stratify the patient into low, intermediate, and high-risk groups and direct the diagnostic work-up.

CLINICAL SKILLS TIP

Dyspnea, pleuritic chest pain, or tachypnea is present in 97% of patients with PE. The absence of all 3 findings is strong evidence that a PE is not present.

VI. Differential Diagnosis (see Chapters 12 and 19)

VII. Diagnostic Findings

A. **Laboratory Studies**
1. **Pulse oximetry** is frequently normal in patients with a PE and cannot be used to exclude the diagnosis.

Table 23–1. Well's criteria for determining the pretest probability of pulmonary embolism.

VARIABLE	POINTS
Clinical signs and symptoms of DVT (objectively measured leg swelling and pain with palpation in the deep vein region)	3.0
Heart rate > 100 beats/min	1.5
Immobilization (bedrest, except for use of bathroom, for > 3 days or surgery within 4 weeks)	1.5
Previous diagnosis of DVT or PE	1.5
Hemoptysis	1.0
Malignancy (currently receiving treatment, treatment within 6 months, or palliative care)	1.0
PE as likely as or more likely than an alternate diagnosis	3.0
Low probability	**< 2**
Intermediate probability	**2–6**
High probability	**> 6**

2. **ABG.** Many patients with PE are hypoxic (PaO_2 < 80 mm Hg), although this is not universally true. The A-a gradient can be used as an indirect measure of V/Q abnormalities, although 15% of patients with PE will have a normal A-a gradient.

3. **D-dimer** is a fibrin degradation product that circulates in a patient with a dissolving fibrin thrombus. It is found in the serum within 1 hour and stops circulating after 7 days. Multiple D-dimer tests exist with varying sensitivities and specificities. A negative D-dimer test is useful to ***exclude PE in low-risk patients.***

B. **Imaging Studies**

1. **ECG.** Useful to rule out a primary cardiac etiology. Sinus tachycardia is present in 44% of patients with PE. Right-sided heart strain seen as T-wave inversions in the anterior (V1-V4) leads may be present in massive PE. S wave in lead I, Q wave in lead III, and T wave inversion in lead III (S1Q3T3) is present in only 12% of patients with a PE.

2. **CXR.** Most common abnormalities seen in patients with PE include atelectasis, parenchymal abnormalities, elevated hemidiaphragm, or pleural effusions. **Hampton's Hump** is a triangular pleural-based infiltrate, representing a pulmonary infarct. **Westermark's sign** is dilatation of pulmonary vessels proximal to the PE with collapse of distal vessels.

3. **Chest CT angiography (CTA).** Accepted diagnostic modality of choice (Figure 23–1). Rapid and sensitive for detecting proximal PEs. The clinical outcome following a negative CTA is favorable, and the likelihood for subse-

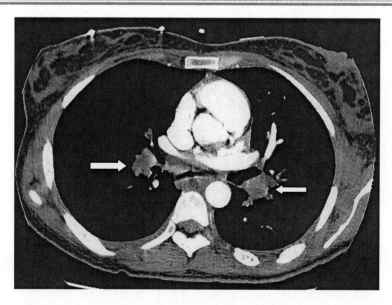

Figure 23–1. Chest CT angiogram demonstrating thrombi in bilateral pulmonary arteries (*arrows*). Arteries will normally appear white.

quent thromboembolic events is extremely low. CTA is also useful to identify alternate diagnoses.

4. **V/Q scan.** Results are interpreted as normal, low, intermediate, or high probability of PE. This test is infrequently used today in favor of chest CTA.

5. **Lower extremity duplex ultrasound.** May be used to look for DVT in a patient with a high clinical suspicion of PE and a negative CTA.

C. **Diagnostic Algorithm**

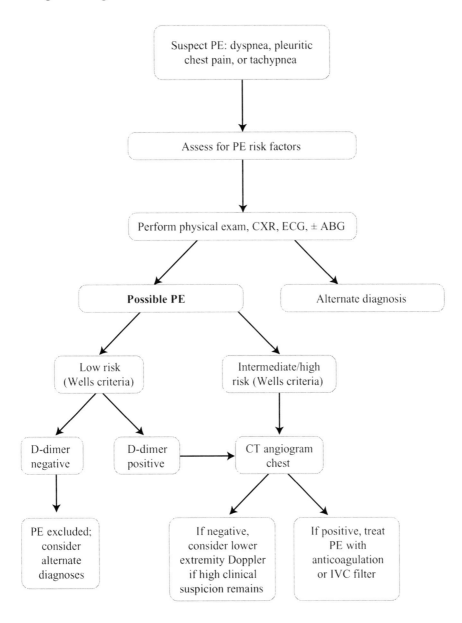

VIII. Treatment

A. **O$_2$** should be administered as needed. Endotracheal intubation may be necessary for cases of refractory hypoxia.

B. **Vasopressors.** Norepinephrine (10 mcg/min) is indicated in patients with hypotension. ***Large IV fluid boluses should be avoided.*** Fluids can exacerbate already elevated right ventricular pressures, leading to further compromise of left ventricular outflow and shock.

C. **Anticoagulation** prevents additional thrombi from forming, but does not dissolve existing clot. Choices include heparin bolus (60 U/kg) IV and infusion (18 U/kg/hr) or SQ enoxaparin (Lovenox) (1 mg/kg q 12 hr). An inferior vena cava filter is indicated in patients with contraindications to anticoagulants (eg, active GI bleeding) or who have failed anticoagulant therapy.

D. **Thrombolytics** are indicated for patients with massive PE in shock. These agents directly lyse the clot. Options include Alteplase (t-PA) 100 mg over a 2-hour period or tenecteplase (TNKase) IV bolus. TNKase dose is based on weight (< 60 kg, 30 mg; 60–70 kg, 35 mg; 70–80 kg, 40 mg; 80–90 kg, 45 mg; > 90 kg, 50 mg).

IX. Disposition

A. **Admission.** All patients with newly diagnosed PE should be admitted to the hospital. Patients with refractory hypoxia or cardiovascular dysfunction should be admitted to an ICU setting.

B. **Discharge.** Patients with a clear alternative diagnosis may be discharged based on the severity of the alternate diagnosis.

CASE PRESENTATION

A 60-year-old man presents to the ED complaining of difficulty breathing for the past few days. He states that 2 weeks ago he had right hip arthroplasty.

1. What other historic information do you want to know?

   • Other risk factors for PE? Recent leg swelling? Chest pain, cough, hemoptysis, diaphoresis, syncope?

2. What should you look for on physical examination?

   • Tachycardia, tachypnea, or fever. Pulmonary rales. Swelling or tenderness of lower extremities.

SUMMARY POINTS

• Always consider PE in patients with complaints of dyspnea, chest pain, hemoptysis, or syncope.

• A D-dimer with good sensitivity and specificity is only useful to exclude PE in low-risk patients.

• Chest CTA is the test of choice for all patients with intermediate to high-risk pretest probability of PE or low-risk patients with a positive D-dimer.

• Administer thrombolytics in hypotensive/unstable patients with PE.

SECTION V
ABDOMINAL EMERGENCIES

CHAPTER 24
ACUTE ABDOMINAL PAIN

I. Defining Features

 A. When evaluating a patient with abdominal pain, the goal of the emergency physician is to first rule out immediate life-threatening conditions. In the hypotensive elderly patient, a ruptured abdominal aneurysm is present until proven otherwise. Similarly, in women of childbearing age, ruptured ectopic pregnancy must be excluded early.

 B. After immediate life-threatening conditions are excluded, other conditions such as appendicitis, cholecystitis, ruptured viscus, mesenteric ischemia, and cholangitis should be considered.

 C. Despite thorough evaluation, 30% of patients are discharged from the ED with a diagnosis of "abdominal pain of unclear etiology."

II. Epidemiology

 A. Abdominal pain is a common presenting complaint and represents 5% of all ED visits.

 B. Elderly patients are at particular risk of harboring serious underlying pathology. Patients > age 65 with acute onset (< 1 week) of abdominal pain require surgery in 40% of cases and have a post-operative mortality rate of 13%. Table 24–1 lists the most common causes of abdominal pain based on patient age.

III. Pathophysiology

 A. Abdominal pain is classified as visceral, parietal, or referred in origin. Depending on the disease process, pain may begin as visceral and become parietal, as in the stretching and subsequent rupture of a hollow viscus.

 B. **Visceral pain** occurs with the stretching of nerve fibers in the walls of hollow organs or the capsules of solid organs. The location of pain is not well localized, but often has an embryologic basis that aids in determining the diagnosis. Epigastric pain occurs in patients with stretching of foregut organs (stomach to duodenum, including biliary tree and pancreas). Periumbilical pain represents pathology of midgut organs (distal duodenum to transverse colon). Suprapubic pain is due to problems of the hindgut organs (distal transverse colon, rectum, and urogenital tract).

 C. **Parietal pain** is due to irritation of the parietal peritoneum. The patient is more readily able to localize the pain (eg, LLQ pain in diverticulitis), but when the entire peritoneal cavity is involved, the pain is diffuse.

137

Table 24–1. Causes of abdominal pain in patients < 50 years and > 50 years.

Age < 50	%	Age > 50	%
Nonspecific abdominal pain	40%	Nonspecific abdominal pain	20%
Appendicitis	32%	Cholecystitis	16%
Cholecystitis	6%	Appendicitis	15%
Obstruction	3%	Obstruction	12%
Pancreatitis	2%	Pancreatitis	7%
Diverticulitis	< 0.1%	Diverticulitis	6%
Hernia	< 0.1%	Cancer	4%
Vascular	< 0.1%	Hernia	3%
Cancer	< 0.1%	Vascular	2%

    D. Referred pain. Abdominal pain may also be referred from organs above the diaphragm (eg, MI causing epigastric pain). Alternatively, abdominal pathology may refer pain above the diaphragm (eg, splenic rupture causing shoulder pain).

IV. **Risk Factors.** Elderly, pregnancy, immunocompromised (eg, HIV/AIDS, diabetes mellitus), prior abdominal surgery, sudden onset of pain, abnormal vital signs, pain before vomiting, trauma, or peritoneal findings may indicate more serious pathology.

V. **Clinical Presentation**

    A. **History**

        1. **Duration.** Pain that began within the preceding week is more likely to be of serious consequence than pain of chronic duration. Sudden onset of pain that awakens a patient from sleep is especially concerning and suggests a ruptured viscus or vascular event.

        2. **Pain pattern.** Patients with visceral pain are usually seen to be "writhing" in pain and cannot find a comfortable position. Patients with parietal pain from peritoneal irritation will report constant pain that is worse with the slightest movement.

        3. **Location.** Pain located in a particular portion of the abdomen frequently suggests the underlying organs that are affected. A classic example is appendicitis. Early in the disease process when the appendix is stretching, the patient feels periumbilical discomfort (midgut organ). When local inflammation or perforation occurs, peritoneal irritation results in pain that becomes localized to the RLQ.

        4. **Radiation.** Pain that radiates to the back suggests pancreatitis, cholecystitis, or aortic aneurysm. Pain radiating to the shoulder reflects irritation of the di-

aphragm and suggests intraperitoneal infection or blood, hepatitis, or cholecystitis. Pain that radiates to the groin may indicate an aortic aneurysm or
nephrolithiasis.

5. **Exacerbating and alleviating factors.** Changes in the intensity of abdominal
pain with eating suggest PUD or biliary colic. It should be noted, however,
that one third of patients with biliary colic do not have onset of pain related
to meals.

6. **Associated symptoms** such as fever, nausea, vomiting, weight loss, diarrhea,
urinary frequency, dysuria, blood in the stool, or loss of appetite should be
elicited.

7. A thorough past medical/surgical history, medications, allergies, and social
history should also be obtained.

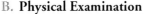KEY COMPLAINTS

*Patients with abdominal pain of acute sudden onset are more likely to harbor serious pathology such as
a ruptured AAA or perforated viscus.*

B. **Physical Examination**
1. **Vital signs** should be noted and any abnormal value rechecked. The presence of fever should raise suspicion of serious pathology, although it may be
present in benign disease processes such as gastroenteritis. Hypotension and
tachycardia suggest sepsis or ruptured AAA and should be addressed immediately before proceeding to perform a thorough history and physical examination.

2. **Abdominal examination** begins with inspection, followed by auscultation of
bowel sounds. Hyperactive sounds are present in bowel obstruction, while
hypoactive sounds are seen with ileus. Palpation of the non-tender quadrants
is initiated first, followed by the tender quadrants. Significant percussion tenderness is present in patients with peritonitis. The patient with peritonitis
also guards the tender abdomen by contracting the abdominal musculature.
Initially the guarding is voluntary, but then becomes involuntary (spasm).
Rebound tenderness lacks sensitivity or specificity as a finding of peritonitis.
A better marker is "cough pain." The patient is asked to cough (Valsalva maneuver) and if the pain worsens, the test is considered positive. A "heel tap"
or shaking the bed will also worsen the abdominal pain of a patient with peritonitis. In addition to signs of peritonitis, the physician should examine for
the presence of a pulsatile mass consistent with an aortic aneurysm.

3. **GU examination** should be performed in both men and women and may
identify an obvious source of pain, including hernias, PID, testicular torsion,
or epididymitis. A rectal examination will detect masses and allow for Hemoccult testing.

VI. **Differential Diagnosis**

A. **Epigastric pain.** Pancreatitis, biliary colic/cholecystis/choledocholithiasis, PUD/
gastritis, or hepatitis.

B. **Periumbilical pain.** Appendicitis (early), enteritis, or inflammatory bowel disease.

C. **Suprapubic pain.** Appendicitis (late and usually RLQ), diverticulitis (usually
LLQ), UTI, PID (bilateral), ectopic pregnancy, or testicular torsion.

D. **Other.** Ruptured AAA (site of pain depends on direction of rupture: back in 50% of cases, LLQ, epigastric), bowel obstruction (diffuse), mesenteric ischemia (diffuse), or nephrolithiasis (flank and lower quadrant).

RULE OUT

In any hypotensive elderly patient, a ruptured AAA should be considered immediately and diagnosed with an ultrasound performed at bedside.

VII. **Diagnostic Findings**

A. **Laboratory Studies**
   1. **WBC count.** The physician should not rely too heavily on the WBC count, because a normal value does not rule out serious underlying pathology. In addition, an elevated WBC count can be consistent with benign conditions such as gastroenteritis.
   2. **Electrolytes and glucose.** Patients with hypercalcemia may present with abdominal pain. A patient with DKA may present with nonspecific abdominal pain.
   3. **BUN and creatinine.** A patient with uremia may present with abdominal pain. In addition, renal function tests may be useful in dehydrated patients and are also necessary before IV contrast is given for CT scan.
   4. **Urinalysis.** This test is useful to determine the presence of ketones in DKA and also provides evidence of a UTI (eg, cystitis or pyelonephritis). Careful interpretation of this test is necessary, as inflammatory processes (ie, appendicitis, diverticulitis) near the ureter may produce pyuria in the absence of a UTI. The absence of urobilinogen on the urinalysis suggests a complete common bile duct obstruction.
   5. **Urine pregnancy test** should be ordered in all females of childbearing age.
   6. **Lipase.** A value 2 times normal is 94% sensitive and 95% specific for pancreatitis.
   7. **Liver function tests** are useful in patients with common bile duct stones and hepatitis.

B. **Imaging Studies**
   1. **Obstructive series** will detect bowel obstruction. These radiographs are not routinely indicated unless there is clinical suspicion of obstruction.
   2. **Upright CXR** is useful to determine whether free air is present under the diaphragm. The sensitivity of this test in patients with perforated peptic ulcer is 60% and may be improved when the patient is upright for 5–10 minutes before the radiograph is taken (Figure 24–1).
   3. **Abdomen and pelvis CT scan** is sensitive and specific for the diagnoses of appendicitis, bowel obstruction, pancreatitis, diverticulitis, nephrolithiasis, and aortic aneurysm. CT scan will also identify dilation of the common bile duct (stones) and can diagnose cholecystitis. Both IV and oral contrast is administered in most cases. If bowel perforation is suspected, diatrizoate (Gastrografin) oral contrast should be substituted for barium. Barium is an irritant to the peritoneal cavity.
   4. **Ultrasound** is used to diagnose cholecystitis and ectopic pregnancy. It will also detect common bile duct dilation, aortic aneurysm, pancreatitis, and hydronephrosis.

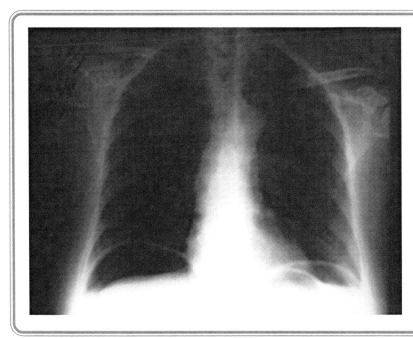

Figure 24–1. Radiograph showing free air under the diaphragm in a patient with a perforated peptic ulcer.

C. **Diagnostic Algorithm**

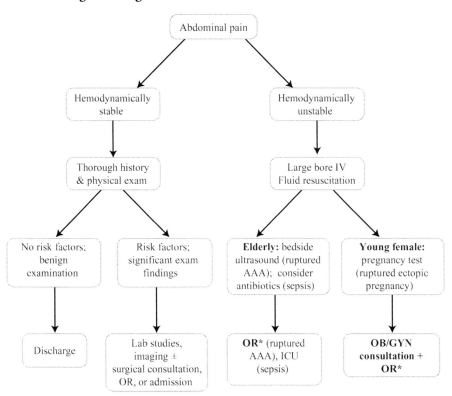

Abdominal pain

Hemodynamically stable

Hemodynamically unstable

Thorough history & physical exam

Large bore IV Fluid resuscitation

No risk factors; benign examination

Risk factors; significant exam findings

Elderly: bedside ultrasound (ruptured AAA); consider antibiotics (sepsis)

Young female: pregnancy test (ruptured ectopic pregnancy)

Discharge

Lab studies, imaging ± surgical consultation, OR, or admission

OR* (ruptured AAA), ICU (sepsis)

OB/GYN consultation + OR*

*OR = Operating room

141

VIII. Treatment

A. Treatment depends on the underlying etiology.

B. **IV fluids** are indicated if the patient has abnormal vital signs or history of fluid losses.

C. **Pain control** depends on the suspected underlying disease process with the following guidelines.

   1. When gastritis/PUD is suspected, a "GI cocktail" (Maalox 30 cc, Donnatal 10 cc, viscous lidocaine 10 cc) may be useful. Histamine-2 blockers are not effective in the acute setting.

   2. Multiple randomized studies have shown that narcotic pain medications (eg, morphine) do not interfere with diagnostic ability. Following the initial examination, these agents should not be withheld in patients with significant pain who do not respond to other measures.

   3. Ketorolac (Toradol) is especially useful in the setting of biliary colic and nephrolithiasis, but should be avoided in patients with gastritis, PUD, or aortic aneurysm.

D. **Antibiotics** are indicated in patients with appendicitis, cholecystitis, sepsis, diverticulitis, PID, and perforated PUD.

E. Consultation with a surgeon or gynecologist is recommended when surgery is indicated or the diagnosis is unclear and there is concern for serious pathology.

F. *Diagnoses that require rapid (minutes) evaluation, treatment, and disposition include ruptured ectopic pregnancy and ruptured AAA.* In these cases, surgical consultants should be contacted once the diagnosis is considered.

IX. Disposition

A. **Admission.** Necessary in patients with a work-up that supports the diagnosis of serious underlying abdominal pathology or in patients with intractable pain or vomiting regardless of the etiology of pain.

B. **Discharge.** Acceptable in patients with resolution of symptoms without suspicion of serious underlying pathology. Follow-up with a primary physician should be ensured, and the patient should be instructed to return if there is progression of symptoms.

CASE PRESENTATION

A 60-year-old man presents with abdominal pain that began suddenly one hour before coming to the ED. He states that the pain is constant and diffuse. He reports one episode of vomiting and denies fevers or diarrhea. The patient reports a history of PUD and pancreatitis from alcohol use.

1. *What important examination findings should be elicited?*

   • *Abnormal vital signs, bowel sounds, peritoneal signs, pulsating mass, and GU examination.*

2. *Examination reveals diffuse tenderness to light percussion with involuntary guarding. The patient has abdominal pain with coughing and also when the heel is tapped. Bedside ultrasound reveals a normal aorta. What are the next appropriate steps?*

   • *This patient has peritonitis, possibly due to a perforated peptic ulcer. IV access should be established, and the patient should receive surgical consultation, pain medications, and antibiotics.*

SUMMARY POINTS

- *Thorough history and physical examination will help rule out serious pathology.*
- *Ruptured AAA must be excluded as soon as possible in elderly hypotensive patients.*
- *Obtain a urine pregnancy test in any female of childbearing age with abdominal pain to exclude ectopic pregnancy.*

CHAPTER 25
APPENDICITIS

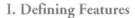

I. Defining Features

A. The appendix is a hollow structure with a closed distal end arising from the cecum. The length of the appendix is from 6 to 10 cm.

B. Appendicitis is an acute inflammatory process due to obstruction of the lumen of the appendix.

C. Anatomically, the appendix may be located in various intra-abdominal positions. A retrocecal location is present in 65% of cases, while a location in the pelvis is found in 30% of cases. The location of the appendix alters the presentation of appendicitis.

D. The typical progression of the disease is vague periumbilical pain; anorexia, nausea, or vomiting; migration to the RLQ; low-grade fever; and leukocytosis.

II. Epidemiology

A. The lifetime risk of appendicitis is between 6% and 8% and is slightly higher in males.

B. The peak incidence of appendicitis in males is between ages 10 and 14. In females, peak incidence is between ages 14 and 19.

C. The rate of appendicitis is slightly higher in the summer months.

III. Pathophysiology

A. Obstruction of the lumen of the appendix is the common initiating event. The cause of obstruction ranges from lymphoid tissue to intraluminal objects, such as fecaliths or tumors.

B. Once obstruction has occurred, intestinal secretions raise the intraluminal pressure and eventually impair venous drainage.

C. The end result is tissue ischemia, bacterial invasion, and ultimately perforation.

IV. Risk Factors

A. There are no true risk factors for appendicitis, and the emergency physician should consider this diagnosis in ***ANY patient with RLQ pain.***

B. Clusters of cases have led some authorities to postulate that an infectious agent that causes lymphoid proliferation within the appendix is a risk factor for appendicitis.

V. Clinical Presentation

A. History

1. Abdominal pain is present in all patients and usually occurs before vomiting (Table 25–1). One half of patients present to the ED within 24 hours of onset of symptoms and another one third present within 24–48 hours of onset of symptoms. Perforation should be suspected in patients who present > 48 hours.
2. The classic presentation is periumbilical abdominal pain that migrates to the RLQ as peritoneal inflammation occurs.
3. When the appendix is located in a retrocecal position, abdominal pain is attenuated and flank pain may be more prominent. A pelvic position may irritate the bladder and cause suprapubic pain.
4. Fever is usually low grade and generally occurs as a late finding.
5. The presence of diarrhea should not be used to exclude the diagnosis of appendicitis.

A. Physical Examination

1. RLQ tenderness is present in almost 100% of patients.
2. **Rovsing's sign** (pain in RLQ with palpation of the LLQ) is present in 25% of patients.
3. **Psoas sign** is elicited in the supine patient by asking the patient to lift the right thigh against resistance. Alternatively, with the patient in the left lateral decubitus position, extend the right hip. Increased pain with either maneuver is suggestive of appendicitis. A positive psoas sign is present when the inflamed appendix is adjacent to the psoas muscle.
4. **Obturator sign** is positive when the appendix is in proximity to the obturator muscle. The sign is elicited by passive flexion of the right hip and knee with internal rotation of the thigh. Increased pain is due to irritation of the obturator muscle and is suggestive of appendicitis.

Table 25–1. Frequency of historical features of appendicitis.

Feature	Frequency
Abdominal pain	100%
Anorexia	92%
Nausea	78%
Vomiting	54%
Migration of pain	50%
Fever	20%
Diarrhea	15%

5. Perforation should be suspected in patients with generalized tenderness, rigidity, or a palpable RLQ mass.

VI. Differential Diagnosis. Diverticulitis, PID, gastroenteritis, Crohn's disease, pyelonephritis, nephrolithiasis, intussusception, endometriosis, ovarian cyst or torsion, regional enteritis, or Meckel's diverticulum.

RULE OUT

Appendicitis is a common condition and is present in 25% of patients < age 60 who present to the ED with acute abdominal pain.

VII. Diagnostic Findings

    A. **Laboratory Studies**

        1. **CBC.** Approximately 70–90% of patients will have an elevated WBC count. The absence of leukocytosis should not be used to rule out the diagnosis.

        2. **Urinalysis** may suggest the diagnosis of pyelonephritis; however, the finding of pyuria should be considered carefully. Inflammation of the appendix in proximity to the ureter or bladder will result in WBCs in the urine.

    B. **Imaging Studies**

        1. **Abdomen and pelvis CT scan** is the imaging modality of choice (Figure 25–1). Sensitivity is 90% without contrast and increases to 98% when contrast is administered (oral, IV, and rectal).

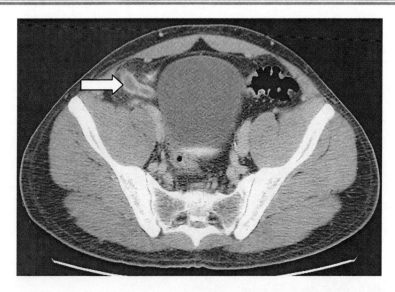

Figure 25–1. CT scan showing appendicitis. Note the increased uptake of IV contrast in the wall of the appendix and the absence of oral contrast in the lumen (*arrow*).

2. **Ultrasound** can be used in pregnant patients. Sensitivity ranges from 75–90%.

C. **Diagnostic Algorithm**

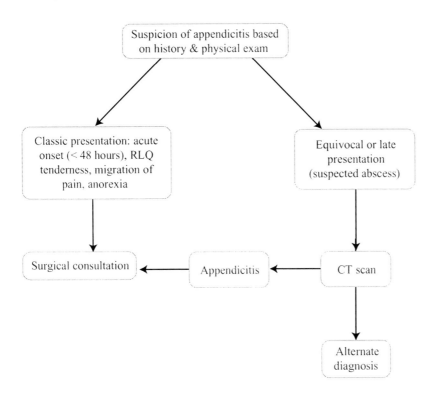

VIII. Treatment

A. **NPO.** The patient should not be allowed to eat or drink in anticipation of surgery.

B. **Pain medications,** including narcotics, are appropriate and have not been shown to decrease diagnostic accuracy. Morphine is most frequently administered, although a short-acting narcotic such as fentanyl is an alternative.

C. **Antibiotics.** If perforation is likely, IV antibiotics (quinolone plus metronidazole) should be administered.

IX. Disposition

A. **Admission.** All patients with the diagnosis of appendicitis should be admitted to the hospital after consultation with a general surgeon. Admission for observation with repeated abdominal examinations is an option for equivocal cases.

B. **Discharge.** Appropriate if an alternate diagnosis is likely based on history, physical examination, or diagnostic testing and the patient is tolerating fluids. Close follow-up should be arranged, and the patient should be educated about symptoms that warrant a prompt return to the ED.

CASE PRESENTATION

A 16-year-old boy presents with abdominal pain. He states that the pain began 12 hours ago. Initially, he felt pain in his periumbilical area, but he now states that it has moved to the RLQ. He has vomited once.

1. *On examination, what findings might you elicit?*
   - *Tenderness, guarding, or rigidity in the RLQ. Pain in the RLQ with compression of LLQ (Rovsing's sign). Psoas or obturator sign.*
2. *What are the keys to management of this patient?*
   - *Keep the patient NPO for possible surgery. Administer analgesics as needed. Provide prompt surgical consultation. CT scan may be indicated if the examination findings are equivocal.*

SUMMARY POINTS

- *Absence of leukocytosis or the presence of diarrhea does not rule out the diagnosis of appendicitis.*
- *Rapid diagnosis and early surgical intervention help to avoid the complications associated with rupture.*
- *If perforation is likely, IV antibiotics should be administered.*

CHAPTER 26
ACUTE CHOLECYSTITIS

I. Defining Features

A. **Cholelithiasis** is the presence of stones within the gallbladder. Approximately 80% of gallstones contain calcium and cholesterol. About 10–20% of gallstones are calcium bilirubinate (pigment) stones.

B. **Biliary colic** occurs when the patient experiences attacks of upper abdominal pain secondary to a gallstone obstructing the neck of the gallbladder.

C. **Acute cholecystitis** is present when gallbladder inflammation occurs in the presence of an obstructing stone.

D. **Acalculous cholecystitis** is defined by inflammation of the gallbladder in the absence of gallstones. It accounts for as many as 10% of cases of cholecystitis. This condition is more common in elderly, critically ill patients and carries a high mortality rate.

E. **Emphysematous cholecystitis** is an uncommon variant occurring in 1% of patients with cholecystitis. In this condition, the gallbladder becomes ischemic and eventually gangrenous due to vascular insufficiency. Air is seen within the gallbladder wall on CT scan. It is more common in elderly patients and diabetics. It is acalculous in 30% of cases. Patients are more likely to present with sepsis.

F. **Choledocholithiasis** (ie, stone in the common bile duct) and **cholangitis** (ie, infection of the biliary tract) can also produce similar signs and symptoms.

II. Epidemiology

A. Cholelithiasis is present in 10–15% of the population of the United States. About 25% of women and 15% of men > age 50 have gallstones.

B. Only 10–20% of people with asymptomatic gallstones will develop complications over a 20-year period.

C. Acute cholecystitis accounts for 3–9% of hospital admissions for acute abdominal pain.

D. The mortality rate of acute cholecystitis is 4%; if emphysematous cholecystitis is present, the mortality rate increases to approximately 20%.

III. Pathophysiology

A. The gallbladder acts as a reservoir for bile produced in the liver. Gallstones form when cholesterol becomes supersaturated and crystallizes on a matrix of calcium.

B. Biliary colic occurs when the gallbladder distends as it contracts against an obstructing stone at the neck of the gallbladder.

C. In acute cholecystitis, persistent obstruction results in increased luminal pressure, mucosal irritation, inflammation, and eventually ischemia. In two thirds of cases, bacteria can be cultured from bile. Infection with gram-negative or anaerobic bacteria is present in half of cases.

IV. **Risk Factors.** Increased age, female gender, obesity, family history, hemolytic anemia (pigment stones), or diabetes mellitus (emphysematous cholecystitis).

V. **Clinical Presentation**

A. **History**
1. Biliary colic causes pain in the epigastric area or RUQ. The pain is constant (not colicky) and usually lasts 30 minutes to 6 hours.
2. Nausea and vomiting are frequently present.
3. If the process continues, pain becomes more severe and localizes to the RUQ.
4. Classically, symptoms start following a fatty meal, although in one third of patients, this history is not elicited.
5. The presence of fever suggests acute cholecystitis, although this finding is not universal, especially in an elderly or diabetic patient.

B. **Physical examination.** Findings suggestive of acute cholecystitis include tenderness in the RUQ, rebound, Murphy's sign, and fever (Table 26–1).

CLINICAL SKILLS TIP

Murphy's sign is elicited by palpating under the patient's right costal margin. The patient is asked to take a deep breath. When an arrest of inspiration occurs due to pain, Murphy's sign is positive.

VI. **Differential Diagnosis.** Biliary colic, choledocholithiasis, cholangitis, gastritis or PUD, pneumonia, hepatitis, perihepatitis (PID), pancreatitis, pyelonephritis, appendicitis, and gastroenteritis.

VII. **Diagnostic Findings**

A. **Laboratory Studies**
1. **CBC.** Leukocytosis is present in 63% of patients with acute cholecystitis.

Table 26–1. Sensitivity and specificity of examination findings in the patient with acute cholecystitis.

Examination Findings for Acute Cholecystitis	Sensitivity	Specificity
RUQ tenderness	77%	54%
Rebound	30%	68%
Murphy's sign	65%	87%
Fever	35%	80%

2. **Chemistry.** Electrolytes should be checked, especially in the presence of significant vomiting.
3. **Liver function tests.** Alkaline phosphatase, liver enzymes, lipase, and bilirubin levels should be obtained to rule out common bile duct obstruction and hepatitis.
4. **Urinalysis** should be obtained to exclude pyelonephritis.

B. **Imaging Studies**
1. **Ultrasound.** Sensitivity 88–94%, specificity 80%. Typical findings include the triad of gallbladder wall thickening (> 3 mm), sonographic Murphy's sign (pain with probe palpation over the gallbladder), and the presence of gallstones. Gallbladder wall thickening is not specific for acute cholecystitis and may be seen in cases of chronic cholecystitis, hepatitis, or CHF. Pericholecystic fluid is very specific for cholecystitis, but is present in only 25% of cases. Bedside ultrasound performed by the emergency physician can be used to exclude cholelithiasis and is also sensitive for cholecystitis.
2. **Hepatobiliary scanning.** Highly sensitive and useful in equivocal cases and to detect the presence of acalculous cholecystitis. The patient receives an IV injection of a radioactive material, called hydroxy iminodiacetic acid (HIDA), which is taken up by the liver and excreted into the biliary tree. In cholecystitis, there will be no uptake in the gallbladder.
3. **Abdominal CT scan** can also be used to diagnose cholecystitis, although it is not as sensitive (range is from 50% to 90%) as ultrasound (Figure 26–1). CT scan has the same sensitivity as ultrasound to detect common bile duct stones

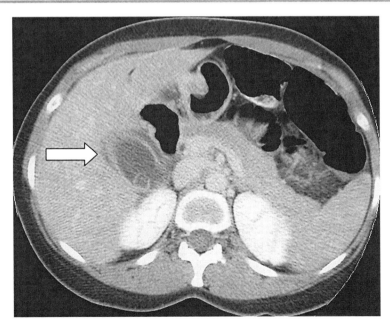

Figure 26–1. Abdominal CT scan showing cholecystitis. Note the gallstone in the presence of pericholecystic fluid and a thickened gallbladder wall (*arrow*).

and common bile duct dilation. It is useful in atypical cases in which other diagnoses are being considered. It is also useful in detecting complications such as gallbladder perforation, pericholecystic abscess, and gangrenous or emphysematous cholecystitis.

C. **Diagnostic Algorithm**

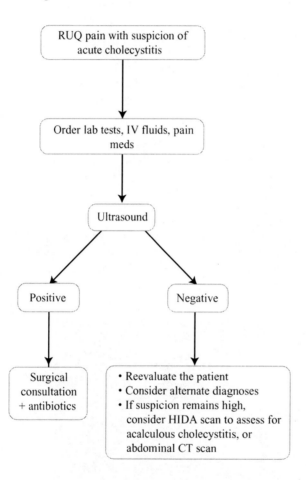

VIII. Treatment

A. **IV fluids** and **antiemetics** in patients with significant vomiting. Prochlorperazine (Compazine) 10 mg IV or promethazine (Phenergan) 25 mg IV.

B. **Analgesics.** Ketorolac (Toradol) 30 mg IV is useful in biliary colic and will not alter operative bleeding times. It should be avoided, along with other NSAIDs, if gastritis or PUD is suspected. Narcotic pain medication such as morphine or fentanyl may also be administered.

C. **Antibiotics.** Ticarcillin/clavulanate (Timentin) 3.1 g q 6 hours or Piperacillin/tazobactam (Zosyn) 3.375 g q 6 hours. In patients who are allergic to penicillin, an aminoglycoside and metronidazole are appropriate.

D. **Surgery consultation.** Definitive treatment includes laparoscopic cholecystectomy, usually within a few days of presentation.

IX. Disposition

A. **Admission.** Admit all patients with acute cholecystitis after obtaining surgical consultation. If sepsis is present, the patient should be admitted to an ICU. In patients with a negative work-up but intractable pain or vomiting, admission for observation is warranted.

B. **Discharge.** Patients with biliary colic (afebrile, normal WBC count +/- negative ultrasound) who are pain-free after treatment and tolerating oral fluids. Give instructions to return to the ED if fever, vomiting, or return of pain occurs.

CASE PRESENTATION

A 40-year-old woman presents to the ED with epigastric pain of 12 hours duration. She has had several bouts of vomiting and states that she has had 1 previous episode of similar symptoms in the past.

1. *What additional questions should you ask the patient?*
   · *Is the pain related to eating? Has she had any fevers? Past medical/surgical history?*
2. *What findings should be elicited on physical examination?*
   · *Tenderness in the RUQ? Murphy's sign? Peritoneal signs?*

SUMMARY POINTS

· *Biliary colic frequently presents with epigastric pain and is not associated with fever or leukocytosis.*
· *No single sign or symptom is adequately sensitive or specific to rule in or exclude acute cholecystitis. For this reason, liberal use of imaging studies, including bedside ultrasound by the emergency physician, is recommended.*
· *Antibiotics should be administered early in ill-appearing patients who are suspected of having acute cholecystitis.*

CHAPTER 27
ABDOMINAL AORTIC ANEURYSM

I. **Defining Features.** An AAA is defined as ≥ 50% increase in the diameter of the aorta or an infrarenal aortic diameter ≥ 3 cm.

II. **Epidemiology**

   A. AAA causes 15,000 deaths in the United States a year.

   B. It is responsible for 1–2% of all deaths in men > age 65.

   C. The incidence of AAA begins to increase in men > age 55. By age 80, 5% of men have an AAA, and 5% of women age 90 have an AAA.

   D. The overall mortality rate of a patient with a ruptured AAA is 90%. In patients who arrive at the hospital, the mortality rate improves to 60%. The mortality rate for elective operative repair is 2–7%.

III. **Etiology.** The etiology of AAA is unclear, although atherosclerosis, chronic hypertension, aging, and a genetic component are thought to contribute.

IV. **Risk Factors.** Elderly (men > 55, women > 70), atherosclerosis, family history of first-degree relative, hypertension, and smoking. Increased diameter of the aneurysm is a risk factor for rupture. Aneurysms < 4 cm have a 1% risk of rupture over the subsequent 6 years. Aneurysms 4–4.9 cm and ≥ 5 cm have a 2% and 20% six year rupture rate, respectively.

V. **Clinical Presentation**

   A. **History**
      1. A patient with an AAA may present asymptomatic, with pain when the aneurysm expands, with pain when the aneurysm ruptures, or with syncope.
      2. The classic triad of **abdominal/back pain, hypotension,** and a **pulsatile abdominal mass** is present in less than one half of patients with a ruptured AAA.
      3. **Pain** is present in 96% of cases of a ruptured AAA. The location may be abdominal (58%), back (70%), or flank/groin (10%).
      4. Syncope (30%), vomiting (20%), or diarrhea (10%) may also be present.

KEY COMPLAINTS

*While the location of the pain varies depending on the direction and extent of rupture, the presence of pain is almost a universal finding in patients with a **ruptured AAA.***

KEY COMPLAINTS

B. **Physical Examination**
1. The patient may be normotensive, hypertensive, or hypotensive. Transient hypotension may also occur and can be erroneously attributed to a vasovagal etiology.
2. Abdominal examination may detect an aneurysm, but the sensitivity depends on the size of the aneurysm and the patient's abdominal girth. Sensitivity is 75% when the aneurysm is > 5 cm.
3. Femoral pulses should be assessed. Lower limb ischemia is present in 5% of cases.

CLINICAL SKILLS TIP

Bedside ED ultrasound allows for the rapid detection of AAA, with > 90% accuracy in diagnosing or excluding the presence of an AAA.

VI. **Differential Diagnosis. Most common misdiagnoses in ruptured AAA** are renal colic (24%), diverticulitis (13%), GI bleed (aortoenteric fistula; 13%), bowel perforation, bowel obstruction, gastroenteritis, acute MI, MVC (if rupture occurs while driving), sepsis, or low back strain.

RULE OUT

AAA *must be ruled out in any elderly patient who presents with abdominal, back, flank, or groin pain.*

VII. **Diagnostic Findings**
A. **Laboratory Studies**
1. None are imperative to make the diagnosis.
2. Hematocrit is < 38 in 40% of patients with ruptured AAA.
3. Elevated lactate level indicates the presence of shock.
B. **Imaging Studies**
1. **Plain abdominal radiographs** are rarely obtained but may reveal aortic calcifications, a soft tissue mass, or curvilinear calcifications.
2. **Ultrasound** has a sensitivity approaching 100% for the presence of an AAA; it is insensitive in detecting rupture, however.
3. **Abdominal CT scan** is indicated only in the hemodynamically stable patient. The sensitivity is 90–94% and the specificity is 92–100% for diagnosing a ruptured AAA (Figure 27–1).
C. **Procedures. Bedside ultrasound** allows for rapid detection of an aortic aneurysm. Rupture is confirmed if fluid is present in the peritoneal cavity, but because most aneurysms rupture into the retroperitoneum, often no free fluid is present. The abdominal probe is placed in the epigastric area in the transverse plane (Figure 27–2). The aorta is visualized anterior and just to the left of the vertebral bodies. The probe is moved inferiorly until the aorta bifurcates at the umbilicus. Next, the probe is rotated 90° and a longitudinal view is obtained.

D. **Diagnostic Algorithm**

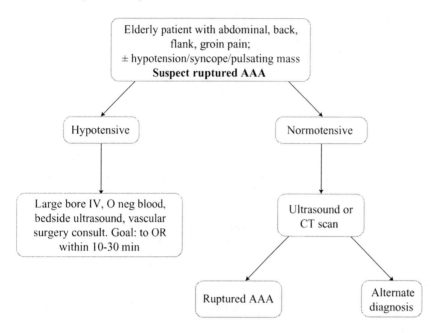

Elderly patient with abdominal, back, flank, groin pain; ± hypotension/syncope/pulsating mass
Suspect ruptured AAA

Hypotensive

Normotensive

Large bore IV, O neg blood, bedside ultrasound, vascular surgery consult. Goal: to OR within 10-30 min

Ultrasound or CT scan

Ruptured AAA

Alternate diagnosis

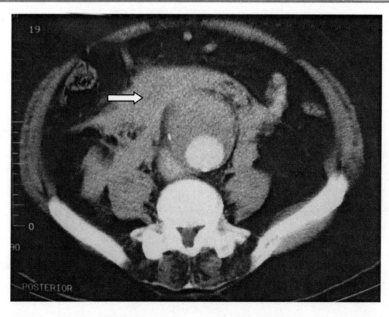

Figure 27–1. CT scan showing a ruptured AAA. This AAA is rupturing into the peritoneal cavity (arrow). The majority of ruptured AAAs are retroperitoneal (70%).

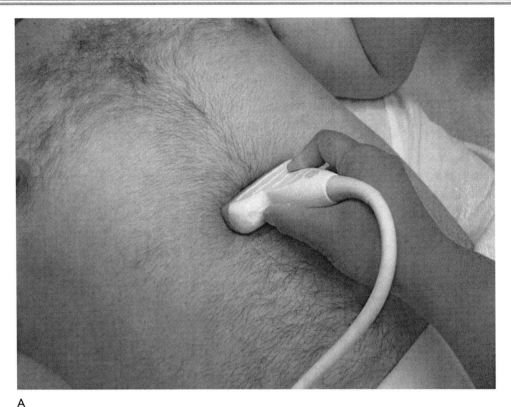

A

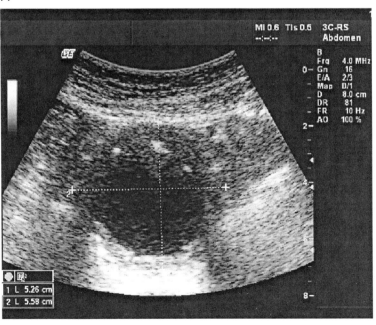

B

Figure 27–2. Ultrasound of an AAA. **A,** Transverse position of probe; **B,** transverse view of AAA.

VIII. Treatment

A. The goal of treatment of a ruptured AAA is rapid volume resuscitation, initially with IV fluids and then with uncrossmatched type O blood as soon as possible. FFP is also frequently necessary because coagulopathy may develop.

B. Two large bore (16-gauge) IV lines in the antecubital veins or a large bore (8 French) central line should be placed immediately.

C. A vascular surgeon should be consulted immediately, and the patient should be taken to the OR as soon as possible to repair the AAA.

IX. Disposition

A. **Admission.** All patients with abdominal/back pain and an AAA should be admitted for observation, further investigation, or surgery. A ruptured AAA mandates immediate surgery.

B. **Discharge.** Patients with an asymptomatic AAA (ie, incidental finding) and an alternate benign cause for their symptoms may be discharged after follow-up with a vascular surgeon has been arranged. However, the physician must be certain that the aneurysm is truly asymptomatic.

CASE PRESENTATION

An 80-year-old hypertensive man presents with abdominal pain of acute onset and a syncopal episode while at home.

1. *What risk factors does this patient have for a ruptured AAA?*

   • *Classic presentation, elderly, male, and hypertension.*

2. *In conjunction with an examination, what are the next appropriate steps?*

   • *Two large bore IVs, order uncrossmatched type O blood, bedside ultrasound while in the ED, and vascular surgery consultation for surgical repair.*

SUMMARY POINTS

• *In 30% of patients with ruptured AAA, the diagnosis is missed or delayed. The most common misdiagnosis is renal colic.*

• *The goal of the emergency physician is to always consider this diagnosis in an elderly patient with a complaint of pain anywhere in the abdomen, back, flank, or groin.*

• *When ruptured AAA is suspected, the evaluation should proceed rapidly with a goal to get the patient to the operating room as quickly as possible.*

CHAPTER 28
GASTROINTESTINAL BLEEDING

I. Defining Features

A. Bleeding can occur anywhere within the GI tract, and can be grossly divided into upper and lower sources.

B. **Upper GI bleeding** is defined as occurring proximal to the ligament of Treitz (the suspensory ligament of the duodenum). **Lower GI bleeding** is defined as occurring distal to the ligament of Treitz.

C. It is not always possible to clinically distinguish between upper and lower GI bleeding in the ED. Some helpful clues are listed below.

D. **Appearance of Gastric Contents**
   1. **Hematemesis** is the vomiting of blood and indicates an upper GI bleed. "Coffee ground" emesis suggests that the blood has partially digested and that bleeding is either slow or has stopped.
   2. **NG tube aspirate** positive for blood also indicates an upper GI source of bleeding. NG lavage can be negative in 25% of patients with an upper GI source of bleeding because the nasogastric tube does not reliably pass the pylorus.

E. **Appearance of Stool**
   1. **Melena** is black, tarry stool that reflects the presence of blood in the GI tract > 8 hours. At least 300 cc of blood must be present to produce melena. Melena is 4 times more likely to be from an upper GI source of bleeding and almost always reflects bleeding proximal to the right side of the colon.
   2. **Hematochezia** is bright red or maroon colored blood per rectum. It is 6 times more likely to be from a lower GI source. An exception is a rapid upper GI source of bleeding. Hematochezia is present in 10% of upper GI bleeds.

II. Epidemiology

A. GI bleeding accounts for 5% of admissions from the ED.

B. An intervention is required to stop ongoing bleeding in 10% of patients.

C. The overall mortality rate of patients admitted for GI bleeding is 10%.

D. Upper GI bleeding is 4–8 times more common than lower GI bleeding.

III. Etiology

A. The 3 most common causes of upper GI bleeding are **peptic ulcers, gastritis, and varices** (Table 28–1).

Table 28–1. Causes of Upper GI bleeding

Cause	Percentage
Peptic ulcer (duodenal 2/3)	40%
Erosive gastritis	25%
Varices (esophageal and gastric)	20%
Mallory-Weiss tear	5%
Other (epistaxis, aortoenteric fistula, carcinoma, caustic ingestion)	10%

B. Lower GI bleeding may be due to multiple causes (Table 28–2). A brisk upper GI bleed should always be considered in the differential of hematochezia. Less common causes include pseudomembranous colitis, infectious diarrhea, aortoenteric fistula, radiation colitis, and mesenteric ischemia.

IV. Risk Factors

A. **Elderly.** GI bleeding can occur at any age, but elderly patients have less ability to compensate for acute hemorrhage.

B. **Cirrhosis.** Patients with a history of cirrhosis should be presumed to have varices as the source of hemorrhage until proven otherwise. These patients are also likely to have an associated coagulopathy.

C. **NSAID, aspirin,** or **cigarette** use. These agents increase the risk of PUD.

D. **Vomiting.** Persistent vomiting or retching may produce a longitudinal tear at the gastroesophageal junction, known as a Mallory-Weiss tear.

Table 28–2. Causes of Lower GI bleeding

Cause	Percentage
Diverticulosis	60%
Inflammatory bowel disease	13%
Hemorrhoids, anal fissure	11%
Neoplasia	9%
Coagulopathy	4%
Arteriovenous malformation (AVM)	3%

V. Clinical Presentation

A. **History**
1. In most cases, patients will report hematemesis, coffee-ground emesis, hematochezia, or melena. The duration and frequency of these symptoms should be elicited.
2. For hematemesis, it is important to determine whether blood was present initially or appeared following several episodes of vomiting. The latter history suggests a Mallory-Weiss tear.
3. A history compatible with cirrhosis (chronic alcohol use, hepatitis, IV drug use) suggests varices.
4. When bleeding has been slow but chronic, the patient may present with lightheadedness, fatigue, chest pain, or shortness of breath due to anemia without any knowledge of GI bleeding.

B. **Physical Examination**
1. Vital signs should be obtained immediately. When abnormalities are present, treatment is frequently necessary prior to obtaining a thorough history.
2. The abdomen should be thoroughly examined, noting areas of tenderness or peritonitis.
3. Rectal examination should be performed with Hemoccult testing. The presence of hemorrhoids should be documented. They may or may not be the source of lower GI bleeding.
4. Examination should also elicit any evidence of the stigmata of cirrhosis including ascites, spider angioma, jaundice, or palmar erythema.

VI. Differential Diagnosis (see Tables 28–1 and 28–2)

VII. Diagnostic Findings

A. **Laboratory Studies**
1. CBC, electrolytes, renal function, and coagulation studies.
2. ***It should be noted that a normal hemoglobin value does not rule out a massive acute hemorrhage.*** Compensatory hemodilution may not occur for 2–3 hours.
3. Blood bank should be contacted for immediate type and cross. Uncrossmatched type O blood is ordered for patients with unstable vital signs and significant blood loss. If a coagulopathy is suspected, FFP is also ordered.

B. **Imaging studies. Upright CXR** is indicated in patients with suspicion of perforation or aspiration.

C. **Procedures. NG aspiration** should be performed on all patients suspected of having an upper GI bleed. Aspirate appearing like gross blood or "coffee grounds" is evidence of an upper GI source. The stomach may then be lavaged with 200–300 mL saline to see if the aspirate clears. Note that false negatives may occur with bleeding distal to the pylorus and false positives may occur from nasal trauma.

D. **Diagnostic Algorithm**

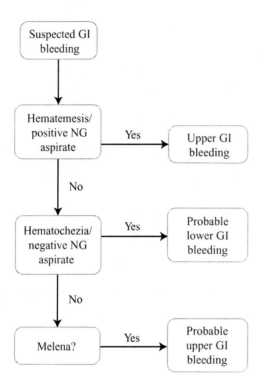

VIII. **Treatment**

A. **General**
   1. Cardiac monitor with O_2 supplementation.
   2. Two large bore (16 gauge) IV catheters for any unstable patient. If these lines cannot be inserted, a large bore central line (8 French) should be placed to maximize volume resuscitation.
   3. IV fluid bolus of 1–2 L NS.
   4. If the patient remains unstable, administer packed RBCs.

B. **Upper GI Bleed**
   1. **Histamine-2 antagonists** are frequently administered, although they have not been shown to be of benefit in the acute setting.
   2. **Proton pump inhibitors** (PPI) decrease the rate of re-bleeding. Pantoprazole 80 mg IV bolus followed by 5 mg/hr infusion is recommended.
   3. **Octreotide** is beneficial in decreasing the rate of bleeding, the incidence of re-bleeding, and mortality by decreasing portal hypertension. It is particularly useful in variceal bleeding, but may also reduce bleeding from non-variceal sources. Give 50 mcg IV bolus followed by 50 mcg/hr IV drip.
   4. **Emergent endoscopy** is indicated for patients with fresh blood in the NG aspirate and hematochezia from an upper GI source. Patients with liver disease also benefit from early endoscopic intervention.

5. Surgical intervention may be required in patients with uncontrolled hemorrhage or patients with liver disease and portal hypertension.

C. **Lower GI Bleed**

     1. In unstable patients, consult gastroenterology and general surgery early.

     2. Diagnostic and therapeutic options include angiography, technetium-labeled RBC scan, colonoscopy, or surgical intervention (partial colectomy).

     3. Angiography. Detects bleeding rates of 0.5–2.0 mL/min, and allows for localization and arterial embolization.

     4. Technetium-labeled RBC scan. Detects bleeding rates of 0.1 mL/min. Allows for localization of bleeding site only.

     5. Colonoscopy. In emergent cases, colonoscopy misses the diagnosis in 40% of cases because of poor bowel preparation. When the site of bleeding is identified, it may allow for therapeutic interventions to stop bleeding, but is unsuccessful in 20% of cases.

     6. Surgical intervention is required in cases of massive lower GI bleeding when other therapies fail.

IX. Disposition

A. **Upper GI Bleed**

     1. Admission. Most patients with an upper GI bleed require admission. Admission to an ICU setting should be strongly considered for patients with unstable vital signs, > age 75, persistent bleeding that does not clear with NG lavage, presence of coagulopathy or severe anemia (Hct < 20%), evidence of portal hypertension, or unstable co-morbid conditions.

     2. Discharge with close follow-up can be arranged for reliable patients who meet all of the following criteria: < age 65, without co-morbidities including coagulopathy, without significant liver disease, normal vitals signs, negative NG lavage and no melena, and hemoglobin > 10 gm/dL.

B. **Lower GI Bleed**

     1. Admission. Most patients with lower GI bleeding will require admission. ICU admission is appropriate for unstable patients. Mortality is higher in elderly patients with co-morbidities, and these features should prompt consideration for admission to an intensive care setting.

     2. Discharge. Young stable patients with normal hemoglobin, no active bleeding, evidence of hemorrhoids or fissures as a possible source, and no evidence of portal hypertension, coagulopathy, or other significant co-morbidities may be discharged with close follow-up.

CASE PRESENTATION

A 75-year-old woman presents with a 2-day history of dark, tarry stools. She has a history of PUD and takes a PPI. Her vital signs reveal a BP of 80/50 mm Hg with an HR of 120 beats/min. NG tube reveals bright red blood that does not clear after lavage.

1. What is your initial management of this patient?

    • IV access with 2 large-bore lines or a central line. Place the patient on a cardiac monitor and administer O_2. Administer NS boluses, and call the blood bank for a type and cross.

2. The vital signs normalize after fluid boluses and 2 units of packed RBCs. What should you do next?

    • Administer a PPI and consider octreotide. Consult GI for emergent endoscopy. Arrange admission to the ICU.

SUMMARY POINTS

- *Aggressive resuscitative measures (IV access, NS, and blood products) are necessary in unstable patients with GI bleeding.*
- *A brisk upper GI bleed should be considered in the differential of patients who present with hematochezia.*
- *Octreotide should be administered in patients with liver disease and significant upper GI bleeding, even when the diagnosis of esophageal varices has not been confirmed.*
- *Emergent endoscopy should be arranged when active upper GI bleeding is present.*

CHAPTER 29
INTESTINAL OBSTRUCTION

I. Defining Features

    A. **Intestinal obstruction** is a mechanical blockage of the flow of intestinal contents that occurs in either the small bowel (80% of cases) or large bowel (20% of cases).

    B. The most common cause of intestinal obstruction is adhesions from prior abdominal surgery. The frequency of the causes of intestinal obstruction is adhesions (60%), colon cancer (20%), hernia (10%), inflammatory bowel disease (5%), volvulus (3%), or other (2%).

    C. Obstruction can be either complete or partial. It is difficult to distinguish an early complete obstruction from a partial obstruction.

    D. **Volvulus** is a closed-loop obstruction that occurs when a loop of bowel twists on its mesenteric pedicle. When this leads to bowel ischemia and necrosis, a strangulated obstruction exists.

    E. **Strangulated bowel obstructions** are also due to adhesions or hernias, and account for 20% of all patients with small bowel obstructions.

    F. **Ileus** is the result of adynamic bowel. It is most commonly present immediately following surgery, but is also seen in the presence of inflammatory conditions of the abdomen (eg, appendicitis, pancreatitis), electrolyte abnormalities (eg, hypokalemia), or from narcotic pain medications.

II. Epidemiology

    A. Bowel obstruction is responsible for approximately 4% of patients who present with acute onset of abdominal pain.

    B. Small bowel obstructions represent 20% of surgical admissions.

    C. Mortality rate from bowel obstruction is 5%, most commonly from strangulation and infarction that lead to sepsis.

III. Pathophysiology

    A. The organs of the GI tract secrete 8–10 L of fluid a day, most of which is resorbed in the colon.

    B. Obstruction to forward propagation results in proximal accumulation of bowel contents and distention of proximal segments of bowel.

    C. Increased intraluminal pressure causes a reduction in lymphatic and venous outflow from the bowel wall, which results in edema formation and third spacing of fluids into the bowel lumen.

D. Secretion into the bowel lumen increases and contributes to intravascular volume depletion.

E. In a strangulated bowel obstruction, arterial flow to the bowel is reduced, resulting in ischemia and infarction. Bacterial overgrowth combined with gangrenous bowel result in perforation, peritonitis, and sepsis.

IV. **Risk Factors.** Prior abdominal surgery, prior bowel obstruction (risk of recurrence is > 50%), inflammatory bowel disease, hernias, malignancy, intussusception, and other (volvulus, feces, foreign bodies, strictures).

V. **Clinical Presentation**

A. **History**
1. **Abdominal pain** that is intermittent and colicky is the initial complaint.
2. If the obstruction is proximal, **vomiting** begins soon after the development of abdominal pain. More distal obstructions will result in delayed onset of vomiting of up to 24 hours.
3. **Flatus, bowel movements, or diarrhea** may be present early in the course of a complete obstruction and should not be used as conclusive evidence that a bowel obstruction is *not* present. These findings are also present in cases of a partial bowel obstruction.

B. **Physical Examination**
1. Patients usually present writhing in **pain,** unable to find a comfortable position (visceral pain). In late presentations or when strangulation has occurred, **peritonitis** may be present.
2. **Abdominal tenderness** is usually diffuse.
3. Abdominal distension, hyperactive bowel sounds, and tympany with percussion all suggest bowel obstruction.
4. The presence of a hernia (inguinal, umbilical, or abdominal wall) is ruled out by a directed examination and should be specifically documented. However, in obese patients, this examination may be insensitive.

CLINICAL SKILLS TIP

Rectal examination may introduce air into the rectum and make interpretation of plain radiographs more difficult. For this reason, rectal examination is often deferred until after obtaining an obstructive series.

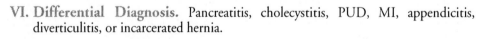

VI. **Differential Diagnosis.** Pancreatitis, cholecystitis, PUD, MI, appendicitis, diverticulitis, or incarcerated hernia.

VII. **Diagnostic Findings**

A. **Laboratory Studies**
1. **Electrolyte** abnormalities due to vomiting and third spacing of fluids.
2. **BUN** or **creatinine** may be elevated due to dehydration.
3. **CBC.** Leukocytosis may be present and suggests infection.

B. **Imaging Studies**
1. **Obstructive series.** Three radiographs: upright CXR, flat plate (supine abdominal radiograph), and upright abdominal radiograph. In patients unable to stand, a lateral decubitus is obtained.
   a. **Mechanical obstruction.** The obstructive series is 50–66% sensitive. The upright abdominal film will reveal dilated loops of bowel (> 3 cm), air-

fluid levels (layering of air and intestinal contents), and/or absence of air in the rectum (Figure 29–1). The "string of pearls" sign is a series of small pockets of gas in a row, and represents a predominance of fluid in the bowel lumen with a small amount of air trapped between the valvulae conniventes of the bowel. CXR is used to screen for free air under the diaphragm, indicating bowel perforation.

  b. **Ileus.** Findings on the obstructive series include dilation of the bowel without a transition point and absence of multiple air-fluid levels.

2. **CT scan.** Sensitivity is 92–100%. CT scan has the added advantage of being able to determine the site of obstruction, the presence of bowel ischemia, and in many cases, the cause of obstruction. If no cause is identified on CT scan, adhesions are likely. CT scanning is the study of choice in patients with fever, localized abdominal pain, or leukocytosis. Bowel wall thickening indicates early strangulation.

C. **Procedures.** Placement of an **NG tube** is uncomfortable for the patient and should be carried out in the following manner to decrease pain and anxiety.

1. Sit the patient upright with the head of the stretcher at 90°. Determine which nostril is less congested by having the patient blow the nose on both sides. Inject viscous lidocaine into the nostril or alternatively spray benzocaine into the nostril and mouth.

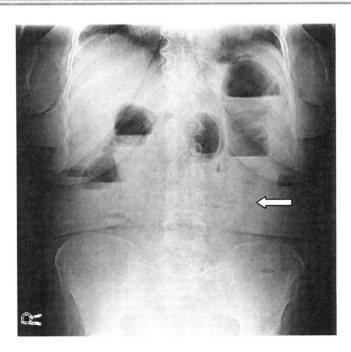

Figure 29–1. Radiograph showing a small bowel obstruction. Note the multiple air-fluid levels and the "string of pearls" sign (*arrow*).

2. Insert the NG tube straight back until the tip is at the posterior pharynx, and then pause. Give the patient a glass of water with a straw. Instruct the patient that as they begin to swallow the water, you will insert the tube.
3. On the count of 3, insert the tube as the patient swallows. The tube is inserted to approximately 30–40 cm. Coughing suggests inadvertent placement in the lung.
4. ***Check the location of the tube by inserting 60 cc of air and listening over the stomach for gurgling.*** Aspiration of stomach contents will also indicate that the tube is in the proper location.
5. Tape the tube securely to the nose. Place the tube to low intermittent suction (LIS).

D. **Diagnostic Algorithm**

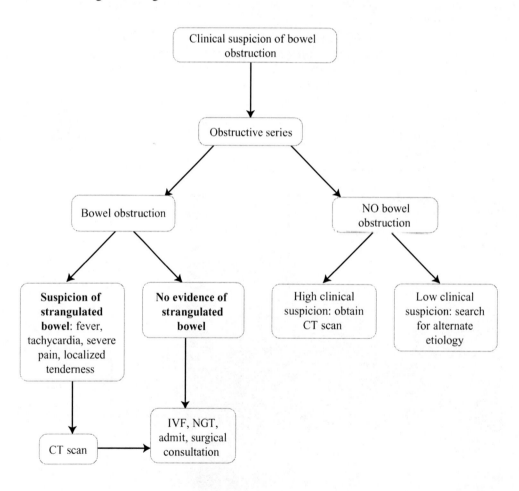

VIII. Treatment

A. **IV line** is placed promptly.

B. **Fluids.** Administer initial bolus of 1 to 2 L 0.9 NS. Patient may be significantly volume depleted because of intestinal third spacing.

C. **Antiemetics.** Prochlorperazine (Compazine) 10 mg IV or promethazine (Phenergan) 25 mg IV.

D. **Pain medications.** Morphine 4 mg IV. Repeat as needed.

E. **NG** tube is inserted and placed on LIS in all patients with a bowel obstruction. This provides symptomatic relief and may avoid the need for surgery.

F. **Broad-spectrum antibiotics** to cover gram-negative and anaerobic organisms are administered in patients with fever, peritonitis, or sepsis.

G. **Surgical consultation** is obtained.

IX. Disposition

A. **Admission.** Indicated in all cases of intestinal obstruction. Admission to the floor is appropriate for most patients. ICU admission is indicated for patients with hypotension despite fluid replacement or sepsis. Surgery may be indicated acutely if peritoneal signs are present. Surgical consultation should be obtained early in acutely ill patients.

B. **Discharge.** None.

CASE PRESENTATION

An 80-year-old man presents to the ED with acute onset of abdominal pain and vomiting. He is seen writhing on the bed, unable to find a comfortable position. Examination reveals a distended, diffusely tender abdomen without signs of peritonitis.

1. *What findings support the diagnosis of intestinal obstruction on plain radiographs?*
   - *Multiple air-fluid levels, absence of air in the rectum, and dilated loops of bowel.*

2. *What is the appropriate ED treatment of patients with intestinal obstruction?*
   - *IV fluids, NG tube placement, anti-emetics and narcotic pain medication, and antibiotics if there is fever, peritonitis, or signs of sepsis.*

SUMMARY POINTS

- *Intestinal obstruction presents with acute abdominal pain, abdominal distension, and vomiting.*
- *An upright abdominal film is diagnostic in most cases, but if negative and clinical suspicion remains, a CT scan should be obtained.*
- *Intestinal obstruction is treated with IV fluids, NG suctioning, anti-emetics, narcotic pain medications, and antibiotics in select cases.*

SECTION VI
INFECTIOUS DISEASE EMERGENCIES

CHAPTER 30
FEVER

I. Defining Features

A. **Fever** is a core temperature > 38° C (100.4 °F) in infants and > 38.3°C (100.9°F) in adults.

B. **Hyperthermia** is an elevated body temperature without a resetting of the hypothalamic temperature center. It is caused by the body's inability to dissipate heat.

II. Epidemiology

A. Fever is the presenting complaint in 5% of adult, 15% of elderly, and 40% of pediatric visits to the ED.

B. Younger patients most often have benign self-limited causes of fever (eg, URI, otitis media); however, they also may present with a serious focal bacterial infection (eg, cellulitis, UTI, pneumonia, meningitis).

C. Respiratory, GU, and bacterial skin infections predominate in the elderly and immunosuppressed, often requiring hospitalization and leading to increased mortality.

III. Etiology.
Endogenous (cytokines) and exogenous (bacterial and viral) pyrogens trigger production of prostaglandin E2 (PGE2) in the hypothalamus. PGE2 raises the hypothalamic temperature set point. The body then generates and conserves heat in order to reach this new hypothalamic set point, thereby raising the body temperature.

IV. Risk Factors

A. Age, malnutrition, and chronic disease blunt the febrile response, making recognition of fever more difficult. These same factors also increase the morbidity and mortality rates from infection.

B. Prior home treatment with antipyretics (acetaminophen and NSAIDs) and the cyclic nature of the febrile response often lead to underestimation of fever in the ED.

V. Clinical Presentation

A. **History.** Important historical information includes onset of fever, duration, pattern, any associated symptoms, travel within the past year, chronic illnesses, recent medication changes, recent hospitalizations, chemotherapy, radiotherapy, or the presence of indwelling vascular access devices or artificial heart valves.

B. **Physical Examination**
1. **Vital signs.** Elderly and immunosuppressed patients may not mount a febrile response despite serious infection. HR and RR increase as fever rises. An

increase in temperature of 1°C results in an increase in HR by approximately 10 beats/minute.

2. **General appearance.** Cachexia or other signs of chronic illness.

3. **Neurologic examination.** Perform a brief mental status examination. In the elderly, AMS may be the only sign of an occult infection.

4. **ENT examination.** Examine for evidence of infection (eg, otitis media, sinusitis, pharyngitis) or abscess. Assess the neck for thyroid enlargement, lymphadenopathy, and meningismus.

5. **Chest examination.** Auscultate for evidence of pneumonia (eg, wheezing, rales, or rhonchi), new murmurs suggesting endocarditis, or the rub of pericarditis.

6. **Abdomen examination.** Palpate for signs of focal or generalized peritonitis. Check for CVA tenderness. Perform a GU examination in males and a pelvic examination in females with abdominal pain.

7. **Skin examination.** Completely disrobe the patient and examine for evidence of rashes (petechiae of meningococcemia) or focal infection (joint inflammation, cellulitis, infected ulcers or abscess), especially about dependent and perineal areas.

CLINICAL SKILLS TIP

Rectal temperature should be taken in infants, children, and adults with significant tachypnea or AMS. Rectal temperatures are most accurate and usually 1°C higher than oral temperatures.

VI. Differential Diagnosis

A. **Infectious Causes**

1. **Neurologic.** Meningitis, cavernous sinus thrombosis, encephalitis, or brain abscess.

2. **Respiratory.** Epiglottitis, retropharyngeal abscess, pneumonia, peritonsillar abscess, otitis media, pharyngitis, sinusitis, or URI.

3. **Cardiovascular.** Endocarditis, myocarditis, or pericarditis.

4. **GI.** Peritonitis, cholangitis, appendicitis, cholecystitis, diverticulitis, intra-abdominal abscess, colitis, or enteritis.

5. **GU.** Fournier's gangrene, UTI (cystitis, pyelonephritis), tubo-ovarian abscess, PID, epididymitis, orchitis, or prostatitis.

6. **Skin and soft tissue.** Necrotizing fasciitis, cellulitis, or abscess.

B. **Noninfectious causes.** Acute MI, PE, intracranial hemorrhage, CVA, neuroleptic malignant syndrome/serotonin syndrome, malignant hyperthermia, thyroid storm, transfusion reaction, or drug fever.

RULE OUT

Most causes of fever originate from infections, and 85% can be diagnosed by completing a history and physical examination.

VII. Diagnostic Findings

A. **Laboratory Studies**

1. **CBC.** Laboratory values of elderly patients with life-threatening infections may be normal. The neutrophil count provides a worthwhile measure of ade-

quacy of response to infection in the elderly or immunocompromised chemotherapy patient.
2. **Urinalysis.** Highly sensitive and specific for infection.
3. **Culture and Gram stain.** Blood, urine, wound, and CSF cultures should be sent to the laboratory on selected patients in the ED and may help guide use of future antibiotic therapy.

B. **Imaging Studies**
   1. **CXR.** Important in the elderly and neonate in whom physical examination findings may be minimal. May be normal despite infection in the dehydrated patient.
   2. **Abdominal CT scan or ultrasound.** For suspected appendicitis, diverticulitis, cholecystitis, and intra-abdominal abscess.
   3. **Head CT scan.** Before LP in patients with focal neurologic findings, seizures, AMS, HIV/AIDS, or signs of increased ICP. Do not delay antibiotic administration while waiting for CT scan or LP to be performed when meningitis is suspected.

C. **Procedures. LP** for cases of suspected meningitis (see Chapter 5).

D. **Diagnostic Algorithm**

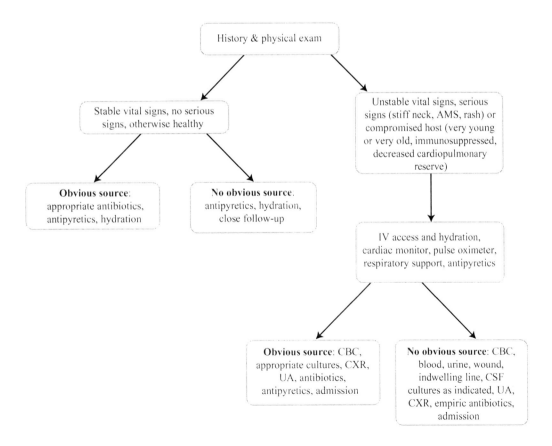

VIII. Treatment

A. **Antipyretics** (eg, acetaminophen or ibuprofen) increase patient comfort and reduce the metabolic demand.

B. Patients with signs and symptoms of shock (eg, AMS, hypotension, tachycardia) require **aggressive fluid resuscitation.**

C. **Intubation** reduces the work of breathing in the septic patient with limited cardiopulmonary reserve.

D. In all critically ill or immunocompromised patients, give **antibiotic therapy** early. If there is no known source of infection, give broad-spectrum antibiotic therapy to cover aerobic (gram-positive and gram-negative) and anaerobic organisms. Special consideration must be given to the neutropenic patient and patients with renal failure or suspected meningitis.

IX. Disposition

A. **Admission.** Unstable patients, the immunocompromised (eg, HIV, elderly, neonate), patients with serious focal bacterial infections (eg, fasciitis, meningitis), and infections with serious co-morbidities (eg, pneumonia and CHF).

B. **Discharge.** Stable patient without co-morbid illness, without serious focal infection, and has improved objectively (eg, vital signs) and symptomatically with ED treatment.

CASE PRESENTATION

A 34-year-old woman presents to the ED complaining of fever of 3 days' duration. She has had fevers as high as 39°C (102.2°F) with shaking chills and sweats. She denies cough, URI symptoms, or rash.

1. *What other historical facts do you want to know?*
   - *Flank pain and dysuria of pyelonephritits, headache and stiff neck of meningitis, RLQ pain and anorexia of appendicitis, vaginal discharge and bilateral lower quadrant abdominal pain of PID. Contacts with ill persons or recent travel. Past medical history.*

2. *What will you look for on physical examination?*
   - *Fever and other vital signs. General appearance. Localizing signs of infection such as photophobia, meningismus, sinus tenderness, tonsillar exudates, cardiac rub or murmurs, rales or rhonchi, abdominal or CVA tenderness, cellulitis, or rash.*

SUMMARY POINTS

- *Fever is a symptom, not a disease.*
- *Be thoughtful in your evaluation of fever to avoid misdiagnosing a serious bacterial illness as "just another viral syndrome."*
- *Provide empiric antibiotics early for moderate to severely ill patients with a possible infectious etiology. Give directed antibiotic treatment in the ED to patients with serious focal bacterial infections.*

CHAPTER 31
SEPSIS

I. Defining Features

A. **Systemic inflammatory response syndrome (SIRS)** is a systemic syndrome manifested by the presence of at least 2 of the following criteria:
1. Temperature > 38°C (100.4°F) or < 36°C (96.8°F).
2. HR > 90 beats/minute.
3. RR > 20 breaths/min or $PaCO_2$ < 32 mm Hg.
4. WBC < 4000/mm^3 or > 12,000/mm^3 or > 10% bands.

B. SIRS can be caused by many different clinical entities (eg, trauma, infection, pancreatitis, burns). When SIRS is caused by an infection, the clinical syndrome is called **sepsis.**

C. **Bacteremia** is the presence of bacteria in the blood.

D. **Severe sepsis** is sepsis with end-organ dysfunction or hypoperfusion as manifested by oliguria, lactic acidosis, or AMS.

E. **Septic shock** is **severe sepsis** with hypotension despite adequate fluid resuscitation.

II. Epidemiology

A. At least 750,000 cases of sepsis occur in the United States every year.

B. Antibiotic resistance, HIV, and an older population all contribute to an increasing incidence of sepsis in the United States.

C. Mortality rates for septic shock remain at 50% despite medical advances.

D. The **lung, abdomen,** and **urinary tract** are the most common sources of infection leading to sepsis.

III. Pathophysiology

A. The clinical syndrome of sepsis results from both the initial infection and the systemic host response.

B. Infectious toxins (bacterial endotoxins) and the resultant inflammatory response (endogenous cytokines) cause diffuse microvascular damage resulting in vasodilation, capillary leak, and DIC. Myocardial depressant factors cause impairment of cardiac contractility. This combination leads to progressive organ dysfunction, resulting in hypoperfusion and hypotension.

IV. Risk Factors. Extremes of age, immunosuppression (eg, HIV, chemotherapy, chronic steroid use, transplantation), severe cardiac and respiratory disease, exposure to multiple drug-resistant organisms (recent or prolonged hospitalization), vascular catheters, indwelling mechanical devices, IV drug use, or burns.

V. Clinical Presentation

   A. History

      1. Patients with sepsis typically present with fever, tachycardia, or tachypnea. They may not have localizing signs of infection.

      2. Patients at the extremes of age and the immunosuppressed often present with subtle signs of early sepsis, such as unexplained AMS in the absence of fever.

   B. Physical Examination

      1. **Vital signs.** Classic findings of sepsis include fever or hypothermia (confirm with a rectal temperature reading), hypotension, tachycardia, and tachypnea.

      2. **General appearance.** Diaphoresis, respiratory difficulty, and mental status.

      3. Search for a focus of infection in the ears, nose, throat, chest, abdomen, and skin.

CLINICAL SKILLS TIP

Check the hands of the septic patient; if warm and well-perfused, then early septic shock is likely. If the hands are cold and clammy, then septic shock is late, under resuscitated, or involves severe cardiac depression.

CLINICAL
SKILLS TIP

VI. Differential Diagnosis (see Chapter 30)

VII. Diagnostic Findings

   A. Laboratory Studies

      1. **CBC** with differential to assess for leukocytosis, bandemia (> 10%), or neutropenia (< 500 neutrophils/mm^3). The absolute neutrophil count is determined by multiplying the total WBC count by the percentage of neutrophils plus bands.

      2. **Chemistry** to assess electrolytes, bicarbonate, anion gap, glucose, and renal function.

      3. **Coagulation studies** (PT/PTT/INR) to assess for coagulopathy.

      4. **Urinalysis** is highly sensitive and specific for infection.

      5. **Culture and Gram stain** of any potential source of infection such as blood, urine, wound or abscess, central line, and CSF or joint fluid. Only 30–60% of patients with clinically evident sepsis syndrome will have positive blood cultures.

      6. **Lactate** acts as a surrogate for end-organ perfusion and allows for the evaluation of the effectiveness of ED resuscitation (declining lactate with fluid and antibiotics).

   B. Imaging Studies

      1. **CXR.** Very important in the elderly and neonate in whom physical examination findings may be minimal. May be normal in the dehydrated patient.

      2. **Abdominal CT scan or ultrasound.** For suspected appendicitis, diverticulitis, cholecystitis, and intra-abdominal abscess.

C. **Procedures. Central line placement:** Large bore catheter (8 French) for patients who need monitoring of central venous pressure (CVP) or rapid infusion
of fluid or blood products. Triple lumen catheter can be threaded through the
large bore catheter later if multiple drips are required after initial resuscitation
(see Chapter 3).

D. **Diagnostic Algorithm**

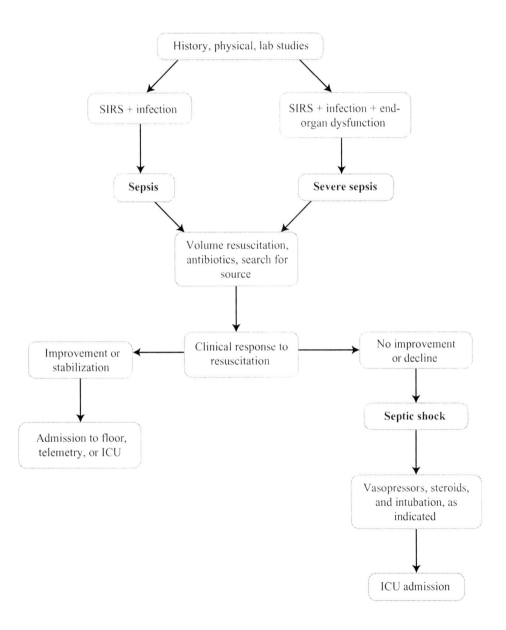

VIII. Treatment

A. **Fluid resuscitation** with 2–4 L NS or LR. Goal is CVP of 8–12 mm Hg and MAP of 65 mm Hg. Other less accurate markers for tissue perfusion include mental status, BP, HR, urine output, and lactate level. In the elderly and patients with known cardiac impairment, give fluid in 250–500 mL boluses, frequently assessing for signs of fluid overload. A Foley catheter allows accurate measurement of urine output (0.5–1 cc/kg/hr is adequate) to measure response to resuscitation and end-organ perfusion.

B. **Antibiotics.** Early use has been clearly demonstrated to reduce the mortality in sepsis. If no known source of infection is present, then give broad-spectrum antibiotic therapy to cover aerobic and anaerobic infections. Special consideration must be given to neutropenic patients and those with renal failure.

    1. **Sepsis of unknown source.** Third-generation cephalosporin and an aminoglycoside.

    2. **Immunocompromised with sepsis of unknown source.** Two broad-spectrum antibiotics with pseudomonal coverage such as piperacillin-tazobactam and an aminoglycoside.

    3. **Neutropenic fever.** Monotherapy with a third-generation cephalosporin with antipseudomonal activity (eg, ceftazidime).

    4. **Vancomycin** should be added to the regimen of any patient with an indwelling catheter, recent hospitalization, or hypotension.

C. **Vasoactive agents.** For patients with persistent hypotension after adequate fluid resuscitation.

    1. **Dopamine** (β1 inotropic > α1 vasoconstriction) at a normal starting dose of 5–10 mcg/kg/min. Use may be limited by resulting tachycardia.

    2. **Norepinephrine** (α1 vasoconstriction >> β1 inotropic) at a normal starting dose of 5 mcg/min. Titrate up as needed.

D. **Endotracheal intubation.** Early intubation decreases work of breathing, improves oxygenation and ventilation, and protects the airway of severely ill patients.

E. **Steroids.** Patients with septic shock with suspected adrenal insufficiency (eg, chronic steroid use) may respond to administration of dexamethasone (10 mg IV), which will not alter results of future adrenal stimulation testing.

IX. Disposition

A. **Admission.** Patients with severe sepsis or septic shock should be admitted to an ICU. Patients with sepsis who have improved with ED resuscitation and have no serious co-morbidities may be admitted to a telemetry or stepdown unit.

B. **Discharge.** None.

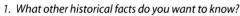

CASE PRESENTATION

A 27-year-old man presents to the ED complaining of fever and productive cough. He says that his symptoms began 4 days ago with sudden onset of fever and soaking sweats. The cough is productive of green sputum. His past medical history is significant for Hodgkin's lymphoma.

1. *What other historical facts do you want to know?*

   · *Timing of last chemotherapy treatment to determine the risk of neutropenia. Presence and type of indwelling ports. Recent hospitalizations to determine risk of nosocomial infection.*

2. *The patient is febrile, and his BP is 70/40 mm Hg. What do you do now?*
   - *ABCs. Manage the airway early and provide aggressive rehydration. Consider vasopressor therapy after administering 4 L NS. Administer broad-spectrum antibiotic coverage early. Culture all potential sites of infection including CSF, sputum, blood, urine, wounds, and lines. Admit to ICU.*

SUMMARY POINTS

- *As the population ages, the number of patients presenting to the ED with septic shock will increase.*
- *Patients at the extremes of age and the immunocompromised require a high index of suspicion to detect serious infection and provide timely management.*
- *Provide aggressive volume resuscitation and administer broad-spectrum antibiotics early to all patients with sepsis.*
- *Closely monitor the patient's response to resuscitation (urine output, mental status, BP), and use vasopressors and mechanical ventilation early if needed.*

CHAPTER 32
MENINGITIS AND ENCEPHALITIS

I. Defining Features

A. **Meningitis** is inflammation of the membranes (meninges) surrounding the brain and spinal cord. It is traditionally classified as bacterial or aseptic.

B. **Aseptic meningitis** refers to patients with clinical and laboratory evidence of meningeal inflammation with negative bacterial cultures. It is usually viral in origin.

C. **Encephalitis** is inflammation of the brain tissue and is usually viral in origin.

D. **Meningoencephalitis** occurs when both the brain and its surrounding membranes are involved.

II. Epidemiology

A. Introduction of the *Haemophilus influenza* vaccine has decreased the number of cases of meningitis caused by this agent by 90%.

B. There is a 59% reduction in the incidence of pneumococcal meningitis in children < age 5 since the introduction of pneumococcal vaccine (Prevnar) in 2000.

C. Over the past 5–10 years, the average age of a patient diagnosed with meningitis has risen from 15 months to 25 years of age.

D. The current mortality rate for bacterial meningitis is 25%, and the morbidity rate is 60%.

III. Etiology

A. *Streptococcus pneumoniae* and *Neisseria meningitides* are the most common causes of **bacterial meningitis.** Less common bacterial causes include *Listeria monocytogenes,* Group B *streptococcus* (neonates and immunocompromised), and *H. influenza* (adults and unimmunized children).

B. Causes of **aseptic meningitis** include viruses (especially enteroviruses), fungi, parasites, TB, inflammation from neoplasms, and autoimmune diseases.

C. **Acute encephalitis.** The most common causes of encephalitis include HSV, enteroviruses, arboviruses (eg, West Nile virus), and HIV.

IV. Risk Factors.
Immunosuppression (eg, chronic steroid use), recent neurosurgical procedures, underlying infections (eg, endocarditis), extremes of age, and overcrowded living conditions (eg, college dormitories).

V. Clinical Presentation

A. History

1. Fever, headache, AMS, and neck stiffness are classic symptoms of meningitis. Up to 20% of patients may have atypical presentations. The triad of fever, neck stiffness, and AMS is only present in 50% of cases.
2. The **duration of symptoms is important** (acute and progressive suggestive of bacterial or serious viral meningitis vs. insidious and stable suggestive of benign viral meningitis or other infectious diagnosis).
3. Seizures (usually generalized) are common.
4. Cranial nerve deficits occur secondary to increased ICP or exudates encasing the cranial nerve root.
5. Encephalitis often produces hypersomnia, focal findings, and seizures, reflecting the part of the brain most affected.

B. Physical Examination

1. **Vital signs.** Fever is almost always present but may be absent in patients who are immunosuppressed, at the extremes of age, or after antipyretic use.
2. Perform careful **ENT, cardiac,** and **respiratory** examinations to look for an initial source of infection.
3. A detailed **neurologic** examination is mandatory, looking for any focal neurologic deficits. Assess for signs of meningeal irritation such as photophobia, nuchal rigidity, or the presence of Kernig or Brudzinski signs. Funduscopy is essential before LP to rule out papilledema (bilateral swollen optic discs with loss of disc margins). Inattention or drowsiness may be the only neurologic sign of encephalitis.
4. Inspect the skin carefully for a petechial rash, which is found in 80% of patients with *Neisseria meningitides.*

CLINICAL SKILLS TIP

***K**ernig sign: Extending the **K**nee with the hip flexed causes stretching of the lumbar roots and pain in the back and hamstrings. **B**rudzi**N**s**K**i sign: **B**ending/flexing the **N**eck results in flexion of the **K**nees.*

VI. Differential Diagnosis.

Brain abscess, migraine, SAH, seizure disorder, toxic ingestion, neuroleptic malignant syndrome, serotonin syndrome, hypoglycemia, heat stroke, and thyroid storm.

VII. Diagnostic Findings

A. Laboratory Studies

1. **CSF analysis** (Table 32–1).
   a. *Tube 1: cell count and differential.* Normal CSF has a WBC < 5 cells/mm^3 with a mononuclear predominance.
   b. *Tube 2: Gram stain, culture.* India ink for fungal infections and acid-fast smears for TB are < 50% sensitive.
   c. *Tube 3: glucose and protein.* Low glucose level is noted in 50% of cases of bacterial, fungal, and tuberculous meningitis. Marked protein elevations are noted in bacterial, fungal and tuberculous meningitis.
   d. *Tube 4: repeat cell count.* To differentiate presence of RBCs present in tube 1. If they clear, traumatic tap is assumed.
2. **Blood cultures.** 50% positive in bacterial meningitis.

Table 32–1. Summary of CSF findings.*

Type of Infection	Gram Stain	Cell Count	Glucose	Protein
Bacterial	Positive in 60–80%	100–10,000 cells/mm³; neutrophilia	Low	High
Viral	Negative	10–1,000 cells/mm³ mononuclear predominance	Normal	Normal to slightly elevated

* Considerable overlap exists between types of infection and CSF findings.

3. **CBC.** Assess immune response and platelets.
4. **Chemistry** for suspected metabolic derangements.
5. **Coagulation studies (PT/PTT).** Obtain in patients who are alcoholics, on anticoagulants, with underlying liver disease, or suspected DIC prior to LP.

B. **Imaging studies.** A non-contrast **head CT scan** prior to LP is indicated in patients with AMS, focal neurologic findings, signs of increased ICP (eg, papilledema), immunocompromise, or seizure.

C. **Procedures.** The patient or family member should be consented before performing an **LP** (see Chapter 5).

D. **Diagnostic Algorithm (see page 185)**

VIII. **Treatment**

A. **Antibiotics.** Goal is to administer within 30 minutes.
1. **0–3 months.** Ampicillin plus ceftriaxone (for *L. monocytogenes,* Group B *streptococcus, E. coli,* and *S. pneumoniae*).
2. **3 months–50 years.** Ceftriaxone plus vancomycin (for *S. pneumoniae, N. meningitidis, H. influenza*).
3. **> 50 years.** Ampicillin plus ceftriaxone plus vancomycin (*S. pneumoniae, L. monocytogenes,* and gram-negative bacilli).

B. **Steroids.** For patients with suspected bacterial meningitis, administer dexamethasone 15 minutes prior to giving antibiotics.

C. **Acyclovir.** For suspected HSV encephalitis, give acyclovir 10 mg/kg IV over 1-hour period.

D. **Prophylaxis** for close contacts of a patient with meningococcal meningitis. Rifampin 600 mg PO q 12 hours for 48 hours. For *H. influenza,* rifampin 20 mg/kg/day for 4 days, maximum of 600 mg/day. For high-risk patients (eg, the asplenic patient) exposed to pneumococcal meningitis, oral penicillin 500 mg PO q 6 hours for 7 days.

E. **Vaccination.** Quadrivalent meningococcal vaccine is recommended for outbreaks on military bases and for college students. Pneumococcal vaccine should be given to any patient > 65.

Diagnostic Algorithm

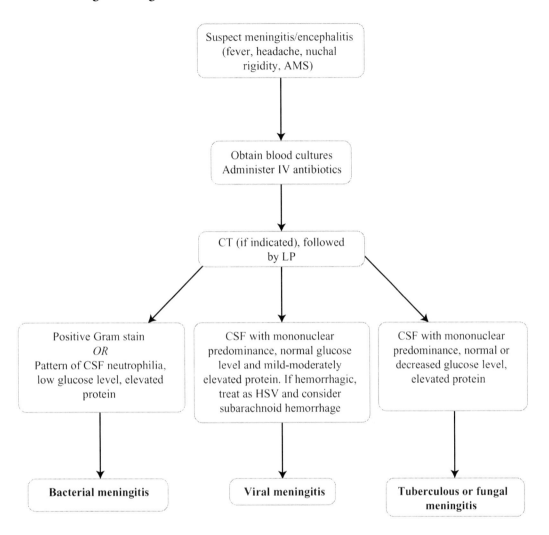

Suspect meningitis/encephalitis (fever, headache, nuchal rigidity, AMS)

↓

Obtain blood cultures
Administer IV antibiotics

↓

CT (if indicated), followed by LP

Positive Gram stain *OR* Pattern of CSF neutrophilia, low glucose level, elevated protein → **Bacterial meningitis**

CSF with mononuclear predominance, normal glucose level and mild-moderately elevated protein. If hemorrhagic, treat as HSV and consider subarachnoid hemorrhage → **Viral meningitis**

CSF with mononuclear predominance, normal or decreased glucose level, elevated protein → **Tuberculous or fungal meningitis**

IX. Disposition

A. **Admission.** Bacterial meningitis, HSV encephalitis, and symptomatic viral meningitis after appropriate therapy in the ED. If meningococcal meningitis is in the differential, admit the patient to an isolation room.

B. **Discharge.** Known viral meningitis with controlled symptoms, a reliable social situation, and appropriate follow-up. ***Considerable overlap may exist in the CSF findings of bacterial meningitis, viral meningitis, and encephalitis.*** When the diagnosis is unclear, the patient should be treated for bacterial meningitis and admitted to the hospital pending results of CSF culture.

CASE PRESENTATION

A 19-year-old college student is brought to the ED complaining of fever and a headache. His past medical history is unremarkable.

1. *What other historical facts do you want to know?*

   • *Duration of symptoms? Meningeal symptoms such as photophobia and stiff neck? Symptoms of encephalitis such as increased sleep, seizures, or cranial nerve palsies? Vaccination history?*

2. *The patient reports that for the past 12 hours he has had a progressively worsening headache associated with neck stiffness, photophobia, and a petechial rash. He appears ill and is febrile, with a temperature to 38.9° C (102° F). A neurologic examination reveals nuchal rigidity. What is your next step in the treatment of this patient?*

   • *Dexamethasone 10 mg IV, ceftriaxone 2 g, and vancomycin 1g IV. LP. Admit to an isolation room. Contact and treat all known contacts to prevent outbreak.*

SUMMARY POINTS

• *Fever, AMS, and stiff neck equals meningitis until proven otherwise.*

• *All cases of suspected meningitis require prompt administration of IV antibiotics.*

• *Obtain a head CT scan before performing LP in patients with AMS, focal neurologic findings, signs of increased ICP, immunocompromise, or seizure.*

CHAPTER 33
SOFT TISSUE INFECTIONS

I. Defining Features

A. **Cellulitis** is a progressive bacterial infection of the dermis and subcutaneous fat and is associated with leukocyte infiltration and capillary dilation.

B. **Erysipelas** is a skin infection that involves the lymphatic drainage system.

C. **Abscesses** are localized pyogenic infections that can occur in any part of the body.

D. **Necrotizing infections** are life and limb-threatening infections that involve the skin, subcutaneous tissue, fascia, and muscle.

II. Epidemiology

A. Cellulitis is more common in men and seen more often on the lower extremities.

B. Approximately 2% of all adult visits to the ED are for the treatment of cutaneous abscesses.

C. Erysipelas is common in infants, children, and older adults. It is usually found on the lower extremities (70%) or face (20%).

D. Necrotizing infections usually occur in the setting of skin trauma, surgical procedures, decubitus ulcers, and immunocompromise.

III. Etiology

A. **Cellulitis** is caused by bacterial invasion of the skin, most often by *Staphylococcus aureus* or *Streptococcus pyogenes*. *Haemophilus influenzae* may be causal in unimmunized children and adults.

B. **Erysipelas** is primarily caused by invasion of the skin by *Streptococcus pyogenes* in areas with impaired lymphatic drainage.

C. **Abscesses** are caused by bacteria that normally colonize the skin. *S. aureus* is the most common organism involved. Mixed infections (aerobes and anaerobes) usually occur in the perineal areas.

D. **Methicillin resistant *S. aureus* (MRSA)** is quickly becoming the infecting agent in many community-acquired cases of abscesses and cellulitis. It should be suspected in children, athletes, prisoners, IV drug users, health care workers, and those who fail to respond to conventional therapies.

E. **Necrotizing soft tissue infections** are caused by a mixture of aerobic and anaerobic bacteria in most cases. Commonly isolated bacteria include *S. aureus*, *S. pyogenes* (ie, "flesh eating bacteria"), *enterococci,* and anaerobes such as *Bacteroides* and *Clostridium perfringens* (ie, gas gangrene).

187

IV. **Risk Factors.** Local trauma, obesity, malnutrition, immunocompromise, IV drug use, vascular or lymphatic insufficiency, surgical procedures, and decubitus ulcers.

V. **Clinical Presentation**

  A. **History**

    1. Ask about trauma (eg, bite, possible foreign body).

    2. Always ask about the time course and presence of any systemic symptoms. Rapidly progressive infections with systemic symptoms require aggressive care in the ED.

    3. Ask about past medical history. Immunocompromise (eg, chronic steroids) predisposes the patient to soft tissue infections and may mask the severity of illness.

    4. Check status of tetanus immunization and any previous antibiotic allergies.

  B. **Physical Examination**

    1. **Vitals signs** provide rapid clues to the severity of infection. Tachycardia and hypotension may indicate sepsis. Fever occurs in < 10% of patients with simple cellulitis or abscess.

    2. **Skin examination.** Completely undress the patient and examine the involved body part. An obvious break in the skin may not always be noted. Assess the involved area for erythema, warmth, edema, and pain. Crepitus suggests gas formation in the soft tissues. Examine for focal areas of fluctuance and induration indicating abscess formation. Note and mark the extent of erythema on the patient with a pen. This will allow for comparison on successive examinations.

    3. **Lymphatics.** Assess for evidence of lymphatic spread (red lines tracking proximally from wound), called lymphangitis.

    4. **Vascular examination.** Always examine pulses for presence of arterial insufficiency.

VI. **Differential Diagnosis**

  A. **Cellulitis.** Thrombophlebitis, viral and drug exanthems, dermatitis, allergic reactions, insect bites, lymphedema, or fungal infections.

  B. **Abscess.** Cutaneous cysts, tumors, foreign body granulomas, or vascular malformations (especially in the axillae and groin).

  C. **Necrotizing soft tissue infections.** Dry gangrene, pressure necrosis, acute DVT, chronic venous insufficiency, acute arterial insufficiency, or compartment syndrome.

RULE OUT

Necrotizing soft tissue infections. *Always remember that such infections present with severe pain but may have few findings on physical examination. The absence of crepitus does not rule out a deep space infection.*

VII. **Diagnostic Findings**

  A. **Laboratory Studies**

    1. **CBC.** In patients with significant areas of cellulitis, suspicion of necrotizing infection, immunocompromise, or systemic symptoms. Not necessary in simple cellulitis and abscess.

2. **Chemistry.** In patients with history suggestive of hyperglycemia or other metabolic abnormalities and in all patients with suspected necrotizing infections.

3. **Gram stain and culture wound.** In patients with suspected MRSA abscess and necrotizing infections, to guide proper antibiotic therapy. Blood cultures add little to the diagnosis and treatment of soft tissue infections.

B. **Imaging Studies**

1. **Plain radiographs** to evaluate for traumatic injury, osteomyelitis, and the presence of gas formation. Radiographs are insensitive for small amounts of soft tissue air.

2. **Ultrasound** is more sensitive for soft tissue air, and it can aid in the diagnosis of deep abscesses and DVT.

3. **CT scan** is very sensitive for soft tissue air, deep space abscesses, and foreign bodies (Figure 33–1).

C. **Procedures. Abscess drainage** (see Chapter 1).

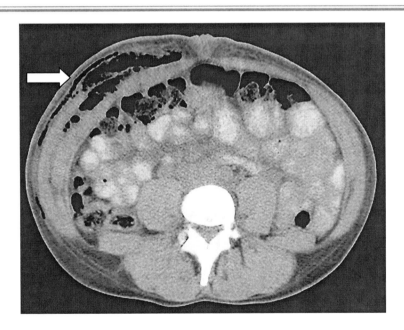

Figure 33–1. Abdominal CT scan in a patient with necrotizing fascitis. Note the presence of air in the abdominal wall (arrow).

D. Diagnostic Algorithm

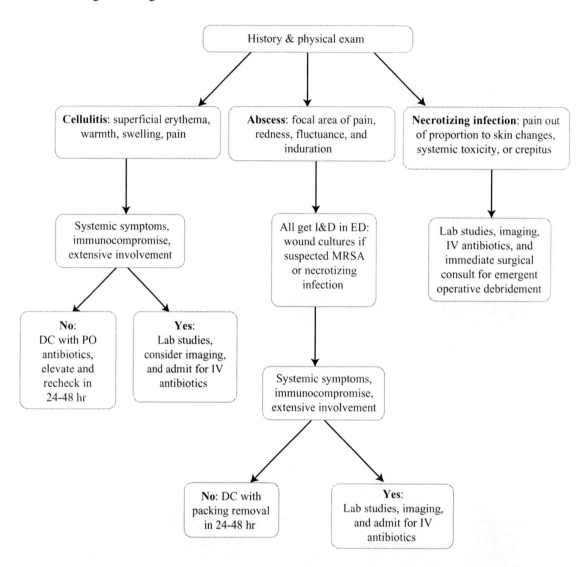

VIII. Treatment

A. **Cellulitis.** If systemic toxicity, immunocompromise, or involvement of high-risk areas such as hands, face, or perineum or circumferential extremity, admit for IV antibiotics (eg, oxacillin) based on presumed infection. If no systemic signs of infection or immunocompromise, and limited areas of involvement, discharge with oral antibiotics (eg, dicloxacillin), continue 3 days past the resolution of symptoms, and recheck in 2 days.

B. **Abscess.** Incision and drainage (I & D) is the treatment for an abscess. Most abscesses do not require antibiotics after I&D. Indications for antibiotics include systemic symptoms, extensive surrounding cellulitis, or immunocompromise.

C. **Necrotizing soft tissue infections.** Fluid resuscitation and other supportive measures. Immediate consultation with a general surgeon for emergent debridement. Empiric broad-spectrum antibiotic coverage for *S. aureus, S. pyogenes,* gram-negative pathogens including *Pseudomonas aeruginosa,* and anaerobes. Piperacillin/tazobactam (Zosyn) is a good single agent therapy. Alternatively, use clindamycin and ceftriaxone.

IX. Disposition

A. **Admission.**
1. **Cellulitis or abscess.** Extensive area of involvement, systemically ill, significant co-morbid illness, or immunocompromise.
2. **Suspected necrotizing infection.** Admit for broad-spectrum antibiotic therapy and operative debridement.

B. **Discharge.** Cellulitis or drained abscess with limited area of involvement, no or minimal systemic symptoms, and no significant co-morbidities.

CASE PRESENTATION

A 59-year-old man presents with pain of 1 week duration in his right leg. He reports subjective fevers at home and states that his "sugars have been running high all week."

1. *What other historical facts do you want to know?*

   · *Timing and progression of illness. Prior episodes of cellulitis, DVT, or symptoms of vascular insufficiency. Significant co-morbidities (HIV, diabetes mellitus).*

2. *He is a diabetic and is febrile, with a temperature > 38°C (101°F). Pulses are present, and there is significant tinea pedis on the right foot with circumferential redness, warmth, swelling, and tenderness to just below the knee. What do you do now?*

   · *CBC, chemistry, urinalysis, imaging, and possible surgical consultation if crepitant or violaceous appearing. IV antibiotics, admission, elevate, and prescribe medications to control pain.*

SUMMARY POINTS

· *Most cases of cellulitis can be safely managed as outpatients with oral antibiotics, elevation, and recheck in 24–48 hours.*

· *All abscesses require drainage. Most patients can be safely discharged without antibiotics, and recheck/repacking in 48 hours.*

· *Patients who are systemically ill, immunocompromised, or who have areas of involvement, including the face, rectum, or perineum, require IV antibiotics, laboratory and imaging studies, and admission.*

· *Patients with pain out of proportion to physical examination findings, crepitus, or rapidly spreading cellulitis may have a life-threatening necrotizing infection requiring aggressive workup, broad-spectrum IV antibiotics, and immediate surgical consultation for operative debridement.*

CHAPTER 34
HIV EMERGENCIES

I. Defining Features

A. **Human immunodeficiency virus (HIV)** is a cytopathic retrovirus that attacks the CD4 T lymphocytes in the immune system.

B. **Acquired immunodeficiency syndrome (AIDS)** is defined as a CD4 count < 200/mm³ or the presence of an AIDS-defining illness. AIDS occurs when HIV-induced loss of CD4 cells and the resulting immunosuppression permit infection from opportunistic pathogens.

C. **AIDS-defining opportunistic infections** include *Pneumocystis carinii* pneumonia (PCP), TB, toxoplasmosis, cryptococcus, cryptosporidiosis, esophageal candidiasis, disseminated mycobacterium avium complex (MAC), and cytomegalovirus (CMV).

II. Epidemiology

A. In the United States, approximately 1.2 million persons are infected with HIV, with up to 50,000 new cases every year.

B. The estimated prevalence of HIV-positive patients seen in urban EDs may be as high as 11.4%.

C. TB is 500 times more common in HIV-infected patients vs. the general population.

III. Pathophysiology

A. **Acute retroviral syndrome** occurs in up to 90% of patients 2–4 weeks after exposure to HIV and may clinically manifest as an acute flu-like illness. **Seroconversion** occurs 3–8 weeks after exposure, and standard HIV tests (ELISA and Western Blot) are negative until this time.

B. An immune response to the virus is then generated, and the viral load falls with a variable period of **clinical latency** (usually 2–10 years). The CD4 count is > 500/mm³ during this period, but cells are being continually destroyed.

C. When the CD4 count is **< 500/mm³,** patients may develop lymphadenopathy, oral candidiasis, idiopathic thrombocytopenic purpura, or hairy leukoplakia.

D. CD4 counts **< 200/mm³** lead to more advanced disease and opportunistic infection. Median survival is 9–12 months if the patient remains untreated.

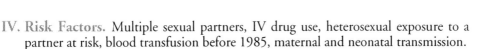

IV. Risk Factors. Multiple sexual partners, IV drug use, heterosexual exposure to a partner at risk, blood transfusion before 1985, maternal and neonatal transmission.

V. Clinical Presentation

A. History

1. All patients presenting to the ED with complaints of infections should be asked about their HIV status and pertinent risk factors.

2. Patients with unknown HIV status, significant risk factors, and symptoms consistent with an opportunistic infection should be assumed to be immunosuppressed.

3. Patients with known HIV should be asked about their latest CD4 count, viral load, medications (including prophylaxis), and history of any opportunistic infections or recent hospitalizations. Patients with counts > 500/mm^3 generally do not get opportunistic infections.

4. **Fever.** Pulmonary and CNS infections are the chief causes of fever. New or worsening headache with CD4 count < 200/mm^3 suggests CNS infection. Any pulmonary complaint suggests pneumonia or TB.

5. **Pulmonary complaints.** Patients should be asked about prior episodes of PCP or TB. They should also be questioned about the use of prophylactic medications (eg, trimethoprim-sulfamethoxazole [Bactrim]) for PCP. The presence of oral candidiasis in a patient with shortness of breath suggests PCP.

6. **Neurologic complaints.** New or worsening headache suggests toxoplasmosis, cryptococcal meningitis, or CNS lymphoma. Painless visual loss occurs with CMV retinitis.

7. **GI complaints.** Difficulty swallowing occurs with candidal esophagitis, and failure to improve with fluconazole (Diflucan) suggests CMV or herpes esophagitis. Acute diarrhea may be caused by bacteria (eg, *Salmonella*), whereas chronic diarrhea may represent a parasitic (eg, *Giardia*) or viral (eg, CMV) cause. Pancreatitis and kidney stones occur as a result of antiretroviral therapy.

B. Physical Examination

1. **Vital signs.** History of fever at home requires a work-up even if the patient is afebrile in the ED. Tachypnea and hypoxia suggest PCP.

2. **General appearance.** Assess for respiratory distress. Wasting, dehydration, and parietal hair loss are common in patients with advanced AIDS.

3. **HEENT examination.** Visual acuity and funduscopic examination for possible CMV retinitis ("tomato and cheese pizza retina"). Oral examination for candidiasis and hairy leukoplakia (Figure 34–1).

4. **Neck examination.** Assess for lymphadenopathy or meningismus.

5. **Lung examination.** Auscultate for rales, rhonchi, or wheezes; however, many patients with PCP will have normal breath sounds.

6. **Heart examination.** Listen for new murmurs, suggesting endocarditis, especially in the IV drug user.

7. **Abdominal examination.** Examine for evidence of peritonitis, pancreatitis, or hepatobiliary disease, which may occur secondary to acute infection or antiretroviral medications.

8. **Neurologic examination.** Assess mental status and any focal deficits, which are present in up to 60% of patients with toxoplasmosis.

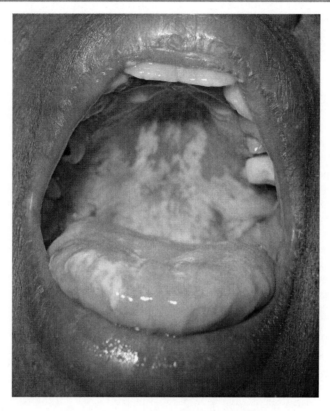

Figure 34–1. Photograph showing patient with oral candidiasis.

9. Skin examination. Examine for Kaposi's sarcoma, cellulitis, abscesses, or drug reactions.

VI. Differential Diagnosis

A. **Fever.** Pneumonia (PCP, bacterial), toxoplasmosis, cryptococcus, bacterial meningitis and sepsis, TB, salmonellosis, sinusitis, lymphoma, CMV, disseminated MAC, or drug reaction.

B. **Cough or dyspnea.** PCP pneumonia, community-acquired pneumonia, TB, fungal pneumonia, Kaposi's sarcoma, or lymphoma.

C. **Neurologic complaint.** Toxoplasmosis, cryptococcal meningitis, bacterial or viral meningitis, encephalitis, or drug reactions.

D. **GI complaint.** Esophagitis (candidal, CMV, herpes), pancreatitis, AIDS cholangiopathy, nephrolithiasis, CMV enteritis, or bacterial/parasitic enteritis.

RULE OUT

TB. Patients with HIV, cough, and fevers are at risk for pulmonary TB. They should be masked and placed in a respiratory isolation room directly from triage. Up to 12% of HIV-infected patients with TB may have a normal CXR.

A. **Laboratory Studies**
1. **CBC.** Use the absolute lymphocyte count as a correlation for the CD4 count.
2. **Chemistry.** Useful in patients with prolonged diarrhea, dehydration, or wasting to assess glucose level, electrolytes, and renal function.
3. **Liver profile and lipase.** In patients with abdominal pain and jaundice. LDH is also useful in patients with suspected PCP. Elevation > 220 IU/L in patients with shortness of breath suggests PCP (94% sensitive), and a normal LDH level suggests an alternative diagnosis.
4. **Blood cultures.** In patients with a fever without a source and for suspected serious bacterial, viral, or fungal infections.
5. **Urinalysis and urine culture.** In all febrile patients without a source. Many AIDS patients have UTIs without symptoms.
6. **Stool.** Check for leukocytes, bacterial culture, ova, and parasites in patients with diarrhea or bloody stools.
7. **ABG** for patients with pulmonary complaints. Patients with PCP and a widened A-a gradient or low PaO_2 are candidates for adjunctive steroid therapy.
8. **LP.** In patients with new headache or fever, especially in patients with CD4 count < 200/mm^3. ***CT before LP is recommended in all patients with HIV*** to rule out mass lesion and increased ICP. Additional CSF studies performed in HIV patients include India ink (cryptococcus), viral and fungal culture, toxoplasmosis, cryptococcus titers or antigens, and VDRL for neurosyphilis.

CLINICAL SKILLS TIP

If the CD4 count is unknown, an absolute lymphocyte count (ALC) can be used to predict the CD4 count. The ALC is equal to the total WBC count multiplied by the percentage of lymphocytes. An ALC of < 1000/mm^3 predicts a CD4 count < 200/mm^3. An ALC of > 2000/mm^3 predicts a CD4 count > 200/mm^3.

B. **Imaging Studies**
1. **CXR.** All HIV patients with pulmonary symptoms or fever without a source. PCP classically shows a diffuse bilateral interstitial infiltrate, but findings vary widely and can be normal (39%) or indistinguishable from bacterial pneumonia (Figure 34–2).
2. **Head CT scan with contrast.** All patients with neurologic symptoms (Figure 34–3).
3. **Abdominal CT scan and ultrasound.** Immunosuppression masks normal inflammatory responses to serious intra-abdominal pathology such as appendicitis and biliary disease. Maintain a low threshold for imaging patients with abdominal pain.
C. **Procedures. LP** (see Chapter 5).

D. **Diagnostic Algorithm**

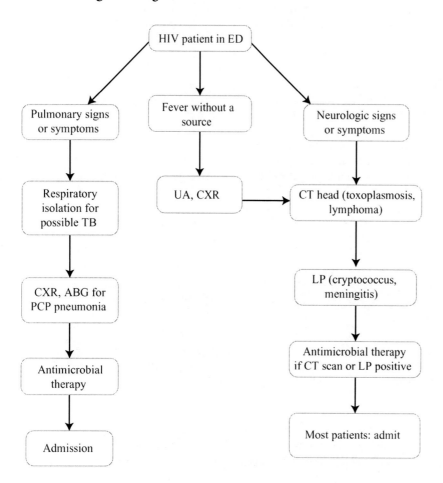

VIII. Treatment

A. **Fever without a Source**

1. Well-appearing patients with CD4 counts > 500 /mm^3 without an obvious source of infection do not need specific antimicrobial therapy and are treated as a normal immunocompetent host.

2. Patients who appear ill and have CD4 counts < 200/mm^3 should be treated with broad-spectrum antibiotic coverage (Piperacillin-Tazobactam plus aminoglycoside).

B. **Pulmonary Complaints**

1. Patients with suspected **PCP** should be treated with trimethoprim-sulfamethoxazole (Bactrim)(5 mg/kg based on trimethoprim). If PaO$_2$ is < 70

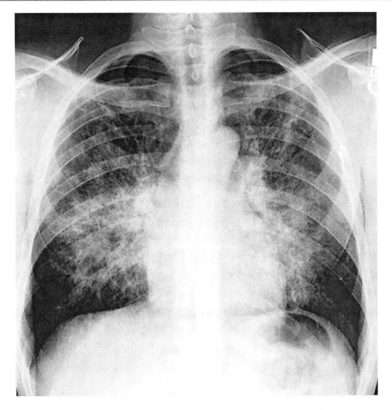

Figure 34–2. Chest radiograph showing classic appearance of PCP pneumonia (bilateral interstitial infiltrates).

mm Hg or A-a gradient is >35 mm Hg, adjunctive steroids should be given (prednisone 40 mg BID).

2. Because PCP is often indistinguishable from **community-acquired pneumonia,** a third-generation cephalosporin (ceftriaxone) or quinolone (levofloxacin) should be added.

3. All patients should be isolated until **TB** has been ruled out.

C. **CNS Complaints**

1. Patients with CT findings consistent with **toxoplasmosis** and mass effect from the CNS lesion require neurosurgical consultation and steroids (dexamethasone 10 mg IV).

2. **Cryptococcal meningitis** is treated with IV amphotericin B after consultation with an infectious disease specialist.

3. Suspected **bacterial meningitis** should be treated immediately with IV ceftriaxone, before both the CT scan and LP.

4. Retinal lesions consistent with possible **CMV retinitis** should be treated with IV ganciclovir in conjunction with consultation with an ophthalmologist and infectious disease specialist.

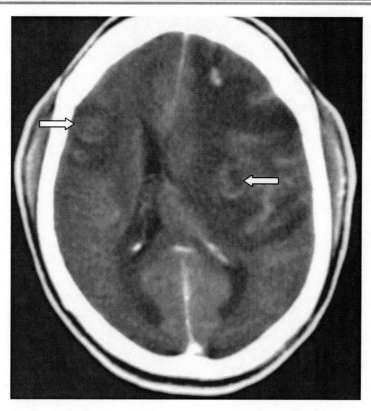

Figure 34–3. Head CT scan showing ring-enhancing lesions of CNS toxoplasmosis in a patient with AIDS.

D. **GI Complaints**
1. Suspected **candidal esophagitis** should be treated with oral fluconazole. Failure to improve suggests drug-resistant candida, CMV, or herpes as the cause.
2. **Acute diarrhea** that is negative for ova and parasites is treated symptomatically (eg, loperamide [Imodium]) in the ED, with outpatient referral.

IX. **Disposition**
A. **Admission.** Fever without a source if the patient is ill-appearing or the CD4 count is < 500/mm^3. Any ill-appearing or dehydrated patient. All patients with pulmonary infections should be admitted to an isolation bed until the possibility of TB is excluded. Admit all patients with focal neurologic findings or abnormal CT scan or LP findings, with CMV retinitis, and with severe drug reactions.
B. **Discharge.** Fever without a source if the CD4 count is > 500/mm^3 and the patient appears well. Patient with a headache who appears well with normal CT and LP. Outpatient follow-up should be arranged to check CSF cryptococcal antigen test.

CASE PRESENTATION

A 27-year-old woman who is HIV positive presents to the ED complaining of dry cough, shortness of breath after walking only a few blocks, and fevers for the past 2 weeks.

1. *What other historical and physical examination findings do you want to know?*
   - *HIV risk factors and prior HIV testing. Recent weight loss, hemoptysis, night sweats, contacts with sick persons. Evidence of thrush, significant pulmonary findings, cardiac murmurs, and rash.*
2. *Temperature is 38°C (101°F) and pulse oximetry is 93%. On examination, there is temporal wasting, thrush, and bilateral scattered rales and rhonchi. CXR shows bilateral interstitial infiltrates. What do you do now?*
   - *Isolate for TB. CBC, chemistry, blood cultures, HIV test, and ABG. Trimethoprim-sulfamethoxazole and prednisone for likely PCP. Admit and administer IV antibiotics.*

SUMMARY POINTS

- *Consider undiagnosed HIV in any patient in the ED with chronic weight loss, fever, or the presence of an AIDS-defining infection, even in the absence of risk factors.*
- *CD4 count determines the likelihood of opportunistic infection.*
- *A meticulous history and physical examination, thorough laboratory and imaging studies, and consultation with an infectious disease specialist are all essential in caring for patients with HIV.*
- *All patients with CD4 count < 200/mm^3 and a respiratory complaint should be put in respiratory isolation until TB has been ruled out.*

SECTION VII
GENITOURINARY EMERGENCIES

CHAPTER 35
NEPHROLITHIASIS

I. Defining Features

A. Nephrolithiasis occurs when urinary solutes precipitate out of the urine and form crystalline stones in the GU tract.

B. Timely evaluation to rule out more life-threatening conditions and administration of pain medications is paramount to proper ED management.

C. Although most patients who present to the ED with symptomatic nephrolithiasis will be discharged, certain complications may warrant more extensive work-up, emergent urologic consultation, and admission.

II. Epidemiology

A. Nephrolithiasis is common in the United States, with an estimated prevalence of 7% in men and 3% in women.

B. Kidney stones most often affect people in the 3rd to 5th decades of life, but can occur at all ages.

C. The recurrence rate is 30% within the first year and 50% at 5 years.

D. Patients with a family history of kidney stones are more likely to develop stones. Caucasians are affected twice as often as African Americans and Asians.

III. Pathophysiology

A. Supersaturation with solute, urine stasis, and relative lack of precipitation inhibitors in the urine all contribute to the formation of kidney stones. The 4 main types of kidney stones are listed in Table 35–1.

B. The GU tract has several anatomic areas of narrowing that may halt passage of a stone. The most common areas are the **renal calyx,** the **ureteropelvic junction** (UPJ), the **pelvic brim** (where the ureter passes over the pelvic bone and iliac vessels), and the **ureterovesical junction** (UVJ).

C. **Ureteral obstruction** occurs when a stone blocks the passage of urine, resulting in hydroureter (dilated ureter) and hydronephrosis (dilated renal pelvis and calices). Obstruction may be **partial** (common) or **complete** (rare). A complete obstruction can cause irreversible renal damage if present > 2 weeks.

IV. Risk Factors.
Dehydration (warm weather, inadequate water intake), hypercalcemia, hyperuricemia (gout), family history, urea-splitting bacteria (Proteus, Klebsiella, Pseudomonas), urinary stasis, and medications (protease inhibitors, diuretics, laxatives).

Table 35–1. Kidney stones by type, frequency of occurrence, and precipitants.

Stone Type	Frequency	Precipitants
Calcium + phosphate/oxalate	75%	Hyperparathyroidism, immobilization
Struvite (magnesium-ammonium-phosphate)	10%	Infection caused by urea-splitting bacteria *Proteus* (most common cause of staghorn calculi)
Uric acid	10%	Hyperuricemia
Cystine	< 5%	Hypercystinuria from genetic disorder

V. Clinical Presentation

A. History

1. Patients will present with rapid onset of severe pain, which is usually episodic and lasts minutes to hours. Pain often originates in the flank and radiates to the anterior, medial, and inferior portions of the abdomen toward the groin and along the course of the ureter.
2. Nausea, vomiting, and diaphoresis are commonly associated.
3. Children may present atypically with only painless hematuria.
4. Urinary frequency and urgency develop when the stone nears the bladder.

B. Physical Examination

1. **Vital signs.** Abnormalities in pulse and BP are common due to severe pain. If fever is present, a concurrent diagnosis such as pyelonephritis should be considered. If hypotension is present, consider sepsis or an alternative diagnosis such as ruptured AAA.
2. **Abdominal examination** should focus on ruling out other causes of abdominal and flank pain. Bruits, pulsatile masses, or pulse deficits suggest a vascular problem. Guarding and peritonitis suggest an alternative diagnosis.
3. **GU examination** should consist of a pelvic examination in females if pain is located in the lower abdomen. In males, note the presence of inguinal hernias, testicular torsion, or infection. CVA tenderness with fever suggests pyelonephritis.

CLINICAL SKILLS TIP

Patients with symptomatic nephrolithiasis are usually writhing and unable to find a comfortable position, in contradistinction to patients with peritonitis who lie perfectly still.

VI. Differential Diagnosis

A. **Immediate life threats.** Ruptured AAA or aortic dissection.

B. **Urologic diseases.** Pyelonephritis or testicular torsion.

C. **Non-urologic diseases.** Biliary colic, ectopic pregnancy, intestinal perforation or obstruction, ovarian cysts and torsion, or herniated disk.

In older, hypertensive patients with no history of nephrolithiasis, always consider an AAA.

VII. Diagnostic Findings

A. Laboratory Studies

1. **Urinalysis.** Performed to assess for hematuria and the presence of concomitant infection. In 15–30% of patients, microscopic hematuria may be absent. Crystals may be present in the urine and aid in the diagnosis of the stone type. Urine pH > 7.6 (normal is 5.5) may indicate infection with urea-splitting organisms.

2. **Renal function.** BUN and creatinine is assessed, especially in patients at risk for renal insufficiency (eg, diabetics, elderly) or patients who may receive IV contrast.

3. **CBC** when infection is suspected.

4. **Urine pregnancy test** in all females of childbearing age to rule out the possibility of ectopic pregnancy.

B. Imaging Studies

1. **Abdomen and pelvis CT scan** is the test of choice for diagnosis of nephrolithiasis (Figure 35–1). It has a sensitivity and specificity of approximately 96% for the diagnosis. CT scan visualizes all 4 types of kidney stones as well as perinephric stranding, hydroureter, and hydronephrosis. It also identifies non-urologic causes of the pain (eg, AAA) in 10% of cases. Non-contrast CT scan does not evaluate renal function or the presence of a complete obstruction.

2. **Intravenous pyelogram** (IVP) is no longer routinely used in the evaluation of kidney stones in the ED. It has lower sensitivity and equal specificity to

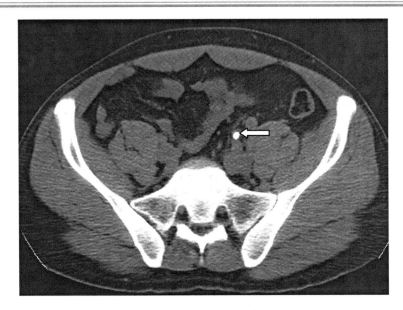

Figure 35–1. CT scan of left ureteral stone (*arrow*).

CT. It provides information on renal function by showing how the kidneys take up and excrete IV contrast.

3. **Renal ultrasound scan** is only moderately sensitive for detecting stones but is highly sensitive for hydronephrosis, which may aid in the diagnosis. It is a useful adjunct in patients who may have contraindications to the above studies (eg, pregnancy).

CLINICAL SKILLS TIP

IV contrast should not be given to patients with a creatinine > 2 mg/dL.

C. **Diagnostic Algorithm**

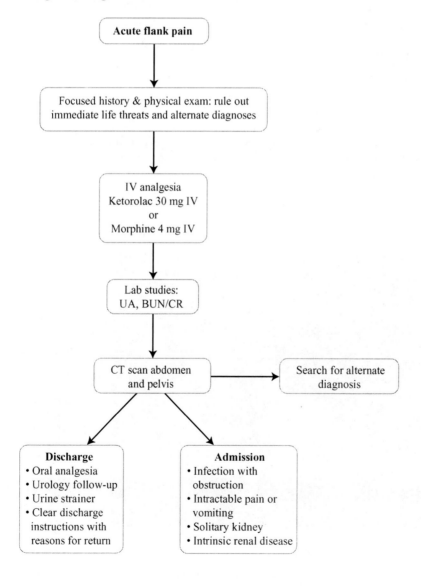

VIII. Treatment

A. **Pain control.** Opioid analgesics (eg, morphine 4 mg) are the mainstay of treatment for acute symptomatic nephrolithiasis. NSAIDs (eg, ketorolac 30 mg IV) are an excellent adjunct to opiates. Avoid in patients with baseline renal impairment, as this drug may worsen renal insufficiency. Antiemetics are useful in treating nausea and vomiting.

B. **Fluids.** IV fluids in patients with nausea and vomiting. A 500–1000 mL bolus NS is usually sufficient in most patients who have no cardiac or renal impairment. Saline boluses are no longer routinely recommended, as they do not help "flush" out the kidney stone.

C. **Infection** with obstruction by a stone is conceptually similar to an abscess. The infection will not improve until it is drained. Patients are at high risk of developing urosepsis. Ureteral stents or percutaneous nephrostomy tubes are used to drain the infection, depending on the location of the stone. Urological consult is mandatory. Antibiotics are administered (eg, ciprofloxacin 400 mg IV).

D. **Stones > 6 mm** in diameter have a low likelihood (< 10%) of spontaneous passage. Proximal location within the ureter worsens the likelihood of spontaneous passage. Urological consultation or referral is necessary in these patients.

IX. Disposition

A. **Admission.** Infection (fever, leukocytosis) with a kidney stone due to the high risk of urosepsis. Intractable pain or vomiting. Solitary kidney or baseline renal disease.

B. **Discharge.** Patients able to tolerate oral fluids and pain medications and have no serious co-morbidities. Urology or primary care follow-up should be arranged within 2 weeks from symptom onset. Prescribe oral opioid analgesics and a urine strainer with instructions to strain all urine until stone passage and to bring passed stones to follow-up appointment. Give instructions to return if fever, persistent vomiting, intractable pain, or inability to urinate.

CASE PRESENTATION

A 60-year-old man is brought to the ED by paramedics and is complaining of right flank pain that occurred suddenly at 5 AM, awakening him from sleep. He has a history of hypertension. He is hypertensive, tachycardic, diaphoretic, and is vomiting.

1. *What other historical facts do you want to know?*
   - *Hematuria? History of kidney stones? Fevers?*
2. *What will you look for on physical examination?*
   - *Pulsatile mass in abdomen. Symmetric femoral pulses. Abdominal pain or guarding. Heart and lung sounds.*

SUMMARY POINTS

- *AAA should be considered in the differential of all at-risk patients being evaluated for kidney stones.*
- *Analgesic administration should not be delayed while obtaining laboratory and radiology studies.*
- *CT scan of the abdomen and pelvis is the test of choice for diagnosing nephrolithiasis.*
- *Urological consultation is mandatory in patients with coexisting infection or renal insufficiency.*

CHAPTER 36
TESTICULAR TORSION

I. Defining Features

A. Testicular torsion is a primary concern in a male with acute scrotal pain, and should be considered in all males with abdominal pain.

B. Torsion is due to twisting of the testicle around the spermatic cord. It compromises venous outflow initially and later arterial blood flow to the testicle, resulting in ischemia and infarction.

C. Testicular torsion is a time-sensitive diagnosis. The longer the torsion persists, the less chance of testicular survival. Thus, the ED work-up must proceed expeditiously.

II. Epidemiology

A. Peak incidence of testicular torsion occurs at **puberty** and during the first year of life.

B. It occurs in about 1 in 4000 males a year.

C. Testicular torsion is 10 times more likely to occur in a male with an **undescended testis.** Thus, torsion should be high in the differential diagnosis of a patient with a painful inguinal mass and an empty scrotum.

III. Pathophysiology

A. The initial effect of torsion is obstruction of venous return. If torsion persists, venous thrombosis followed by arterial thrombosis and ischemia develop. Necrosis and infarction occur quickly after arterial thrombosis.

B. The amount of venous obstruction is related to the degree of rotation of the testis on the spermatic cord and vascular supply. Incomplete rotation causes a lesser degree of edema and vascular congestion, whereas complete rotation leads to immediate complete obstruction and arterial thrombosis.

C. The amount of testicular damage is related to the degree and duration of venous and arterial obstruction. If pain has been present for **< 6 hours,** the testicular salvage rate is 80–100%.

IV. Risk Factors

A. Incomplete or undescended testis.

B. Absence of scrotal ligaments that anchor the testicle to the scrotum, allowing the testicle to hang freely in the scrotum like the clapper of a bell (Figure 36–1).

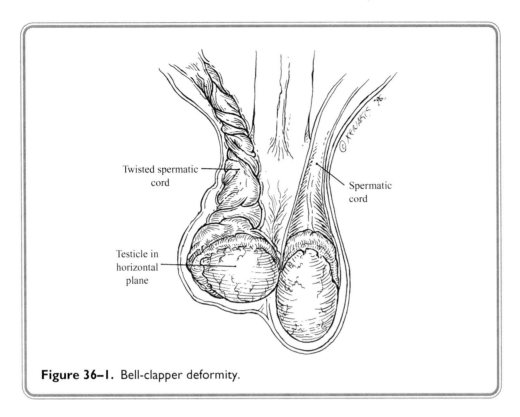

Figure 36–1. Bell-clapper deformity.

C. Abnormal testicular alignment along a horizontal rather than a vertical axis.

D. Testicular atrophy.

E. Scrotal trauma.

V. Clinical Presentation

A. **History**

1. Patients will present with acute onset scrotal pain. The pain is usually severe and noted in the lower abdominal quadrant, the inguinal canal, or the testes. The pain is not positional initially because it is an ischemic vascular event. Later, with significant testicular and scrotal edema, the pain may become positional.

2. Nausea and vomiting are often associated.

3. Torsion usually presents after trauma or strenuous physical activity; however, many occur during sleep.

B. **Physical Examination**

1. Examine the patient in both the supine and standing positions.

2. The involved testicle will be firm, swollen, tender, and the scrotum will often be edematous. With the patient standing, the testicle will lie higher in the scrotum than the opposite side. The size of the scrotal mass is an unreliable indicator of the underlying etiology, and the examination may be unremarkable.

3. The **cremasteric reflex** is typically absent.

4. Examination of the opposite testis may be helpful because anatomic abnormalities are often bilateral.

5. Prehn's sign (relief of pain with elevation and support of the scrotum) is more indicative of epididymoorchitis than testicular torsion; however, this distinction is unreliable.

CLINICAL SKILLS TIP

*The **cremasteric reflex** is tested by lightly scratching the inner aspect of the thigh. A positive reflex is elicited when the ipsilateral testicle retracts upward.*

VI. **Differential Diagnosis.** Epididymitis, orchitis, testicular tumor, torsion of testicular appendage, testicular trauma, acute hernia, or acute hydrocele.

VII. **Diagnostic Findings**

A. **Laboratory Studies**

1. The diagnosis of testicular torsion can be made clinically and no test, either laboratory or imaging, should delay an immediate urological consult when the diagnosis is being strongly considered.

2. **Urinalysis** will usually be normal.

3. **CBC** most often reveals an absence of a leukocytosis.

B. **Imaging Studies**

1. **Color Doppler ultrasound** is the preferred diagnostic study and has a sensitivity of 85–100% and a specificity of 100%.

2. **Nuclear radioisotope scanning** has similar sensitivity to ultrasound; however, the specificity of nuclear scans is much lower than ultrasound. In addition, nuclear scans are more time consuming than ultrasound.

C. **Diagnostic Algorithm (see page 211)**

VIII. **Treatment**

A. **Manual detorsion.** Most testicular torsions occur in the same direction. Therefore, manual detorsion should be performed by rotating the affected testis in the opposite direction 1½ rotations (540°). To remember the direction to detorse, think of **opening a book** (Figure 36–2). The endpoint of the maneuver is relief of pain. If pain becomes more severe, attempt detorsion in the opposite direction. If manual detorsion is successful (ie, relief of pain), emergent consultation with a urologist is still required.

B. **Surgical exploration.** When manual detorsion is unsuccessful, immediate surgical exploration and detorsion is indicated. Patients usually require surgical fixation of both the affected and the unaffected testes to avoid future torsion.

IX. **Disposition**

A. **Admission** for operative urological intervention is indicated in testicular torsion or suspected torsion with an equivocal ultrasound.

B. **Discharge** if no torsion is noted on ultrasound with alternative diagnosis.

Diagnostic Algorithm

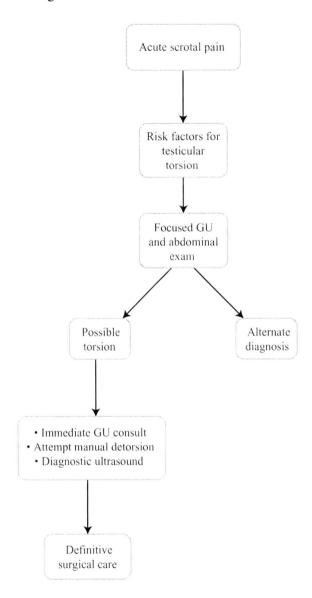

Acute scrotal pain

Risk factors for testicular torsion

Focused GU and abdominal exam

Possible torsion

Alternate diagnosis

- Immediate GU consult
- Attempt manual detorsion
- Diagnostic ultrasound

Definitive surgical care

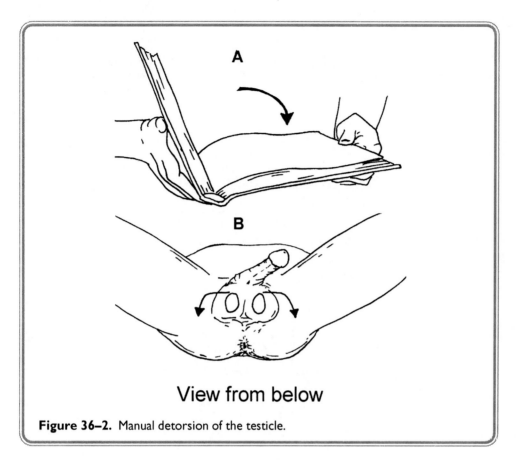

Figure 36–2. Manual detorsion of the testicle.

CASE PRESENTATION

A 14-year-old boy presents to the ED complaining of abdominal pain. The pain awoke him from sleep 2 hours prior to his arrival at the ED. His mother notes that he has had several episodes of vomiting but no diarrhea. During your physical examination, you ask the mother to step outside the room. While you are examining the patient's abdomen, he tells you with some embarrassment that the pain is actually in his scrotum.

1. *What other historical facts do you want to know?*
   - *Trauma? Previous torsion? Duration of pain?*
2. *What will you look for on physical examination?*
   - *Scrotal tenderness and swelling. Abnormally elevated or horizontal lie of the testicle. Lack of a cremasteric reflex. Minimal abdominal findings.*

SUMMARY POINTS

- *Consider the diagnosis of testicular torsion in any male with abdominal pain.*
- *Perform a GU examination on males complaining of abdominal pain, even if they have no GU complaints. This is especially important in adolescent males.*
- *When considering testicular torsion as a diagnosis, never allow an imaging study or laboratory test to delay an emergent urological consultation.*
- *When attempting manual detorsion, remember the direction to turn the testicle is like opening a book.*

CHAPTER 37

PENILE DISORDERS

I. Defining Features

A. **Balanoposthitis** is inflammation of both the glans penis (balanitis) and foreskin (posthitis).

B. **Phimosis** is the inability to retract the foreskin proximally over the glans penis. Phimosis is a urologic emergency when it causes urinary retention.

C. **Paraphimosis** is the inability to reduce a retracted foreskin distally over the glans penis to its naturally occurring position. This is a *true* urologic emergency.

II. Epidemiology

A. Balanoposthitis occurs in up to 3% of uncircumcised males and is more common in diabetics. It may be the first presenting symptom in a patient with new onset diabetes mellitus.

B. Phimosis may be normal in pre-pubertal males **(physiologic phimosis).** By age 4, 90% of foreskins are fully retractable. A foreskin that is not fully retractable by the end of puberty is considered **pathologic phimosis.**

C. Paraphimosis is a common **iatrogenic complication** in debilitated patients after examination or catheter insertion when the caretaker fails to replace the foreskin to its natural position.

III. Pathophysiology

A. The primary cause of **balanoposthitis** is infection. The most common organisms involved are *Candida, Gardnerella, Streptococcus pyogenes,* and anaerobes.

B. Infection and trauma lead to inflammation and scarring that prevent normal retraction of the foreskin, resulting in **phimosis.** It may infrequently cause urinary retention from either constriction at the urethral meatus or painful urination.

C. **Paraphimosis** results when a retracted foreskin is not replaced to its normal physiologic position. The retracted foreskin has a constricting effect, resulting in impairment of venous return from the distal glans penis. This can lead to progressive inflammation, ischemia, and necrosis of the distal penis.

IV. Risk Factors

A. **Diabetics** are at risk for balanoposthitis.

B. Any uncircumcised male with **balanoposthitis** or **trauma** is at risk for phimosis.

213

V. Clinical Presentation

A. **Balanoposthitis.** Patients present with penile pain and swelling and foreskin discharge without systemic symptoms. On examination, the patient is afebrile with an edematous, erythematous, excoriated penis and foreskin. Purulent discharge is present between the glans and foreskin. The foreskin should be in its normal position and easily retractable.

B. **Phimosis.** Adults complain of inability to retract a previously retractable foreskin. They may also complain of urinary retention. On examination, they have a normal appearing foreskin with a distal stricture preventing normal retraction over the glans (Figure 37–1).

C. **Paraphimosis.** Patients present with anxiety, severe penile pain, and swelling. The foreskin is retracted proximal to the glans penis and is edematous (Figure 37–2). The glans may be erythematous or ischemic in appearance. A thick constricting band can be palpated on the foreskin.

CLINICAL SKILLS TIP

Smegma is formed when epithelial cells slough during normal separation of the foreskin in pre-pubescent males. This whitish discharge may be mistaken for infection. Unlike balanoposthitis, there is no associated edema or erythema of the glans and foreskin.

VI. Differential Diagnosis

A. **Balanoposthitis.** STDs (HSV, syphilis, HPV), allergy or dermatitis, psoriasis, penile cancer, or paraphimosis.

B. **Phimosis.** Physiologic phimosis or balanoposthitis.

C. **Paraphimosis.** Hair tourniquet, balanoposthitis, or Fournier's gangrene.

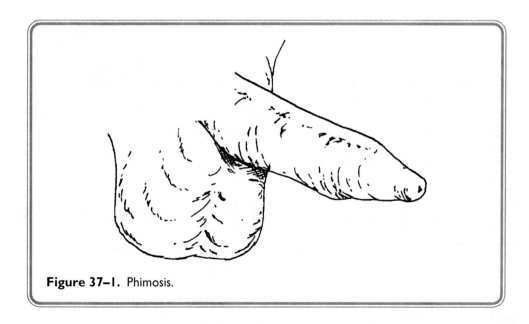

Figure 37–1. Phimosis.

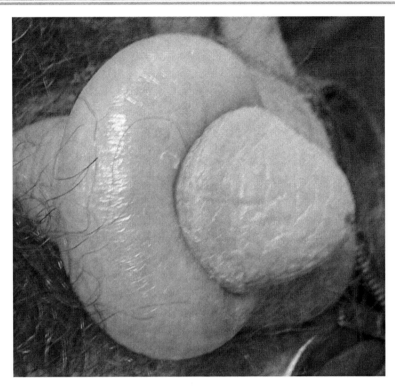

Figure 37–2. Paraphimosis.

RULE OUT:

Do not mistake paraphimosis for balanoposthitis. They both present with pain and swelling, but the foreskin will be retracted and is non-reducible in paraphimosis.

VII. Diagnostic Findings

A. Bedside glucose test in balanoposthitis to rule out diabetes mellitus. When fever and penile warmth are present, a bacterial culture of the discharge may be useful.

B. **Diagnostic Algorithm (see page 216)**

VIII. Treatment

A. **Balanoposthitis.** The mainstay of treatment is **regular cleansing** with soap and water, with the foreskin retracted. Topical **antifungal cream** should also be used. In cases where the penis is warm and the discharge is purulent, an antibiotic should be prescribed. The foreskin should always be reduced over the glans to its natural position after cleansing. Painful urination can be avoided by having the patient urinate in a warm bath.

B. **Phimosis.** Asymptomatic patients can be treated with a topical steroid such as **triamcinolone** 0.025% BID for 6–8 weeks. If urinary retention is present, dilation of the phimotic area with a hemostat will temporarily improve symptoms. If unsuccessful, a **dorsal slit procedure** is performed.

Diagnostic Algorithm

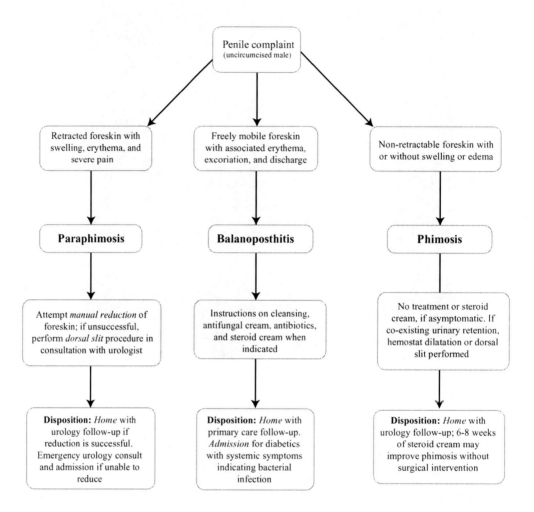

D. **Paraphimosis. Manual reduction** of the foreskin is attempted; if unsuccessful, a **dorsal slit procedure** is performed (Figure 37–3).

IX. Disposition

    A. **Admission.** Patients with non-reducible paraphimosis will require emergent urological consult and sometimes admission. Patients with balanoposthitis with systemic symptoms and co-morbid illness (eg, diabetes mellitus) should be admitted and given IV antibiotics.

    B. **Discharge.** Most patients with balanoposthitis can be discharged home. Patients with phimosis can be discharged home as long as they are able to urinate. They should follow up with a urologist. Patients with paraphimosis, successfully reduced either manually or surgically, can be discharged home as long as they are able to urinate.

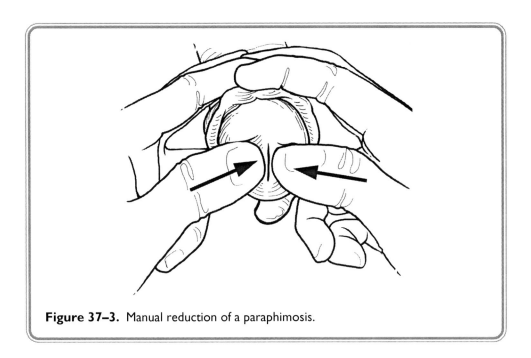

Figure 37–3. Manual reduction of a paraphimosis.

CASE PRESENTATION

A 25-year-old man presents with a complaint of penile pain. He had sexual intercourse the previous evening and awoke 8 hours later with a swollen, painful penis. He is uncircumcised. On examination, you find a swollen foreskin that is retracted behind the glans penis.

1. *How will you perform manual reduction of the foreskin?*
   - *Provide gentle pressure to the foreskin to reduce edema. Hold the tip of the penis with the index and middle finger and thumb of both hands. Push the glans with both thumbs posterior, while pulling the foreskin over the glans with the fingers.*

2. *If manual reduction is unsuccessful, how will you perform a dorsal slit of the foreskin?*
   - *The patient should have IV access for analgesia and sedation. Anesthesia of the penis is achieved with local infiltration of the tissue with 1% lidocaine. Two straight hemostats are used to clamp across the constricting tissue where it is anesthetized. A scalpel is used to cut the band between the 2 hemostats, carefully avoiding the glans and penis. The foreskin is then reduced over the glans penis.*

SUMMARY POINTS

- *The mainstay of balanoposthitis treatment is meticulous hygiene.*
- *Balanoposthitis may be the first presenting sign of diabetes mellitus.*
- *Phimosis may be physiologic until puberty.*
- *Paraphimosis is a true urologic emergency requiring reduction of the foreskin by manual or surgical techniques.*

SECTION VIII
OBSTETRIC
AND GYNECOLOGIC
EMERGENCIES

CHAPTER 38
VAGINAL BLEEDING

I. Defining Features

A. Menarche occurs in girls at approximately age 12. Normal menstruation continues until menopause, which occurs on average at age 51.

B. **Menorrhagia** is an increased volume or duration of bleeding that occurs at the typical time of menstruation. **Metrorrhagia** is bleeding that occurs at irregular intervals outside of the normal menstrual cycle. **Menometrorrhagia** is irregular bleeding that is also of increased duration or flow.

C. Pregnancy must be excluded in women of child-bearing age who present with vaginal bleeding.

II. Epidemiology

A. Vaginal bleeding complicates 20% of early pregnancies. When bleeding occurs, 50% of patients will have a spontaneous abortion.

B. In the United States, about 2% of all pregnancies are ectopic pregnancies. Mortality in these women is due to shock from intra-abdominal hemorrhage.

C. In postmenopausal women with vaginal bleeding, 10% will be diagnosed with cancer, the majority being endometrial cancer.

III. Pathophysiology

A. The adult menstrual cycle is usually 28 days (+/- 7 days), with menstruation lasting 4–6 days.

B. Normal menstrual blood flow is approximately 30–60 mL; > 80 mL of bleeding is considered abnormal.

C. Dysfunctional uterine bleeding (DUB) is due to prolonged or excessive estrogen stimulation or ineffective progesterone production.

D. Ectopic pregnancy exists when implantation occurs at a site outside of the endometrium. In most cases, the ectopic site is the lateral two thirds of the fallopian tube. Other sites include the medial third of the fallopian tube, cornu (junction of the tube and uterus), ovary, fimbria, cervix, and abdomen (Figure 38–1).

IV. Risk Factors.
Risk factors for ectopic pregnancy include history of salpingitis, use of intrauterine device, prior ectopic pregnancy, increased maternal age, and history of tubal ligation. Up to 42% of women with an ectopic pregnancy have no risk factors.

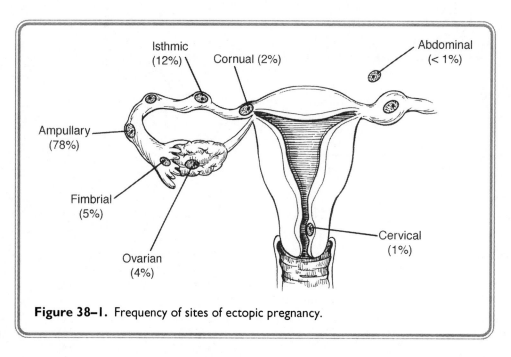

Figure 38–1. Frequency of sites of ectopic pregnancy.

V. Clinical Presentation

A. History

1. Pain may or may not be present. If pain is present, determine pain characteristics such as location, quality, and duration. Approximately 10% of patients with ectopic pregnancy will present with bleeding only.

2. Determine the onset of bleeding, date and duration of the last normal menstrual period, number of previous pregnancies, and previous history of vaginal bleeding.

3. Inquire about past gynecologic problems, including risk factors for ectopic pregnancy.

4. Attempt to have the patient quantify the amount of bleeding. Although not reliable, a tampon or pad absorbs approximately 30 mL of blood. The presence of clotted blood suggests brisk vaginal bleeding.

5. Symptoms of weakness, lightheadedness, shortness of breath, or syncope suggest anemia from prolonged blood loss or acute intra-abdominal hemorrhage (ruptured ectopic pregnancy).

B. Physical Examination

1. **Vital signs.** Note BP and pulse.

2. Before performing a pelvic examination, perform a focused general examination, including the abdomen and flank. Peritoneal signs suggest infection or intraperitoneal blood.

3. **Pelvic examination.** Perform with the patient in the lithotomy position. Male examiners should have a female chaperone present. **Inspect** the external genitalia. On **speculum examination,** determine the presence of blood, blood clots, tissue (products of conception), or discharge in the vaginal vault.

Visually inspect the cervix. On **bimanual examination,** determine whether the cervical os is open or closed. Estimate the size of the uterus (12 weeks at the symphysis, 20 weeks at the umbilicus). Assess the adnexa for tenderness or masses. Tenderness on pelvic examination is present in over 80% of patients with a ruptured ectopic pregnancy.

CLINICAL SKILLS TIP

Determining whether the os is open or closed is achieved during the bimanual examination. An open os is present when the tip of the examiner's index finger can pass through the cervix. Women with a closed internal os should be considered to have a closed os, even if the external portion of the os is open.

VI. Differential Diagnosis

A. **Pregnancy.** In the first trimester of pregnancy, the diagnostic possibilities include continuation of what will be a normal pregnancy or an abnormal pregnancy (spontaneous abortion; ectopic pregnancy; trophoblastic disease) (Table 38–1).

B. DUB, fibroids (occur in 20% of women of reproductive age), malignancy (eg, cervical, uterine or vaginal), infection (eg, PID, vaginal infections), trauma, foreign body (eg, IUD, tampon, sexual devices), and coagulopathy (eg, genetic disorders or secondary to medications).

VII. Diagnostic Findings

A. **Laboratory Studies**

1. **Urine pregnancy test** is 99.4% sensitive for diagnosing pregnancy at the time that a woman "misses" her period.

2. **Serum pregnancy test (βhCG).** In a normal pregnancy, βhCG level doubles every 2 days, peaking at 100,000 mIU/mL. Higher levels suggest trophoblastic disease. An ectopic pregnancy can be present at any βhCG level; therefore, the initial βhCG level cannot be used to exclude ectopic pregnancy. Patients with repeat βhCG levels that decrease by > 50% are at low risk for ectopic pregnancy, while those with levels that do not increase > 66% are at high risk.

3. **Urinalysis** is ordered to rule out a UTI.

4. **CBC** is indicated in patients with resting tachycardia, lightheadedness, or prolonged duration of bleeding (≥ 3 weeks).

5. **Rh status (type and screen).** In pregnant patients with vaginal bleeding.

Table 38–1. Classification of spontaneous abortion.

Type	Internal Cervical Os	Products of Conception
Threatened	Closed	Not passed
Inevitable	Open	Not passed
Incomplete	Usually open	Partially passed
Complete	Closed	Completely passed

B. **Imaging studies. Pelvic ultrasound** is the most useful imaging modality, especially in the setting of pregnancy. Ectopic pregnancy is excluded when an intrauterine pregnancy (IUP) is visualized. A heterotopic pregnancy (IUP and ectopic pregnancy) is rare except in women receiving treatment for infertility. *Patients with a non-cystic adnexal mass, significant fluid in the cul-de-sac, an extrauterine gestational sac, or an empty uterus (with βhCG > 1000 mIU/mL) should be considered high risk for ectopic pregnancy.* In 15–20% of patients, the initial pelvic ultrasound will be indeterminate (no evidence of an IUP or an ectopic pregnancy). Of these indeterminate ultrasounds, 20% eventually will be diagnosed with an ectopic pregnancy.

C. **Diagnostic Algorithm**

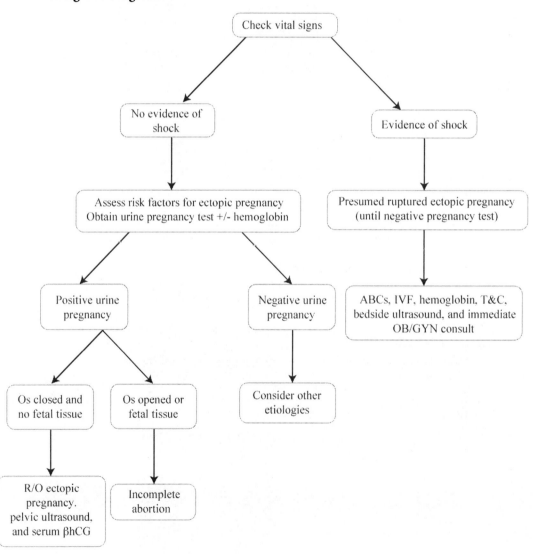

VIII. Treatment

A. When **shock** is present in a young woman with a positive pregnancy test, ruptured ectopic pregnancy is presumed. Perform immediate interventions, including IV fluids, type and cross, bedside ultrasound, and gynecology consultation for surgical intervention. A similar work-up is pursued in women with a positive pregnancy test and an acute abdomen (presumed ruptured ectopic pregnancy), even when the initial vital signs are normal.

B. **Pregnancy**
   1. **Complete and threatened abortion.** If the woman is Rh-negative (15% of the white population), administer RhoGAM 50 mcg IM. Incomplete abortion and ectopic pregnancy will also require RhoGAM if the patient is Rh-negative.
   2. **Incomplete abortion.** Bleeding will continue until all products of conception have passed. Dilatation and curettage (D&C) may be indicated.
   3. **Ectopic pregnancy.** Patients with a ruptured ectopic pregnancy require surgery. Some patients with unruptured ectopic pregnancy are candidates for nonsurgical treatment by the gynecologist with use of methotrexate and leucovorin (IV, PO, or IM as a single dose).

C. **Vaginal bleeding unrelated to pregnancy.** Consider blood transfusion in patients with symptomatic anemia, especially when the hemoglobin is < 7 gm/dL. When bleeding is severe in patients with chronic anovulatory bleeding, relief may be obtained with hormonal therapy (medroxyprogesterone 10 mg PO for 10 days or Ortho-Novum 1/35 1 tablet QID for 5 days).

IX. Disposition

A. **Admission.** Patients with hemodynamic instability, peritoneal findings, severe anemia (Hb < 7 gm/dL), or a confirmed ectopic pregnancy on ultrasound should be admitted. Pregnant patients with a closed cervical os, no fetal tissue passed, no IUP visualized on ultrasound, and βhCG > 1000 mIU/mL should be admitted for observation to rule out ectopic pregnancy.

B. **Discharge** patients with mild to moderate vaginal bleeding, who are hemodynamically stable, and in whom ectopic pregnancy has been excluded. Discharge with gynecology follow-up, and a repeat βhCG level in 48 hours is also appropriate for reliable patients with no IUP seen on ultrasound when the βhCG is < 1000 mIU/mL. This assumes the patient is hemodynamically stable, has no significant abdominal tenderness, and has no other ultrasound findings that suggest an ectopic pregnancy (moderate to large amount of free fluid or a noncystic adnexal mass). In patients with postmenopausal bleeding, refer to a gynecologist for endometrial biopsy.

CASE PRESENTATION

A 16-year-old girl presents to the ED with her mother with a complaint of vaginal bleeding for the past 4 days. She states that her last period was approximately 2 months ago, but she "occasionally misses." When you inquire about previous pregnancies, the mother vehemently denies that her daughter is sexually active. The girl's vital signs are BP 100/65 mm Hg, HR 105 beats/min, RR 14 breaths/min, and temperature 37°C (98.6°F).

1. What other historical information do you want to know?

- *Politely ask the mother to step out of the room during the examination and review the history. Sexual history (sexual activity, previous STD, contraceptive use). Previous gynecologic history (past pregnancies). Ectopic pregnancy risk factors. Amount of bleeding.*
2. *What will you look for on physical examination?*
    - *Abdominal tenderness. Adnexal mass/tenderness. Blood or tissue in vaginal vault. Opened or closed cervical os. Uterine enlargement.*

SUMMARY POINTS

- *Obtain a pregnancy test in any female of childbearing age who presents with vaginal bleeding or abdominal pain.*
- *Risk factors are absent in > 40% of women who have an ectopic pregnancy.*
- *Ruptured ectopic pregnancy is a surgical emergency requiring prompt intervention and gynecologic consultation.*
- *Patients with postmenopausal bleeding should be referred to a gynecologist for endometrial biopsy to exclude malignancy.*

CHAPTER 39
PREECLAMPSIA AND ECLAMPSIA

I. Defining Features

A. **Pregnancy-induced hypertension** is defined as BP > 140/90 mm Hg or a rise in systolic BP of 20 mm Hg or in diastolic BP of 10 mm Hg above baseline (pre-pregnancy) BP. Therefore a "normal" BP does not exclude the diagnosis.

B. **Preeclampsia** is defined as hypertension and proteinuria in a pregnant patient > 20 weeks' gestation. Edema may or may not be present.

C. **Severe preeclampsia** is present when BP is > 160/110 mm Hg on 2 separate occasions, with large proteinuria, oliguria, persistent neurologic symptoms, epigastric/RUQ pain, pulmonary edema, or a platelet count < 100,000/µL. **Eclampsia** is preeclampsia with seizures.

D. **HELLP** (hemolysis, elevated liver enzymes, low platelets) syndrome is a more severe variation of preeclampsia and is more common in multigravida women.

II. Epidemiology

A. Hypertension occurs in approximately 10% of all pregnancies.

B. Preeclampsia complicates 6–8% of pregnancies. In most patients, it occurs after 20 weeks' gestation, but may occur earlier in the presence of a molar pregnancy or with multiple gestations.

C. Eclampsia occurs in 0.05% of all pregnancies. One third of cases occur postpartum (usually within the first 24 hours and rarely after 48 hours).

D. Eclampsia is the second leading cause of maternal death, with a mortality rate of approximately 5%. Multiple convulsions lead to fetal death in 10–28% of cases.

E. HELLP syndrome occurs in 10% of women with severe preeclampsia and 30–50% of women with eclampsia.

III. Pathophysiology

A. The exact etiology of preeclampsia is unknown.

B. In women who develop preeclampsia, there are fewer placental cytotrophoblasts, which ultimately fail to take on the characteristics of normal blood vessels. This abnormal blood vessel development results in placental vasospasm, endothelial injury, and decreased placental blood flow.

C. Cerebral vasospasm, edema, ischemia, and electrolyte shifts are believed to cause the seizures of eclampsia.

227

D. Untreated, HELLP syndrome results in severe end-organ damage, coagulopathy (DIC), and death.

IV. **Risk Factors.** Nulliparity, > age 40, pre-existing hypertension or renal disease, diabetes mellitus, multiple gestations, gestational trophoblastic disease, obesity, African-American race, or previous preeclampsia.

V. **Clinical Presentation**

A. **History**
   1. Presentation is variable, and symptoms are not necessarily related to severity.
   2. Symptoms may include headache, visual disturbances, epigastric or RUQ pain, or edema (peripheral, facial).
   3. Generalized tonic clonic seizures in a woman with preeclampsia are pathognomonic for eclampsia and may occur (although rarely) up to 1 month after delivery.

B. **Physical Examination**
   1. Check vital signs, paying particular attention to BP. If previous records are available, compare BP to previous determinations. The degree of BP elevation is not a dependable predictor of disease severity.
   2. Examine the abdomen, noting tenderness in the RUQ and epigastric areas.
   3. Check the height of the uterine fundus. A fundal height at the umbilicus represents (approximately) a 20-week gestation (Figure 39–1). Listen for fetal heart tones using a stethoscope or a hand-held Doppler.
   4. Peripheral and facial edema may be present.
   5. A complete neurologic examination is indicated. New, persistent neurologic deficits are an ominous sign.

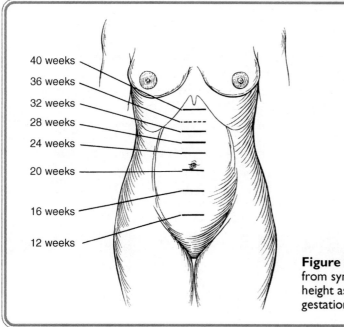

40 weeks
36 weeks
32 weeks
28 weeks
24 weeks
20 weeks
16 weeks
12 weeks

Figure 39–1. Measurement from symphysis pubis to fundal height as a clinical estimator of gestational age.

VI. **Differential Diagnosis.** Pancreatitis, hepatitis, pyelonephritis, renal failure, gastroenteritis, stroke, epilepsy, essential or gestational hypertension.

VII. **Diagnostic Findings**

A. **Laboratory Studies**
1. **CBC.** Hemoglobin, peripheral smear (schistocytes in HELLP syndrome), platelet count (< 150,000/μL in HELLP syndrome).
2. **Electrolytes** with **BUN** and **creatinine.**
3. **Urinalysis** for proteinuria or infection. Significant proteinuria is classically defined as > 300 mg during a 24-hour urine collection. This corresponds roughly to ≥ 1+ proteinuria on the urine dipstick.
4. **PT/PTT, liver enzymes,** and **liver function tests** may be abnormal in HELLP syndrome.
5. **Type and crossmatch.**
6. **Magnesium and phosphate levels** are drawn as baseline levels in patients who may receive treatment with magnesium.

B. **Imaging Studies**
1. **Head CT scan** should be performed in patients with seizures or other neurologic complaints.
2. **Fetal monitoring** should be performed, continuously looking for any sign of fetal distress. Abruptio placentae can complicate severe preeclampsia.

C. **Diagnostic Algorithm (see page 230)**

VIII. **Treatment**

A. **O_2.** Add supplemental O_2 and place the mother in the left lateral decubitus position to take the weight of the uterus off the inferior vena cava and increase venous return to the heart.

B. Establish **IV access,** but do not over hydrate the patient, as this may lead to pulmonary or cerebral edema. Place a Foley catheter to measure urine output (goal is to maintain urine output at 1 mL/kg/hr).

C. **BP control.** Indicated when diastolic BP is > 105 mm Hg. The goal is to reduce diastolic BP to 90–100 mm Hg. Overly aggressive BP reduction may result in placental hypoperfusion. **Hydralazine** is the agent of choice in preeclampsia. Dose is 5 mg bolus over 1–2 minute period, then additional doses in 5 to 10 mg IV increments every 20–30 minutes, to a total of 80 mg over a 12-hour period. Other agents include labetalol (20–40 mg IV), nifedipine (10–20 mg IV), or nitroprusside. Nitroprusside is reserved for patients unresponsive to conventional treatment.

D. **Seizure control. Magnesium** (eclampsia): 4–6 g IV over a 15-minute period, followed by an infusion at 1–2 g/hr to maintain a serum magnesium level of 5–8 mg/dL. Complications of magnesium treatment include flushing, loss of deep tendon reflexes, slurred speech, and double vision, which occur at levels from 8–12 mg/dL. Respiratory depression and muscle paralysis are seen at levels from 15 to 17 mg/dL, while cardiac arrest may be seen when levels reach as high as 30 to 35 mg/dL. Magnesium is also used in severe preeclampsia as prophylaxis. It has been shown to decrease the incidence of eclampsia from 1.2% to 0.3%. Dilantin can be used as an alternative agent, but it is not as effective as magnesium.

Diagnostic Algorithm

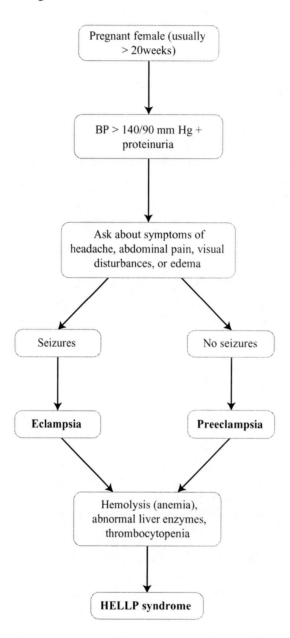

E. **Delivery** is the treatment of choice for severe preeclampsia and eclampsia. Emergent obstetrical consultation is essential to assess risks and benefits to the mother and fetus.

IX. Disposition

A. **Admission.** All cases of eclampsia should be admitted to an ICU, pending emergent delivery. Patients diagnosed with preeclampsia should be admitted to a monitored setting for BP control.

B. **Discharge.** Pregnancy-induced hypertension or early preeclampsia may be managed on an outpatient basis after consultation with an obstetrician. The threshold to admit these patients for monitoring should be low.

CASE PRESENTATION

A 38-year-old woman presents with a complaint of headache and "pain in her side" for the past week. The patient states that she is pregnant and that her last menstrual period was approximately 6 months ago. She has not had any prenatal care. She denies nausea, vomiting, or fever. She denies medications or allergies.

1. *What other information do you want to know?*
   - *History of hypertension? Previous pregnancies? Visual disturbances?*
   - *Lower extremity edema? Estimate gestational age. Neurologic examination.*
2. *BP is 180/105 mm Hg, urinalysis shows 2+ proteinuria, and her lower extremities are edematous. The abdomen is soft with vague RUQ tenderness. Her uterine fundus is 8 cm above the umbilicus. When you have made the diagnosis of preeclampsia, what is your next step?*
   - *Initiate BP control.*
   - *Contact OB/GYN for emergent delivery.*

SUMMARY POINTS

- *Pregnancy-induced hypertension, preeclampsia, and eclampsia represent a spectrum of potentially life-threatening disease that must be diagnosed and treated aggressively.*
- *Consider the diagnosis in any pregnant patient with an elevated BP.*
- *The severity of disease is not directly related to the elevation in BP.*
- *Delivery of the fetus is the definitive treatment of preeclampsia and eclampsia.*

CHAPTER 40
EMERGENCY DELIVERY

I. Defining Features

   A. Emergency deliveries carry a high potential risk of complication and morbidity for the mother and infant.

   B. Although most EDs are equipped to provide the basics needed for an emergency delivery, they cannot provide the same degree of specialized equipment and personnel as a dedicated obstetrics unit.

   C. Emergency physicians must make decisions to optimize outcomes for both the mother and fetus.

II. Epidemiology

   A. Emergency deliveries are rare, representing < 1% of all deliveries.

   B. Maternal mortality rates are estimated at 8.5/100,000 deliveries in whites. This rate is 3 times higher in African Americans.

   C. Cephalic presentations account for 93% of births; breech presentation occurs in 2.7%, and face presentation occurs in 0.05%.

   D. Shoulder dystocia occurs in 0.5–1% of births.

III. Pathophysiology

   A. **Stages of labor. Stage I:** from the onset of organized uterine contractions to full cervical dilation. This stage may last from hours to several days. Once cervical dilation has begun, the patient is considered to be in active labor. **Stage II:** from full cervical dilation to the delivery of the infant. **Stage III:** from the delivery of the infant to the delivery of the placenta.

   B. **True labor vs. false labor.** False labor is defined as disorganized uterine contractions **(Braxton-Hicks contractions)** that do not lead to cervical changes. True labor consists of regular, repetitive contractions that steadily increase in duration and intensity, move the fetus into the pelvis, and cause dilation and effacement of the cervix.

IV. Risk Factors.
Maternal factors that increase the likelihood of emergency delivery are lack of prenatal care, lack of education, lower socioeconomic status, preterm labor, and adolescents.

V. Clinical Presentation

A. **History**

1. All pregnant patients with an estimated gestational age ≥ 20 weeks should be thoroughly evaluated to assess the status of the mother and fetus.

2. Obtain gynecologic, obstetric, and medical histories, including last menstrual period, estimated gestational age or due date, previous pregnancies, prenatal care, and previous obstetrical complications.

3. **Contractions.** Patients will generally complain of crampy lower abdominal or back pain. Ascertain when the contractions began and, if possible, their frequency and duration.

4. **Vaginal bleeding.** Frank vaginal bleeding during early labor is an ominous sign and may represent placenta previa (placenta covers the cervical os) or placental abruption (placental separation from the uterus with hemorrhage).

5. **Spontaneous rupture of membranes** (SROM). The presence of clear, blood-tinged, or meconium-stained vaginal fluid strongly suggests that the chorionic and amniotic membranes have ruptured and predicts the onset of labor.

B. **Physical Examination**

1. **Vital signs.** Pay particular attention to BP, temperature, and pulse oximeter.

2. **Fetal monitoring** should be utilized. If unavailable, use a hand held Doppler to ascertain fetal heart rate, which should be between 120 and 160 beats/minute. A sustained fetal heart rate < 100 beats/minute indicates fetal distress.

3. **Abdominal examination.** Examine the abdomen, checking carefully for tenderness. Measure or estimate the fundal height from the pubic symphysis to the fundus of the uterus in centimeters.

4. **Pelvic examination** is performed with the patient in the lithotomy position.

   a. *Inspect the perineum.* Is delivery imminent (crowning)? Is the umbilical cord visible?

   b. *Speculum examination.* Determine the presence of blood, discharge, or fluid in the vaginal vault. If pooling vaginal fluid is present, note its color and turbidity and perform a Nitrazine test. Nitrazine paper turns dark blue (positive) when exposed to amniotic fluid (pH 7.0–7.4). Normal vaginal secretions have a pH of approximately 4.5–5.5. Obtain vaginal and cervical cultures for gonorrhea, Chlamydia, and Group B Streptococcus.

   c. *Bimanual examination.* Assess for the presence of cervical effacement (thinning) or cervical dilation. The normal non-dilated cervix is closed with a fingertip-sized opening. The fully dilated cervix has an opening of 10 cm. **Station** is determined by the relationship of the presenting part of the fetus to the mother's ischial spines. When the presenting part of the fetus is palpable at the ischial spines, the station is 0. With the presenting part at the introitus, the station is +3. **Check for the presenting part.** Is the head palpable?

CLINICAL SKILLS TIP

If the cord is palpable during the bimanual examination, do not remove the examining hand from the vagina. Instead, elevate the presenting part of the fetus to prevent further compression of the umbilical cord. Contact obstetrical service for an emergency cesarean section.

VI. **Differential Diagnosis.** Preterm labor, false labor, preeclampsia/eclampsia, placental abruption, and premature rupture of membranes.

RULE OUT

*If vaginal bleeding is present, a pelvic ultrasound should be performed to rule out **placenta previa** prior to performing the pelvic examination. Examination may worsen the bleeding.*

VII. **Diagnostic Findings**

   A. **Laboratory studies.** For emergent delivery, no laboratory tests are necessary. A hemoglobin and PT/PTT may be useful if there is significant postpartum bleeding. Additionally, ABO and Rh are useful to determine the need for RhoGAM.

   B. **Imaging studies.** Bedside pelvic ultrasound may be useful in the assessment of fetal heart rate, gestational age, lie, and placental position.

   C. **Diagnostic Algorithm**

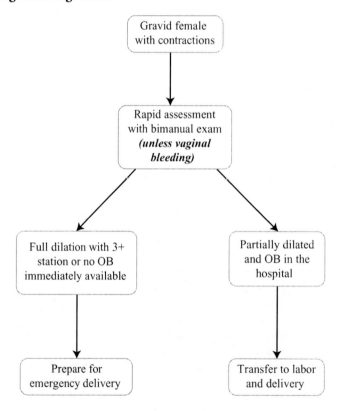

VIII. **Treatment**

   A. The physician must first determine if adequate resources are available to safely perform the delivery in the ED and whether or not the patient can be safely transferred to a delivery suite. An emergency delivery requires teamwork. If available, notify additional personnel to provide assistance.

B. Provide supplemental O$_2$ via 100% non-rebreather mask if the mother has unstable vital signs or if there are signs of fetal distress.

C. Establish IV access with an 18-gauge needle and administer 0.9 NS.

D. **Preparation.** Place the mother on cardiac and BP monitoring. Initiate external fetal monitoring, if available. Position the mother in the lithotomy position. If time allows, prep the perineum with povidone-iodine (Betadine) and drape with sterile towels. Use a mask, eye protection, gown, and gloves. Secure basic delivery equipment, including cord clamps, scissors, bulb syringe, sterile towels, incubator, and neonatal resuscitation equipment.

E. **Deliver the infant,** assuming normal vertex presentation in a fully dilated patient with a station of +3.
   1. Support the perineum inferiorly by placing 2 fingers with a gauze pad or towel on either side of the perineum in a pinching fashion. Use the other hand to control delivery of the head and prevent rapid, forceful expulsion of the head (Figure 40–1a). Controlling the delivery is essential to reduce tearing.
   2. Once the head is delivered, pause. Ask the patient not to push. Suction the infant's nose and mouth with a bulb syringe. Palpate for a nuchal umbilical cord on the infant's posterior neck. If present, reduce the cord by pulling it over the infant's head. If unable to reduce the cord, clamp it with 2 cord clamps and cut in the middle.
   3. With a secure grip on the infant, deliver the body with gentle downward traction to deliver the anterior shoulder. After the shoulder is delivered, guide the infant upward to deliver the posterior shoulder, torso, and lower extremities (Figures 40–1b and 40–1c). Double clamp the umbilical cord, and cut it with scissors.

F. **Care for the newborn.** Suction the infant again, dry with sterile towels, and move to a warm incubator. Administer O$_2$ and continue stimulating the infant. Determine the infant's APGAR scores at 1 and 5 minutes (Table 40–1). If meconium is present and the infant has depressed respirations, decreased muscle tone, or an HR of < 100 beats/minute, intubation with tracheal suctioning should be performed. Routine intubation and tracheal suctioning of vigorous infants in the presence of meconium is no longer recommended.

G. **Deliver the placenta.** Allow the placenta to deliver spontaneously. Traction on the umbilical cord may cause a uterine inversion. After the placenta has been delivered, methods to decrease bleeding include massaging the uterus or administering oxytocin (Pitocin) 20 U in 1 L NS IV to aid in uterine contraction.

H. **Complications** include cord prolapse, postpartum hemorrhage, shoulder dystocia, and breech presentations. Although rare, these complications generally require the assistance of an obstetrician.
   1. **Postpartum hemorrhage** may occur in the presence of retained products of conception, uterine atony, uterine inversion, coagulopathy, or trauma.
   2. **Shoulder dystocia** is caused by the entrapment of the infant's anterior shoulder at the pubic symphysis. The infant is at risk for brachial plexus injury (from traction on the head) and hypoxemia from prolonged delivery. The mother's hips should be maximally flexed, the bladder emptied, and an assistant should apply suprapubic pressure to attempt to facilitate delivery (McRoberts maneuver).

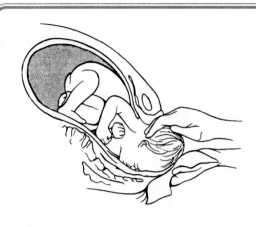

Figure 40–1a. Delivery of the head is performed while putting gentle pressure over the perineum.

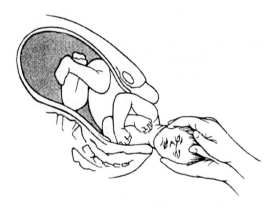

Figure 40–1b. Delivery of the anterior shoulder.

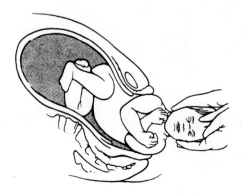

Figure 40–1c. Delivery of the posterior shoulder is performed with gentle upward traction, while supporting the head.

Table 40–1. APGAR scoring.

Sign	0 points	1 point	2 point
Activity	Absent	Arms and legs flexed	Active movement
Pulse	Absent	< 100 beats/min	> 100 beats/min
Grimace	No response	Grimace	Sneeze, cough, pulls away
Appearance	Blue-gray or pale	Normal, except extremities	Normal over entire body
Respiration	Absent	Slow, irregular	Good, crying

> 3. **Breech presentation.** Cesarean delivery for breech presentation has been shown to be safer than vaginal delivery; however, an obstetrician is not always readily available. Frank (buttocks presenting with feet at infant's face) or complete breech (buttocks presenting with hips and knees flexed) should be allowed to progress normally, as the infant's buttocks allow dilation of the cervix so that vaginal delivery will occur. Incomplete (footling) breeches are at increased risk for cord prolapse and occasionally will not allow the cervix to fully dilate, making delivery of the head extremely difficult.

IX. **Disposition.** The mother should be admitted to a post-delivery recovery area. The infant should be admitted to a nursery for routine newborn screening and observation.

CASE PRESENTATION

A 38-year-old woman presents with a complaint of back pain for the past 6 hours. The patient states that she is pregnant and that her last menstrual period was approximately 8 months ago. She has not had any prenatal care. She denies nausea, vomiting, or fever. The patient adds that while she was waiting to be seen, she felt something wet on her leg.

On your physical examination, you note that she is obviously pregnant. Her vital signs are BP 110/60 mm Hg, HR 100 beats/min, RR 12 breaths/min, temperature 37°C (98.6°F), and pulse oximeter is 98%. Her abdomen is soft with mild lower abdominal tenderness. Her fundal height is approximately 36 cm.

1. *What other historical information do you want to know?*
   - *Previous pregnancies? Contractions? Vaginal bleeding or other discharge?*
2. *What will you look for on physical examination?*
   - *Signs of imminent delivery (inspect perineum), active labor (sterile speculum and bimanual examination), rupture of membranes, or fetal distress (bradycardia, meconium stained amniotic fluid).*

SUMMARY POINTS

- *Delivery should be performed in the ED when it is imminent and there is no time to transfer the patient to the labor and delivery suite.*
- *Rule out ruptured membranes in all pregnant patients > 20 weeks' gestation who present with complaints of vaginal discharge.*
- *Know your limitations: remember that teamwork is essential, and request early obstetrical support when complications arise.*

SECTION IX
PEDIATRIC EMERGENCIES

CHAPTER 41
THE PEDIATRIC PATIENT

I. Defining Features

   A. In legal terms, children are considered minors until 18 years of age.

   B. **Emancipated minor status** allows a minor to consent for medical care without parental knowledge, consent, or liability. The specific law varies from state to state, but generally a person < age 18 is considered an emancipated minor if any of the following conditions are met: married, divorced, separated, widowed, member of the armed forces, parent or pregnant, lives willingly separate and apart from parents or guardian, or demonstrates the ability to manage own financial affairs.

   C. Physicians are considered mandated reporters when there is reasonable cause to suspect that a child has been abused, neglected, or placed in imminent risk of serious harm.

II. Epidemiology

   A. Infants and children account for 25–30% of all patient visits to an ED.

   B. The following conditions account for > 50% of pediatric visits to the ED: otitis media, URI, gastroenteritis, asthma, fractures and sprains, soft tissue trauma, and minor head trauma.

III. Pathophysiology

   A. **Pediatric Airway**

      1. The larynx is more cephalad and anterior.

      2. The tongue is proportionally larger.

      3. The epiglottis is tilted and more collapsible, making intubation more difficult.

      4. The narrowest portion of the pediatric airway is at the level of the cricoid cartilage. This mandates the use of uncuffed ET tubes in patients < age 8.

   B. **Pediatric Body**

      1. The skeleton and surrounding ligaments and tissues are more flexible and less protective.

      2. The pediatric head is proportionately larger, increasing the risk of head injuries. In addition, greater white matter content in the brain increases the risk of injury secondary to axonal shearing and cerebral edema.

      3. Infants and children are at risk of hypothermia due to the high surface area to volume ratio.

      4. Growth plates are the weakest portion of the bone and the most prone to injury. As a result, ligamentous injury in children is rare.

5. Pediatric patients are at risk for spinal cord injury without radiographic abnormalities (SCIWORA), because horizontal alignment of facet joints and more elastic intervertebral ligaments predispose to subluxation without bony injury.

IV. **Risk Factors.** Children are at an increased risk for injury or disease because they are unable to communicate, dependent on parent/guardian, anatomically different, and immunologically immature.

V. **Clinical Presentation**

A. **History**

1. Obtain as much information as possible from the child. Questions should be direct and stated in terms the child can understand.

2. Further details and clarifications should be sought from the parents, guardians, or caregivers. The younger the child, the greater reliance on history obtained from the parents.

3. Inquire about birth history, immunizations, prior medical problems, medications, allergies, and developmental milestones.

4. When dehydration is a concern, ask about activity level, oral intake, number of wet diapers, frequency of diarrhea or vomiting, and the ability to make tears.

5. Normal oral intake for an infant depends on age (Table 41–1). Changes from baseline are most important to note. One ounce is equivalent to 30 mL. Solids usually are not initiated until the infant is 6 months of age.

6. Children can become anxious when separated from parents during times of stress. Separate children from parents only when the patient is an adolescent (sensitive or personal issues can be addressed) or abuse/neglect of the child is suspected.

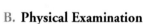

A complaint of headache or back pain in a small child is unusual and should always prompt concern for underlying pathology.

B. **Physical Examination**

1. A calm, gentle approach to the child during the examination can help alleviate the fears inherently associated with a visit to the ED.

Table 41–1. Normal oral intake, in ounces, in an infant based on age.

Age	Volume/Feeding (every 3–4 hours)
I week	1–2 oz
I month	3–4 oz
2–6 months	4–6 oz
> 6 months	6–8 oz

2. Repeated examinations in a crying, uncooperative child may be necessary to ensure an accurate assessment.
3. Normal vital signs vary according to patient age (Table 41–2).
4. Infants can have open fontanelles until 18 months of age.
5. Children have open growth plates in the long bones. Injury to the growth plates is classified by Salter-Harris (Figure 41–1). Tenderness at the growth plate without evidence of fracture is indicative of a Salter-Harris I fracture.

RULE OUT

Child abuse when the history is inconsistent with physical or radiographic findings.

VI. Diagnostic Findings

    A. **Laboratory Studies**
       1. Laboratory testing in children should be reserved for confirming a diagnosis that is already suspected clinically.
       2. There are few instances in which laboratory testing is part of the standard of care when evaluating a pediatric patient in the ED. These include febrile neonates, DKA, sickle cell crises, and patients with fever who are neutropenic.
    B. **Imaging studies.** In order to complete a CT scan or MRI in children, it is often necessary to use sedation (eg, versed).

Table 41–2. Normal vital signs from neonate to age 14.

Age	Weight (kg)	RR	Average HR (beats/min)	Systolic BP (mm Hg)
Neonate	2–3	40	140	50–70
1 month	4	24–35	135	65–95
6 months	7	24–35	130	60–115
1 year	10	20–30	120	65–120
2–3 years	12–14	20–30	115	75–120
4–5 years	16–18	20–30	100	80–120
6–8 years	20–26	12–25	100	85–120
10–12 years	32–42	12–25	75	95–130
> 14 years	> 50	12–18	70	100–140

C. **Diagnostic Algorithm**

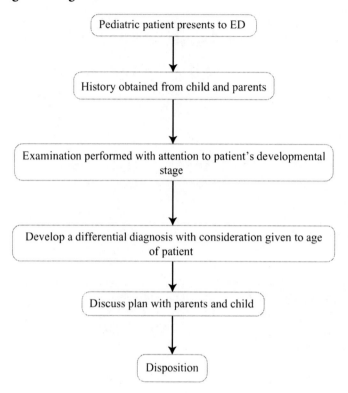

VII. Treatment

A. Treatment must be discussed with the parents, who can then assist with the explanation to the child. It is important to involve the parents in the decision-making process.

B. All medication dosages must be calculated on mg/kg basis: 1 kg is equivalent to 2.2 lb; 1 tsp is equivalent to 5 mL. Use of a Broselow tape can be extremely helpful in an emergent situation.

C. Performance of procedures can be a challenge with children. Attempts should be made to minimize pain and suffering. Use topical anesthetics during laceration repair, suprapubic bladder tap, LP, or IV access. During complex laceration repair or fracture reduction use ketamine, versed, morphine, or fentanyl.

VIII. Disposition

A. **Admission.** Suspected or confirmed surgical abdomen. Medical condition requiring further monitoring and treatment. Diagnosis uncertain and further work-up necessary. Parent unable to provide the necessary care for the child at home. Suspected child abuse.

B. **Discharge.** Medical condition diagnosed and treatment plan initiated. Chronic condition exists and work-up can be completed by primary care physician.

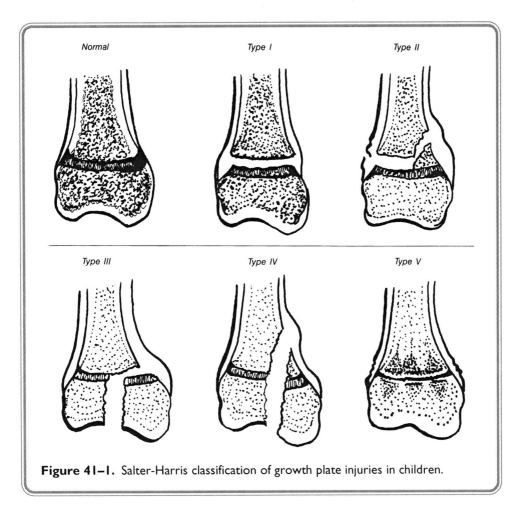

Figure 41–1. Salter-Harris classification of growth plate injuries in children.

CASE PRESENTATION

A 7-year-old boy is brought to the ED after being struck by an automobile. He arrives in a C-spine collar and complains of severe neck pain. Plain films and CT scan of the C-spine are negative for fracture.

1. *What further information do you want to know?*
   - *Pain in posterior neck. Weakness or paresthesias. AMS. Neurologic deficits.*
2. *The child has weakness in the left leg despite no obvious injury to the extremities. What is your next step?*
   - *Maintain C-spine immobilization. Assume SCIWORA. Obtain MRI and neurosurgical consultation.*

SUMMARY POINTS

- *Inherent differences exist between pediatric and adult patients.*
- *Physicians have to treat both the parent and the child.*
- *The older the child, the more reliable the clinical impression becomes as a predictor of serious illness.*
- *Disposition can be affected by unique family situations.*

CHAPTER 42
PEDIATRIC FEVER

I. Defining Features

   A. **Fever** in children is defined as a rectal temperature > 38.0°C (100.4°F).

   B. **Sepsis** is an overwhelming systemic syndrome caused by infection.

   C. **"Toxic appearing"** febrile infants and children require a complete evaluation for sepsis, including LP. Administration of antibiotic should never be delayed in order to complete the work-up.

   D. **Serious bacterial infection** (SBI) includes meningitis, bacteremia, osteomyelitis, septic arthritis, UTI, pneumonia, and bacterial gastroenteritis.

   E. **Occult bacteremia** is the presence of pathogenic bacteria in the blood of the well-appearing febrile child in the absence of an identifiable focus of infection.

   F. **Decisions regarding evaluation and management of the febrile child < age 3 are based on clinical impression and physical examination and are guided by age-dependent recommendations.**

      1. **Neonates (< 1 month)** have immature immune systems and are assumed to have dissemination of SBI with any fever. Initial management of fever includes complete evaluation for bacterial illness, including LP, empiric antibiotic administration, and hospitalization.

      2. **Infants 1–3 months** are classified as high or low risk for SBI. Management recommendations are based directly upon this risk stratification. To qualify as low risk, the infant must be previously healthy, without co-morbidity, nontoxic appearing, without a focus of infection (excluding otitis media), from a reliable social situation, and have normal laboratory values (see VII A 2).

      3. **Children 3–36 months** are at low risk for disseminated infection, and management of fever is generally based on the nature of the infection. In well-appearing febrile children in this age group, there is a small incidence of occult bacteremia. There are several acceptable practice variations for the management of potential occult bacteremia.

      4. **Children > age 3** with fever are managed according to their specific focus of infection.

II. Epidemiology

   A. Fever accounts for approximately 20% of all pediatric visits to the ED, and 20% of these children will have no identifiable source of the fever.

   B. The most common pathogens in childhood sepsis are listed in Table 42–1.

Table 42–1. The most common bacterial pathogens in pediatric patients.

Age Group	Pathogens
0–1 month	Group B Streptococcus, *E. coli*, and *Listeria monocytogenes*
1–3 months	*Streptococcus pneumoniae*, Group B Streptococcus, *Staphylococcus aureus*
3–36 months	*S. pneumoniae*, *Neisseria meningitides*, *Salmonella*, *S. aureus*

    C. Previous studies have shown that 3–5% of children without a focus of infection and a temperature > 39.5°C (103.1°F) were bacteremic (occult bacteremia) with the following pathogens: *Streptococcus pneumoniae* 85%, *Haemophilus influenzae* 10%, and *Neisseria meningitides* 3%.

    D. Since the initiation of the *H. influenza* vaccine, the incidence of occult bacteremia has decreased to 1–2%. A further decrease is expected with routine use of the conjugate pneumococcal vaccine. In 95% of cases, *S. pneumoniae* bacteremia will spontaneously resolve without antibiotic treatment.

III. Pathophysiology

    A. The febrile response is a dynamic process that is part of the larger host response to infection.

    B. Pyrogens, released from leukocytes and other phagocytic cells, cause an increase in prostaglandin synthesis, resulting in an elevated thermoregulatory set point.

    C. Fever results when the hypothalamus produces physiologic changes involving endocrine, metabolic, autonomic, and behavioral processes in response to this increased set point.

    D. The increased O_2 consumption, protein breakdown, and gluconeogenesis associated with fever quickly deplete already limited physiologic reserves of infants and children.

IV. Risk Factors for SBI

    A. **Toxic appearance** is the most obvious risk factor for an SBI. These patients require prompt evaluation and treatment.

    B. **Infants < age 1–2 months** have immature immune systems and are at increased risk of SBI with fever.

    C. **High fever.** Occult bacteremia occurs most commonly in patients with a temperature > 39°C (102.2°F); above 39°C, the height of fever directly correlates with the risk of bacteremia.

V. Clinical Presentation

    A. **History**

        1. Infants < age 2 months may present with nonspecific complaints of excessive crying, irritability, lethargy, or decreased feeding.

        2. Older children usually have more specific complaints such as cough, rhinorrhea, sore throat, vomiting, diarrhea, dysuria, joint pain, or headache.

        3. Jaundice in neonates may indicate the presence of sepsis.

Irritability and a bulging fontanelle in infants and a stiff neck and headache in older children are suggestive of **meningitis.**

B. **Physical Examination**
   1. **Vital signs.** HR is elevated by approximately 10 beats/minute for every 1°C increase in temperature. Poor peripheral perfusion is often the first sign of impending circulatory collapse. Pulse oximetry can be a reliable indicator of occult pulmonary infection.
   2. **General appearance.** Infants who are lethargic or demonstrate paradoxical irritability (inconsolable or worsen when held by parents) may have CNS infection and should be fully evaluated and treated for sepsis.
   3. **Head to toe physical examination** should be performed. *Any infection identified, except for otitis media, is considered to be an SBI.*
   4. **Lung examination.** Forced expiration or percussion of the chest during auscultation can help identify areas of consolidation.
   5. **Skin examination** to identify rashes, petechiae, or purpura. A febrile, ill-appearing child with a petechial or purpuric rash should be considered to have meningococcemia until proven otherwise.
   6. **Extremity examination.** Osteomyelitis and septic arthritis are more common in infants and children than in adults. Assess for erythema, swelling, warmth, and decreased ROM.

Differentiation of SBI and benign viral infections in infants < age 2 months, based on clinical examination alone, is unreliable.

VI. **Differential Diagnosis.** Viral infection/exanthem, URI, Kawasaki's disease, otitis media, sepsis, meningitis, soft-tissue infection, bacteremia, pneumonia, UTI, osteomyelitis, or septic arthritis.

VII. **Diagnostic Findings**
   A. **Laboratory Studies and Imaging Studies**
      1. **Febrile infants < 1 month or toxic-appearing children of any age** without an obvious source of infection should have an evaluation that includes a "full" septic work-up, including
         a. **CBC** with **manual differential.**
         b. **Urinalysis** and **urine culture.** Urinalysis may be normal in infants who subsequently demonstrate bacterial growth on culture. Urine collection must be obtained by bladder catheterization or suprapubic aspiration, since a bag sample can be contaminated with skin flora.
         c. **Liver function tests.** Only performed on patients who clinically appear jaundiced. An elevated direct bilirubin in a neonate may indicate sepsis.
         d. **CXR** if signs or symptoms of lower respiratory tract disease.
         e. **Blood culture.**
         f. **LP.** CSF studies (cell count, glucose level, protein, Gram stain, culture).
         g. **Stool WBC** and **culture** if diarrhea is present.
      2. **Non-toxic appearing infants 1–3 months with fever** should have a similar work-up ± LP. Laboratory and imaging studies used to classify such an infant as low risk for SBI include:

a. WBC count > 5,000/mm^3 and < 15,000/mm^3.
    b. Band/neutrophil ratio < 0.2.
    c. CSF with WBC count < 8 /mm^3 and negative Gram stain (if performed).
    d. Urinalysis with < 8 WBC/HPF.
    e. CXR without infiltrates (if lower respiratory tract signs or symptoms).
    f. Stool with < 5 WBC/HPF and heme-negative (if diarrhea present).

3. **Non-toxic appearing children 3–36 months.** Laboratory evaluation includes urinalysis and urine culture for girls < age 2 and boys < age 1. CXR if signs of lower respiratory tract infection. If a source of infection is still not identified, possible strategies include
    a. No further work-up.
    b. For patients with a temperature > 39.0°C, screening CBC and selective blood culture. If WBC > 15,000/mm^3, then blood culture and antibiotics. If WBC < 15,000/mm^3, then no blood culture or antibiotics.

B. **Diagnostic Algorithm**

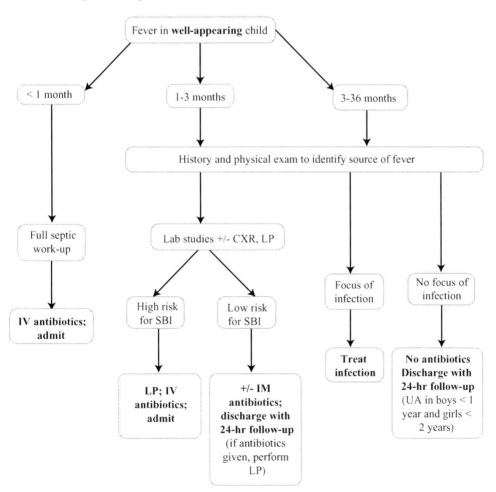

VIII. Treatment

A. **Antipyretic.** Acetaminophen (15 mg/kg) q 4 hr or ibuprofen (10 mg/kg) q 6–8 hr.

B. Encourage **fluid intake** (eg, Pedialyte) to avoid dehydration. IV fluids should be used if significant dehydration is present.

C. **Antibiotic** choices are based on the patient's age.
   1. **Infants < 1 month** should all be treated with ampicillin plus cefotaxime or gentamicin IV.
   2. **Infants 1–3 months** who meet low-risk criteria may be given ceftriaxone 50 mg/kg IM before discharge to treat any occult SBI (pneumonia, UTI). This IM dose will not fully treat meningitis; therefore, an LP should be performed on all patients who receive IM antibiotics before discharge. These infants should receive follow-up within 24 hours. Low-risk children may also be managed expectantly without IM antibiotics. Infants who do not meet low-risk criteria should have a full sepsis work-up and receive IV ceftriaxone.
   3. **Infants and children 3–36 months** with a temperature > 39°C (102°F) and elevated WBC count > 15,000 mm³ should be treated with ceftriaxone 50 mg/kg IM (for possible occult bacteremia). Blood cultures should be sent. Children who have a UTI and who are otherwise well appearing may be treated as an outpatient with antibiotics (third-generation cephalosporin PO). Children with a temperature < 39°C (102.2°F) and a normal urinalysis may be discharged without antibiotics, and a 24-hour follow-up should be arranged.
   4. If meningitis is highly suspected or CSF Gram stain identifies organisms, then ceftriaxone 100 mg/kg/day and vancomycin should be given in the ED.

IX. Disposition

A. **Admission.** All ill-appearing infants and children. All infants < 1 month with documented fever or history of fever at home. Well-appearing infants 1–3 months with a high risk for SBI or with a focal bacterial illness. Immunocompromise with fever.

B. **Discharge.** Well-appearing, vaccinated, febrile children > 3 months (or 1–3 months if low risk) may be discharged with appropriate follow-up.

CASE PRESENTATION

A 6-week-old infant is brought to the ED by his mother, who states that the infant has been fussy today and vomited twice. The mother says that she does not have a thermometer in the house but that the infant felt warm to the touch. In triage, the temperature taken per rectum is 38.3°C (101°F).

1. What other historical facts do you want to know?

   • *Cough or rhinorrhea? Diarrhea? Decreased feeding? Sleeping more? Birth history?*

2. The child is feeding well and is otherwise well appearing. No focus of infection is present on examination. What is your next step?

   • *Use screening criteria to determine if the infant is high or low risk for SBI. If high risk, perform LP, treat with empiric antibiotics, and admit. If low risk, perform LP if antibiotics are to be administered. Conservative management of low-risk infants includes antibiotics and hospitalization. Arrange 24-hour follow-up if discharged.*

SUMMARY POINTS

- All toxic-appearing infants and children require a full septic evaluation and admission.
- Initial management of fever in infants < 1 month includes a complete evaluation for SBI, including LP, empiric antibiotic administration, and hospitalization.
- Treatment of well-appearing febrile infants aged 1–3 months is guided by classifying as low or high risk for SBI.
- Follow-up should be arranged for all well-appearing, low-risk, febrile patients without a focus of infection who are discharged from the ED.

CHAPTER 43
RESPIRATORY DISTRESS

I. Defining Features

A. **Respiratory failure** is the inability of the respiratory system to meet the metabolic demands for oxygenation or CO_2 elimination (ventilation).

B. **Upper airway obstruction** is defined as blockage of airflow in the larynx or trachea. It is characterized by **stridor,** an inspiratory sound caused by airflow through a partially obstructed upper airway.

C. **Croup (laryngotracheobronchitis)** is a URI affecting the subglottic region. The patient presents with a barking cough, inspiratory stridor, and fever.

D. **Bronchiolitis** is a respiratory infection that causes inflammation of the bronchioles. Edema and mucous production lead to obstruction of the airways with V/Q mismatch and hypoxia. It is most common in infants aged 2 to 6 months and is associated with increased likelihood of asthma developing.

E. **Laryngomalacia** and **tracheomalacia** are congenital conditions that affect the structural integrity of supporting structures in the upper airway. This leads to collapse of affected tissues into the airway during respiration.

II. Epidemiology

A. Respiratory distress accounts for 10% of pediatric visits to the ED, 20% of pediatric admissions, and 20% of deaths in infants.

B. **Airway obstruction** is the leading cause of life-threatening acute respiratory distress. Croup is the most common cause of upper airway obstruction and stridor in children aged 6 months to 6 years. It occurs in 5% of children during their second year of life. Upper airway obstruction from foreign body aspiration is most common in children aged 1 to 4 years. About 3000 patients die each year from asphyxia related to foreign body aspiration.

C. **Asthma** is the most common chronic disease in children, affecting 5–10% of the population.

D. **Bronchiolitis** is most commonly caused by respiratory syncytial virus (RSV), although other pathogens include parainfluenza, influenza, and adenovirus.

E. **Pneumonia** incidence varies inversely with age, while the etiology changes based on the season and age of the patient. **Viral pathogens:** fall (parainfluenza), winter (respiratory syncytial virus), and spring (influenza). **Bacterial pathogens:** birth–2 weeks (Group B Streptococcus, *E. coli, and Listeria*); 2 weeks–2 months

(*Staphylococcus aureus, Haemophilus influenzae, Streptococcus pneumoniae, and Chlamydia trachomatis*); 3–12 years (*Mycoplasma pneumoniae, S. pneumoniae*).

III. Pathophysiology

A. Respiratory function is controlled by respiratory centers in the medulla and pons and chemoreceptors in the carotid and aortic bodies that respond to changes in O_2, CO_2, and pH of arterial blood.

B. O_2 and CO_2 exchange occurs at the alveolocapillary membrane and is dependent on adequately matched V/Q.

C. The narrowest area of the upper airway is where most foreign bodies become lodged. The location of the narrowest part of the airway differs for adults (vocal cords) and children (cricoid cartilage).

IV. Risk Factors (anatomic and physiologic)

A. Infants < 4 months are obligate nose breathers. Nasopharyngeal obstruction significantly increases the work of breathing.

B. The diameter of the pediatric airway is a third that of adults. Narrowing of the airway leads to a greater relative increase in resistance to airflow (1 mm occlusion decreases cross-sectional diameter by 20% in adults vs. 75% in children).

C. Abdominal musculature is a primary contributor to respiratory effort in children. Abdominal distention and muscle fatigue can negatively impact ventilation.

D. Pediatric lungs have a lower functional residual capacity (FRC) with less reserve potential. PaO_2 decreases more rapidly when ventilation is interrupted.

V. Clinical Presentation

A. **History**
1. **Initial treatment** may be required for stabilization before a complete history and physical examination can be performed.
2. Ask for a description of respiratory problems including onset, duration, and progression of symptoms.
3. Respiratory distress can present as difficulty with bottle feeding in infants and decreased activity or feeding in toddlers.
4. Inquire about precipitating or exacerbating factors.
5. Review all **prior medications** (chronic and acute use) and note the time of administration.
6. **Past medical history.** Infants born prematurely may have bronchopulmonary disease (BPD), placing them at risk for reactive airway disease, respiratory infections, hypoxia, and hypercarbia. When treating children with asthma, ask about frequency of exacerbations, previous admissions (especially intensive care), and need for intubation. A history of chronic cough or multiple previous episodes of pneumonias may be suggestive of a congenital condition, undiagnosed reactive airway disease, or foreign body aspiration.

KEY COMPLAINTS

Acute onset of choking, gagging, or stridor suggests foreign body aspiration. Cough is the presenting symptom in at least 80% of patients with foreign body aspiration.

B. **Physical Examination**
1. **General appearance.** The assessment should be conducted in a calm, efficient manner, with assistance from the parents. Allow the child to assume a position of comfort.
2. **Vital signs.** RR (breaths/min) varies in relation to age: newborn (30–60); 1–6 months (30–40); 6–12 months (25–30); 1–6 years (20–30); > 6 years (15–20).
3. **Stridor.** The phase of the respiratory cycle in which stridor occurs is a clue to the location of the obstruction. **Inspiratory stridor** is seen with subglottic/glottic obstruction above the larynx (eg, epiglottitis). Nasal flaring, dysphonia, and hoarseness also suggest upper airway obstruction. **Expiratory stridor** is consistent with obstruction below the larynx, in the bronchi or lower trachea.
4. **Chest examination.** Inspect the chest for depth, rhythm, and symmetry of respirations. Retractions indicate accessory muscle use. Supraclavicular, suprasternal, and subcostal retractions indicate upper airway obstruction, while intercostals retractions indicate lower airway obstruction.
5. **Lung examination.** Pneumothorax is suggested by unilateral decreased or absent breath sounds. Wheezing and a prolonged expiratory phase indicate lower airway obstruction. Crackles, rhonchi, and decreased or asymmetric breath sounds are found with alveolar disease. Grunting prevents alveolar collapse and preserves FRC. Its presence implies severe respiratory distress.
6. The remainder of the physical examination should focus on localizing the underlying source of distress, especially if there is no evidence of airway disease. Poor respiratory effort or apnea with depressed airway reflexes suggest CNS disease. CHF can present with diminished heart sounds, a murmur or gallop, venous distention, or hepatosplenomegaly. Pallor or cyanosis suggest anemia. Consider sepsis or metabolic acidosis with isolated tachypnea.

VI. **Differential Diagnosis**

A. **Respiratory**
1. **Upper airway.** Laryngotracheobronchitis (croup), epiglottitis, laryngomalacia, peritonsillar abscess, retropharyngeal abscess, tracheomalacia, allergy (angioedema).
2. **Lower airway.** Asthma, bronchiolitis, pneumonia, aspiration, pneumothorax.

B. Peripheral nervous system (eg, botulism).

C. Cardiovascular (eg, myocarditis/congenital heart defect).

D. Hematologic (eg, anemia).

VII. **Diagnostic Findings**

A. **Laboratory Studies**
1. ABG may be useful for moderate/severe respiratory distress or DKA. Respiratory failure is defined as PaO_2 < 60 mm Hg despite supplemental O_2 of 60% or $PaCO_2$ > 60 mm Hg.
2. CBC identifies anemia and provides supportive evidence of an infectious process when the WBC count is elevated.

3. Respiratory syncytial virus (RSV). Antigen tests of nasal washings provide rapid (30 min) confirmation of RSV and are 90% sensitive and 96% specific. Nasal washings should be obtained from children with bronchiolitis who require hospitalization.

B. **Imaging Studies**

1. **CXR**

   a. May reveal an infiltrate, pleural effusion, hyperinflation, or atelectasis.

   b. The location (esophagus vs. trachea) of an aspirated coin in a child can be determined by the orientation of the coin on the radiograph. When the coin is in the esophagus, it lies in the frontal (coronal) plane and is round on PA view (Figure 43–1). The opposite is true when the coin is in the trachea, because it appears round on the lateral radiograph.

   c. Radiolucent foreign bodies represent 80% of all aspirations. A radiolucent foreign body (eg, peanut) may still provide clues to its presence. Complete bronchial obstruction produces resorption atelectasis distally. Pulmonary infiltrates may be seen due to an inflammatory reaction to the foreign body. Partial obstruction in a bronchus is identified on an expiratory film when there is air-trapping and limited expiration on the affected side.

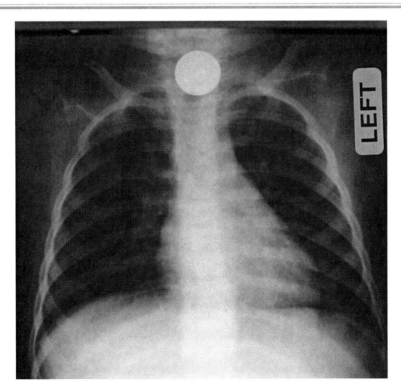

Figure 43–1 Coin in the esophagus of a child. PA view.

2. **Soft-tissue neck radiograph** may reveal a thumbprint sign of epiglottitis (Figure 43–2), the steeple sign of croup, or a widened retropharyngeal space seen in retropharyngeal abscess (Figure 43–3).
3. **Neck CT scan** may be required for definitive diagnosis of a retropharyngeal abscess.
4. **ECG** may reveal decreased QRS amplitude (pericardial effusion), conduction delay (myocarditis), or ST segment and T wave changes (pericarditis).

C. **Diagnostic Algorithm**

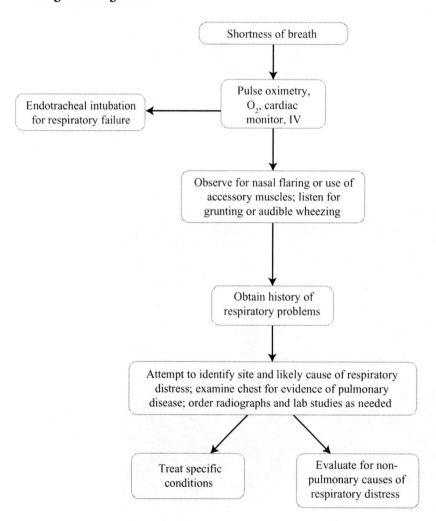

VIII. **Treatment**

A. **Primary survey.** Attention to ABCs is the first priority. Pulse oximetry, cardiac monitor, and IV fluids. Allow child to assume a position of comfort and avoid

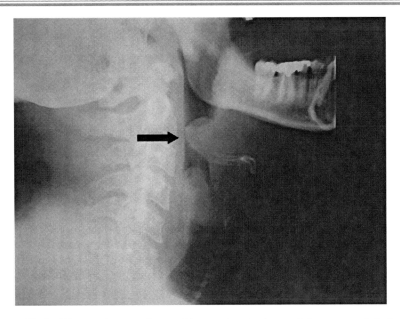

Figure 43–2. The epiglottis is located by tracing the base of the tongue inferiorly until it reaches the vallecula. The structure immediately posterior is the epiglottis. If the epiglottis is enlarged (*thumb print*) and the vallecula is shallow, then epiglottitis is present (*arrow*).

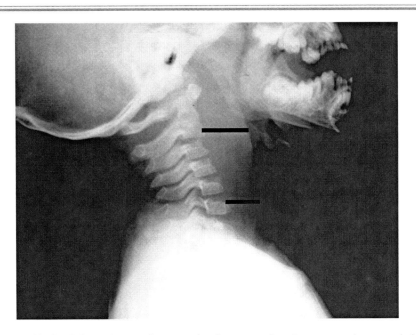

Figure 43–3. Enlarged retropharyngeal soft tissues showing a retropharyngeal abscess (*lines*). The normal retropharyngeal soft tissue space is < 7 mm at C2 and < 22 mm at C6.

unnecessary procedures. Jaw thrust and suction for airway obstruction, supplemental O_2, BVM, and intubation if indicated.

B. **Specific Conditions**

1. **Croup**
   a. *Humidified O_2.*
   b. *Dexamethasone* 0.6 mg/kg/dose IM or PO.
   c. *Racemic epinephrine* 0.05 mL/kg of a 2.25% solution in 3 mL NS via a nebulizer for children with stridor at rest.

2. **Foreign body aspiration**
   a. Definitive management is **removal in the OR** by laryngoscopy or bronchoscopy.
   b. In the setting of critical airway obstruction or impending/actual respiratory arrest, attempt to **force the foreign body out** with back blows or chest or abdominal thrusts. These are all safer methods than the blind finger sweep, which can convert a partial obstruction to a complete obstruction. Other life-saving measures include laryngoscopy with Magill forceps, passing the ET tube beyond the obstruction, or needle cricothyrotomy.

3. **Pneumonia**
   a. *0–1 month:* ampicillin + gentamicin or cefotaxime.
   b. *1–3 months:* ampicillin + cefotaxime.
   c. *3 months–5 years:* cefuroxime, cefotaxime, or ceftriaxone.
   d. *> 5 years:* macrolide.

4. **Asthma**
   a. β-Adrenergic agonists: albuterol 0.15 mg/kg/dose in 2 mL NS delivered q 20 min.
   b. Anticholinergics ipratropium bromide (Atrovent): 500 μg q 20 min for 3 doses, then q 2–4 hr PRN.
   c. Prednisone 2 mg/kg/day.
   d. Consider subcutaneous epinephrine 0.01 mg/kg/dose 1:1000; terbutaline 2–10 μg IV loading dose, and magnesium sulfate 5.0–7.5 mg/kg, if symptoms persist or worsen.

5. **Bronchiolitis**
   a. β-Adrenergic agonist or nebulized epinephrine trial; if no response to treatment, then discontinue.
   b. Ribavirin 20 mg/mL initial solution, with continuous aerosol administration for high-risk groups (chronic pulmonary conditions and congenital heart disease) with RSV.
   c. Clinical trials demonstrate that corticosteroids are of no benefit in the treatment of bronchiolitis. Corticosteroids may be useful in patients with a history of reactive airway disease.

IX. **Disposition**

A. **Admission** is indicated in respiratory failure, requiring mechanical ventilation; respiratory distress not reversible with definitive therapy or requiring intensive monitoring; pneumonia in patients < age 6 months; foreign body aspirations with respiratory symptoms; or new O_2 requirements.

B. **Discharge** if respiratory distress is responsive to treatment. If racemic epinephrine is administered in a child with croup and the child remains asymptomatic after 2 hours of ED observation, then discharge is appropriate.

CASE PRESENTATION

A 1-year-old girl is rushed to the ED in respiratory distress.

1. *What is your initial response?*

   - *Evaluate the patency of airway. Apply pulse oximetry, supplemental O_2, and cardiac monitor. Gain IV access. Observe for accessory muscle use or nasal flaring. Listen for stridor, wheezing, rhonchi, crackles or decreased breath sounds. Ask about fever, past medical history, and choking episodes.*

2. *The parents report that the child has had a recent cold with a barking cough over the past 2 days. On examination, you hear stridor at rest. What is your next step?*

   - *Racemic epinephrine, dexamethasone (IM or PO), and frequent reassessment.*

SUMMARY POINTS

- *Respiratory disorders are always potentially life threatening and must be identified and treated rapidly.*
- *Patient assessment should be conducted in a calm, efficient manner, attempting to localize the underlying source of distress.*
- *Encourage assistance from the parents and avoid unnecessary procedures.*
- *Patients in respiratory distress must be monitored continuously and reassessed frequently because respiratory status can change acutely.*

CHAPTER 44
ABDOMINAL PAIN

I. Defining Features

A. Causes of a surgical abdomen include necrotizing enterocolitis, midgut volvulus, intussusception, and appendicitis. The most common "medical" cause of pediatric abdominal pain is **gastroenteritis.**

B. **Appendicitis** is the most common surgical cause of abdominal pain. It is associated with perforation in 20–30% of children. Perforation is most common in patients < age 5.

C. **Necrotizing enterocolitis** (NEC) is an inflammatory process of intestinal tissues leading to variable degrees of intestinal damage, including infarction. Neonates present with feeding intolerance, vomiting, abdominal distention, ileus, and bloody diarrhea. NEC is typically present within the first week of life and affects the terminal ileum and colon.

D. **Midgut volvulus** occurs in patients who have incomplete embryologic rotation of the midgut (malrotation), leaving the midgut and its vasculature suspended on a narrow pedicle. Volvulus is caused by rotation of the gut on its own mesenteric axis, producing intestinal obstruction and midgut gangrene.

E. **Intussusception** occurs when one portion of the bowel telescopes into an immediately adjacent segment, creating an obstruction.

F. **Colic** is fussiness with prolonged periods of crying following feeding. It usually begins at 2–3 weeks and persists until 3 months. The child is well between episodes and has no other systemic symptoms. This is a diagnosis of exclusion.

II. Epidemiology

A. Common viral pathogens that produce gastroenteritis include rotavirus, Norwalk virus, and adenovirus. Bacterial infection is usually caused by *Esherichia coli, Yersinia, Campylobacter, Salmonella,* or *Shigella.*

B. The peak incidence of appendicitis occurs in children aged 10–12 years.

C. Ileocolic is the most common location of intussusception. About 80% of cases occur in children < age 2.

D. About 50–75% of cases of midgut volvulus occur within the first month of life.

III. Pathophysiology

A. **Visceral pain.** Distention or spasm of an abdominal organ stimulates nerves locally, resulting in visceral abdominal pain. Overlap of local nerve fibers from

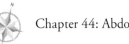

different organs leads to pain that is poorly localized and colicky in nature. Visceral pain is often accompanied by nausea and vomiting.

B. **Parietal pain.** The affected viscus initiates an inflammatory process, which stimulates the parietal peritoneum, producing abdominal pain. Parietal pain is well localized.

C. **Referred pain.** Stimulation of shared nerve segments from other areas of the body results in referred abdominal pain; for example, diaphragmatic irritation from pneumonia can present as right-sided abdominal pain.

IV. Risk Factors

A. **Prematurity.** NEC and inguinal hernias are more common in premature infants.

B. **Male gender.** Volvulus, intussusception, and inguinal hernias are more common in males.

C. **Day-care.** Gastroenteritis is 3 times more common in children who are in day-care facilities.

D. **Henoch-Schönlein purpura** (HSP). Occasionally, patients with HSP develop submucosal hematomas in the bowel wall, which act as lead points that can cause intussusception.

V. Clinical Presentation

A. **History**
1. Obtain as much information as possible from the child before turning to the parent or guardian.
2. **Duration, location, intensity, quality, and radiation of the pain.** Paroxysmal abdominal pain (with pulling up of legs) followed by asymptomatic intervals is suspicious for intussusception.
3. **Associated symptoms.** Ask about symptoms such as vomiting, diarrhea, fever, or weight loss. Constipation is a deviation from established bowel patterns and includes a change in frequency and consistency of stool. Bilious vomiting in an infant suggests midgut volvulus. Inquire about recent trauma. Blood in the stool is concerning for conditions such as NEC and invasive gastroenteritis.
4. **Chronology of events.** Abdominal pain that begins before vomiting is more suggestive of appendicitis. Vomiting before pain suggests a more benign etiology, such as gastroenteritis.

B. **Physical Examination**
1. **Vital signs.** Recheck any abnormal vital signs obtained at triage.
2. **General appearance** provides a great deal of information. A child who is eating, playing, or jumping up and down is unlikely to have a serious cause of abdominal pain.
3. **Abdomen** should be inspected for distention. Assess for tenderness, bowel sounds, rebound, or guarding. Absent bowel sounds (ileus) often accompanies surgical conditions, sepsis, or infectious enterocolitis. Repeated examinations may be necessary in a crying, irritable child to ensure accuracy.
4. **Genital examination** must be performed to rule out incarcerated inguinal hernia or penile hair tourniquet as the cause of the pain.

5. **Rectal examination.** If a surgical abdomen is suspected or there is a history of GI bleeding, a rectal examination is indicated and stool guaiac testing should be performed.

VI. **Differential Diagnosis.** The likely cause of abdominal pain can be grouped based on the age of the child (Table 44–1).

RULE OUT

Intussusception in patients with intermittent abdominal pain and currant-jelly-like stool.

VII. **Diagnostic Findings**
   A. **Laboratory Studies**
      1. No one test is 100% accurate or reliable in establishing the diagnosis in most cases of abdominal pain.
      2. **CBC.** A mildly elevated WBC count with a left shift is supportive evidence when appendicitis is suspected clinically. A highly elevated WBC count is more suggestive of perforated appendicitis.

Table 44–1. Causes of abdominal pain by age.

Age	Diagnosis	Age	Diagnosis
< 2 years	Necrotizing enterocolitis (< 1 month)	**> 12 years**	Appendicitis
	Colic (< 3 months)		Bowel obstruction
	Malrotation with midgut volvulus		UTI
	Intussusception		Pregnancy
	Incarcerated inguinal hernia		PID
	Gastroenteritis		Cholecystitis
	Constipation		Renal caliculi
	Lead poisoning		PUD
			DKA
2–12 years	Appendicitis		Mesenteric adenitis
	UTI		Psychosocial
	Inflammatory bowel disease		
	Henoch-Schönlein purpura		
	DKA		
	Constipation		
	Child abuse		
	Streptococcal pharyngitis		
	Mesenteric adenitis		
	Lead intoxication		
	Psychosocial		

3. **Urinalysis** with positive leukocytes and nitrites is suggestive of a UTI, although up to 20% of young children with documented UTI will have a normal urinalysis. A catheterized specimen in young children and a clean catch specimen in older children should be sent for urine culture to confirm infection.
4. **Urine pregnancy test** is indicated in females of childbearing age.
5. **Chemistry** is obtained in patients with dehydration.
6. **Type and screen** if surgical intervention may be necessary.
7. **Stool WBC** and **bacterial culture** if bacterial enteritis is suspected.

B. **Imaging Studies**
1. **Flat and upright abdominal radiographs** are indicated when obstruction is suspected. The double-bubble sign (air-fluid levels in the stomach and duodenum with no gas in the remainder of bowel) is found with volvulus. Absence of air in the RLQ and RUQ with a RUQ soft-tissue density is present in 25–50% of patients with intussusception.
2. **Abdominal CT scan** has a sensitivity of 85–100% and a specificity of 83–100% for the diagnosis of appendicitis and aids in the diagnosis of intussusception and volvulus.

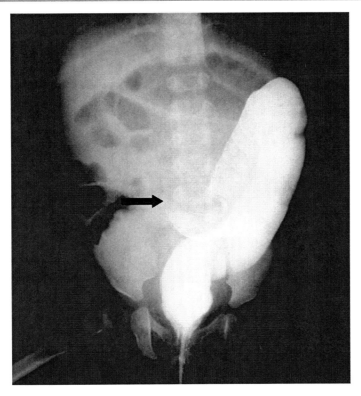

Figure 44–1. Barium enema in a child with intussusception. Note the lead point (arrow) outlined by the contrast agent.

3. **Upper GI series** provides the most conclusive evidence of midgut volvulus, and is the diagnostic test of choice for this condition.

4. **Ultrasound** is sensitive for diagnosing intussusception and may also be useful to diagnose appendicitis. It is the preferred diagnostic study for ovarian or testicular pathology.

5. **Barium or air enema** can be both diagnostic and therapeutic in cases of intussusception (Figure 44–1).

C. **Diagnostic Algorithm (see page 265)**

VIII. Treatment

A. Suspected or confirmed surgical conditions (eg, volvulus). NPO, IV fluids to correct dehydration, consider NG tube, and surgical consultation.

B. **Appendicitis.** Most cases of appendicitis will require appendectomy. In well-appearing patients with perforation and abscess formation that is localized to the RLQ, CT-guided percutaneous drainage is performed, followed by appendectomy 8–12 weeks later.

C. **Intussusception.** Nonoperative reduction (barium or air enema) is successful in most cases. Peritonitis or evidence of perforation on plain radiographs are absolute contraindications to an attempt at nonoperative reduction.

D. **Gastroenteritis.** In children who appear dehydrated, IV bolus of 0.9 NS 20 mL/kg should be administered. An oral challenge with clear fluids such as apple juice or electrolyte-containing fluids (eg, Pedialyte) is attempted before discharge. Children with only diarrhea and no vomiting can be given a regular diet.

E. **Antibiotics** are indicated for children with evidence of UTI or perforated appendicitis.

IX. Disposition

A. **Admission** is warranted for suspected or confirmed cases of a surgical abdomen; patients with a successfully reduced intussusception (recurrence occurs in 10–20% of patients, usually within 24–72 hours); dehydrated patients or those unable to tolerate fluids; or the diagnosis is uncertain and further work-up is necessary.

B. **Discharge** if a medical condition is diagnosed and the treatment plan is initiated, or a chronic condition exists and work-up can be completed by the primary care physician.

CASE PRESENTATION

A 10-month-old boy is brought to the ED with a complaint of lethargy. The parents report that the child has had several episodes of excessive crying and pulling up of the legs. Between episodes, the infant has appeared well. During the examination, the infant vomits. When you remove the diaper, you notice a dark red jelly-like stool.

1. *What other information do you want to know?*

   • *Fever? Trauma? History of prematurity? Vomiting or diarrhea? Abdominal tenderness? Toxic appearance? Stool guaiac?*

2. *When you suspect the diagnosis of intussusception, what are your next steps?*

   • *Surgical consultation, correct dehydration, and ultrasound or air enema.*

Diagnostic Algorithm

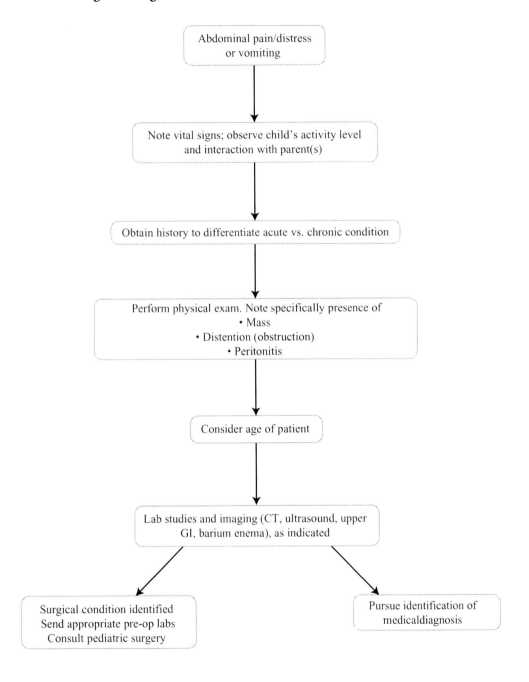

Abdominal pain/distress or vomiting

↓

Note vital signs; observe child's activity level and interaction with parent(s)

↓

Obtain history to differentiate acute vs. chronic condition

↓

Perform physical exam. Note specifically presence of
- Mass
- Distention (obstruction)
- Peritonitis

↓

Consider age of patient

↓

Lab studies and imaging (CT, ultrasound, upper GI, barium enema), as indicated

↓   ↓

Surgical condition identified
Send appropriate pre-op labs
Consult pediatric surgery

Pursue identification of medicaldiagnosis

SUMMARY POINTS

- *The main priority in the ED is the identification of a surgical condition.*
- *Appendicitis does not always present in the classic fashion. A work-up is indicated if either the history is highly suggestive of appendicitis or if RLQ pain is consistently present on abdominal examination.*
- *Serial abdominal examinations may be necessary to identify an evolving process or to accurately assess the condition of a crying, irritable child.*

CHAPTER 45
DEHYDRATION

I. Defining Features

   A. Dehydration is defined as a negative water balance. It may result from increased losses or from reduced intake.

   B. Dehydration is categorized based on initial serum sodium level: hypotonic (Na < 130 mEq/L); isotonic (Na 130–150 mEq/L); or hypertonic (Na > 150 mEq/L).

   C. Severity of dehydration is judged by the amount of fluid or the percentage of body weight lost: mild (< 50 mL/kg or < 5% of body weight); moderate (50–100 mL/kg or 5–10% of body weight); or severe (> 100 mL/kg or > 10% of body weight).

   D. Total body water (TBW) = intracellular fluid (ICF) + extracellular fluid (ECF). ECF = intravascular + extravascular compartments.

II. Epidemiology

   A. GI loss is the most common cause of dehydration in children.

   B. **Viruses** are responsible for 80% of gastroenteritis in children, with rotavirus accounting for 30–50% of cases.

   C. Most children present to the ED with **isotonic dehydration.**

III. Pathophysiology

   A. ECF consists primarily of sodium, chloride, and bicarbonate and is closely associated with TBW. ICF is composed of potassium, phosphate, and proteins. Cellular membranes are impermeable to osmotically active particles such as sodium and potassium but are freely permeable to water. Osmolar equilibration is maintained between compartments by movement of water in response to changes in osmolarity.

   B. Sodium concentration is regulated by antidiuretic hormone (ADH).

   C. Potassium concentration is maintained by the Na-K+ ATPase pump.

   D. Osmolarity (mOsm/L) = 2 (Na) + BUN/2.8 + glucose/18.

IV. Risk Factors. Children have higher morbidity and mortality rates associated with dehydration than adults due to higher body surface area/kg, larger TBW content, higher maintenance fluid requirements, increased metabolic turnover rate of water, immature kidneys with a relative inability to produce appropriately concentrated urine, and reliance on caregivers for basic needs.

V. Clinical Presentation

A. History

1. Obtain a detailed history of all intake and output (ie, type of liquids and solids attempted and quantity tolerated, number of episodes, amount, and character of emesis and diarrhea). Estimate urine output by the number of wet diapers in infants and young children. Ask about the color and odor of urine. Inquire about weight loss. Note the time interval of symptoms.

2. Last episode of vomiting is important in determining when oral trial is advisable.

3. Ask about associated symptoms, including throat pain, dysuria, and urinary frequency.

4. Note underlying diseases that could contribute to dehydration (kidney disease, diabetes mellitus, cystic fibrosis, metabolic disorders).

B. Physical Examination

1. Examination begins with assessment of the general appearance of the child.

2. Vital signs are an important objective measure. The first sign of mild dehydration is tachycardia. Hypotension is a late sign of severe dehydration.

3. Examine the throat for erythema, ulcerations, or tonsillar exudates, and assess hydration of mucus membranes.

4. Assess the abdomen for tenderness, rebound, or guarding.

5. Assess hydration status (Table 45–1).

Table 45–1. Clinical assessment of severity of dehydration in the pediatric patient.

Signs and Symptoms	Mild (3–5% body weight)	Moderate (5–10% body weight)	Severe (>10% body weight)
Mental status	Alert/restless	Irritable and drowsy	Lethargic
Respirations	Normal	Deep ± rapid	Deep and rapid
Pulse	Normal	Rapid and weak	Weak to absent
Blood pressure	Normal	Normal to low	Low
Anterior fontanelle	Normal	Sunken	Very sunken
Mucous membranes	Moist	Dry	Very dry
Tears	Present	Absent	Absent
Skin turgor	Pinch and retract	Tenting	Tenting to doughy
Urine output	Normal	Decreased	Absent
Eyes	Normal	Sunken	Sunken
Capillary refill	< 2 sec	2–3 sec	> 3 sec

Any 2 of the following findings are predictive of clinically significant dehydration in children: ill appearance, absence of tears, dry mucous membranes, and delayed capillary refill (> 2 sec).

VI. **Differential Diagnosis.** Gastroenteritis, stomatitis, pharyngitis, UTI, appendicitis, metabolic disease (eg, DKA, diabetes insipidus, hyperthyroidism), congenital adrenal hypoplasia, renal disease (eg, acute tubular necrosis, chronic renal disease, Bartter's syndrome, sodium-losing nephropathy, nephrotic syndrome), burns, fluid restriction (eg, CNS depression, child abuse).

VII. **Diagnostic Findings**

A. **Laboratory Studies**
  1. Most children with uncomplicated gastroenteritis do not require laboratory studies.
  2. Electrolytes, glucose level, and BUN/creatinine, if rehydration is required.
  3. Urinalysis for glucose level, ketones, and specific gravity.

B. **Diagnostic Algorithm**

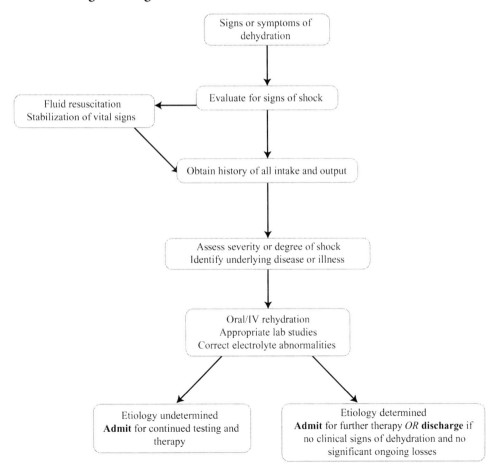

VIII. Treatment

A. Identify patients with signs of shock and resuscitate with fluid immediately (20 mL/kg NS or LR over a 20–30 minute period). Reassess and repeat fluid bolus until perfusion is adequate and vital signs normalize (fluid bolus × 3 if necessary). Urine output is the most important indicator of restored intravascular volume (minimum = 1 mL/kg/hr).

B. Oral rehydration should be considered with mild to moderate dehydration if the child is well enough to take oral fluids. Oral rehydration solutions for infants and toddlers should contain 45–50 mEq/L sodium and 25–30 g/L glucose (Pedialyte, Infalyte). Give 5–10 mL fluid q 5–10 min and increase as tolerated, with the goal of 30–50 mL/kg over a 4–hour period. If vomiting, wait 1 hour after last episode before reinitiating oral fluids.

C. In general, the rate of fluid administration for treatment of moderate/severe dehydration is determined by the estimated fluid losses plus ongoing maintenance fluid requirements (Table 45–2).

D. Specific management of dehydration varies, depending on the type of dehydration present.

   1. **Hypotonic dehydration (Na < 130 mEq/L).** Calculate sodium deficit for replacement fluids. Sodium deficit (mEq) = (135-measured Na) × (pre-illness weight in kg) × 0.6. Sodium deficit should be replaced over a 4-hour period but should not exceed 1.5–2.0 mEq/hr; 0.9 NS is an appropriate solution.

   2. **Hypertonic dehydration (Na > 150 mEq/L).** The free water deficit is calculated as free water deficit (mL) = (measured serum Na-145) × 4 mL/kg × pre-illness weight (kg). Because of the risk of cerebral edema, correct the free water deficit over a 48-hour period, with a goal of reducing serum sodium by no more than 10–15 mEq/L/day; D5 ¼ to D5 ½ NS are appropriate solutions.

   3. **Isotonic dehydration.** Administer maintenance fluid requirements plus half the fluid deficit over the first 8 hours and the remaining fluid deficit over the following 16 hours. Fluid deficit = % of dehydration x weight of the child (kg). D5 1/2 NS is an adequate solution.

IX. Disposition

A. **Admission** is indicated in severe or moderate dehydration with acidosis (serum bicarbonate level of ≤ 13 is predictive of return to ED for failure of treatment as outpatient). Other indications include significant ongoing fluid losses, inability

Table 45–2. Calculations for maintenance fluid in the pediatric patient.

Patient Weight	4/2/1 Method	Holiday-Segar Method
First 10 kg	4 mL/kg/hr	100 mL/kg/day
Second 10 kg	2 mL/kg/hr	50 mL/kg/day
Each additional 10 kg	1 mL/kg/hr	20 mL/kg/day

to tolerate oral fluids, hypotonic or hypertonic dehydration, or undetermined etiology in need of further assessment.

B. **Discharge** if no clinical evidence of dehydration or mild/moderate isotonic dehydration after treatment.

CASE PRESENTATION

A 2-year-old girl presents after having 5 episodes of non-bilious vomiting and 6 bouts of watery diarrhea over the past 12 hours.

1. *What further information is important?*
   - *Fever, urine output, liquids and solids attempted, and underlying disease.*
   - *Vital signs, general appearance, presence of tears, dry mucous membranes, and capillary refill time.*
2. *You suspect moderate dehydration secondary to gastroenteritis. How should you manage the child?*
   - *Attempt oral challenge if last vomiting episode was > 1 hour ago. If actively vomiting, order IV fluid bolus (20 mL/kg NS). Consider electrolytes, glucose and BUN/creatine. Reassess clinical status.*

SUMMARY POINTS

- *Dehydration is not a disease; the underlying cause must be identified and treated.*
- *Severity of dehydration can be classified using clinical assessment.*
- *Management priorities in the ED are stabilization of vital signs, replacement of intravascular volume deficit and ongoing losses, and correction of electrolyte abnormalities.*
- *Frequent reassessment of clinical status is necessary in order to monitor the response to treatment.*

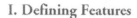

CHAPTER 46
OTITIS MEDIA

I. Defining Features

A. Clinical distinction between **acute otitis media** (AOM) and **chronic otitis media with effusion** (OME) is important and determines the need for antibiotic treatment.

B. **AOM** involves the acute onset of middle-ear inflammation (fever, ear pain, or red tympanic membrane) accompanied by the presence of middle-ear effusion (air fluid level, poor mobility, or altered landmarks).

C. **Suppurative complications of AOM** are rare but include mastoiditis, epidural abscess, lateral and sigmoid sinus thrombosis, meningitis, brain abscess, and subdural abscess.

D. **Mastoiditis** is a complication of inadequately treated otitis media (OM), and is due to extension of infection into the mastoid air cells. In the United States, it occurs most often in the pediatric age group.

E. **Lateral and sigmoid sinus thrombosis** is a rare complication of OM caused by extension of infection into the lateral and sigmoid venous sinuses of the brain.

II. Epidemiology

A. OM is the 2nd most common childhood illness, with URIs being the most common.

B. Peak incidence of OM is in children aged 3 to 24 months. About 62% of children are treated for OM by age 1 and 83% by age 3.

C. The common pathogens responsible for infection are *Streptococcus pneumoniae*, nontypeable *Haemophilus influenzae*, and *Moraxella catarrhalis*.

D. β-Lactamase resistance is well established with *H. influenzae* and *M. catarrhalis* isolates. *S. pneumoniae* isolates demonstrate increasing resistance to penicillin.

III. Pathophysiology

A. Dysfunction of the eustachian tube contributes to the development of OM.

B. Obstruction of the eustachian tube leads to accumulation of fluid behind the tympanic membrane (TM).

C. The effusion provides optimal conditions for bacterial growth from the colonized nasopharynx.

IV. Risk Factors

A. **Anatomic differences in young children.** Short eustachian tubes and frequent supine positioning allow reflux of nasopharyngeal pathogens into the middle ear. Also, horizontal orientation of the eustachian tubes impairs middle ear drainage.

B. **Risk of recurrent OM.** Age at first episode < 6 months, > 3 episodes of AOM in past 6 months, day-care attendance, smokers in home, supine bottle-feeding (breast feeding from 3–6 months of age reduces the incidence of OM by 13%), and pacifier use.

V. Clinical Presentation

A. **History**
1. Children typically present with **ear pain** or **ear drainage.**
2. **Irritability** or **fever** in infants and young children may be the only complaint.
3. Non-specific **URI symptoms** are often associated.
4. Persistent ear pain or discharge in a patient with a history of OM should prompt concern for mastoiditis.

B. **Physical Examination**
1. **Vital signs.** Fever is present in the majority of children with AOM, but is > 40°C (104°F) in only 4% of patients. When the fever is > 40°C, consider other diagnoses, including bacteremia.
2. **Visual inspection.** Inspect the pinna, external auditory canal, and postauricular region for signs of inflammation. A patient with mastoiditis will have swelling and tenderness over the mastoid process, and frequently the pinna will be displaced anteriorly.
3. **TM examination.** Gently pull the pinna in an upward and outward direction to straighten the external auditory canal. This improves visualization of the TM. Pain when performing this maneuver or when compressing the tragus suggests the diagnosis of otitis externa.
4. If cerumen is obstructing otoscopic visualization of the TM, stop the examination and use an ear curette to gently remove the obstruction.
5. Evaluate the color, position, and mobility of the TM.
   a. *Color.* The normal TM is partially translucent and appears gray. When AOM is present, the TM becomes less translucent and is yellow, dark pink, or red. The color of the TM is less predictive of the presence of AOM than the position and mobility (Figures 46–1 and 46–2).
   b. *Position.* In AOM, the TM is usually bulging. This is in contrast to OME, in which the position of the TM is retracted.
   c. *Mobility.* Impaired mobility of the TM during pneumatic otoscopy occurs in both OME and AOM.

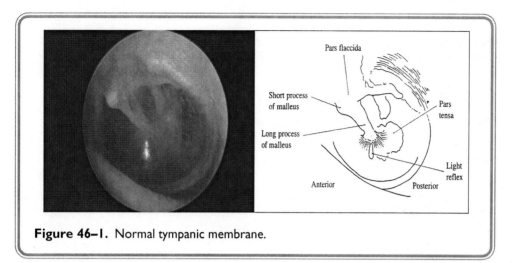

Figure 46–1. Normal tympanic membrane.

VI. Differential Diagnosis. OME, otitis externa, pharyngitis, dental abscess, parotitis, mastoiditis, lateral sinus thrombosis, URI.

RULE OUT

Complications of OM *(mastoiditis, brain abscess, sinus thrombosis) should be ruled out in patients with persistent and progressive symptoms, posterior auricular pain, AMS, or focal neurologic symptoms.*

VII. Diagnostic Findings

    A. **Laboratory Studies**

        1. The diagnosis of AOM is made clinically, and no laboratory tests are necessary for confirmation.

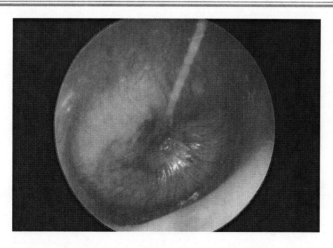

Figure 46–2. Image showing patient with acute otitis media.

2. In infants < age 3 months with fever, OM is not considered a source of infection and further laboratory work-up is required to exclude an SBI (pneumonia, meningitis). Infants < age 1 month with AOM require a full septic work-up due to the possibility of hematogenous spread of infection.

B. **Imaging Studies**
   1. Head CT scan is used to diagnose suspected cases of mastoiditis and to rule out other intracranial processes (abscesses).
   2. MRI is indicated for suspected cases of sigmoid and lateral sinus thrombosis.

C. **Diagnostic Algorithm**

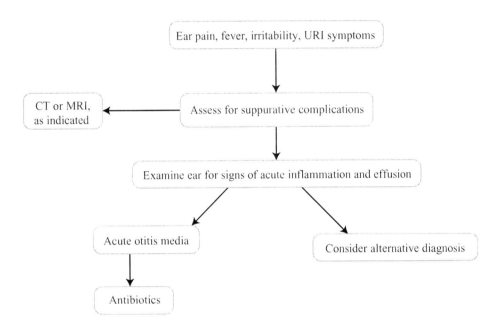

VIII. Treatment
   A. **Initial Antibiotic Treatment**
      1. Amoxicillin (80–90 mg/kg divided BID).
      2. Type I penicillin allergy (urticaria or anaphylaxis). Azithromycin (10mg/kg QD day 1, then 5 mg/kg QD for the next 4 days) or erythromycin-sulfisoxazole (50 mg/kg/day of erythromycin QID).
      3. Non-type I PCN allergy. Cefdinir (14 mg/kg/day QD or BID) or cefuroxime (30 mg/kg/day QD).
   B. **Clinically Defined Treatment Failures at 48–72 Hours**
      1. Amoxicillin-clavulanate (90mg/kg/day of amoxicillin component BID).
      2. Ceftriaxone (50mg/kg/dose IM QD), up to 3 doses may be necessary.
   C. **Length of Treatment**
      1. Give 10 days for severe disease or children < age 6.
      2. Give 5–7 days for children > age 6 with uncomplicated infection.

D. Observation without antibiotic treatment can be considered in patients without fever or vomiting, if parents agree to a trial of symptomatic therapy and appropriate follow-up is assured. If the patient is still symptomatic at day 3, antibiotics should be started.

IX. Disposition

A. **Admission** is indicated in an infant < age 1 month with temperature > 38.0°C (100.4°F), when suppurative complications (meningitis, brain abscess, mastoiditis, lateral sinus thrombosis, or focal neurologic deficit) are present, or in febrile or ill-appearing immunocompromised patients.

B. **Discharge** all other patients who have uncomplicated OM.

CASE PRESENTATION

A 3-year-old child is brought to the ED by her parents who say the child has had fever and earache for the past 2 days.

1. *What other information do you want to know?*
   - *Ear drainage? Previous history of ear infections? Preexisting conditions?*
   - *Red, opaque, and bulging TM; decreased or absent mobility of TM; absence of more serious illness.*
2. *The TM is opaque, red, and bulging. There is decreased mobility. There are no focal neurologic deficits or altered mental status. What is your next step?*
   - *Treat with antibiotics for 10 days. Arrange follow-up.*

SUMMARY POINTS

- *Identify patients with potential suppurative complications of infection.*
- *Antibiotic treatment is indicated for AOM, not OME.*
- *Both AOM and OME can present with air fluid levels or decreased TM mobility.*
- *Clinical distinction is based on the appearance of a red, purulent, bulging TM in AOM, in contrast to a dull and retracted TM in OME.*

SECTION X
TOXICOLOGY

CHAPTER 47
THE POISONED PATIENT

I. Defining Features

A. Knowledge of basic toxicology and a sound approach to the poisoned patient are fundamental expertise required by all emergency physicians.

B. Regional poison centers (1-800-222-1222), medical toxicologists, Poisondex®, textbooks, and the medical literature are essential resources utilized when caring for poisoned patients.

C. **Toxidrome** is a syndrome complex that is specific for a certain class of poison. Understanding and recognizing basic toxidromes aids in making the appropriate diagnosis.

D. Treating a poisoned patient involves supportive care, decontamination, and antidotal therapy when possible.

II. Epidemiology

A. According to Toxic Exposure Surveillance System data, every year for the past 10 years, > 2 million exposures and poisonings have been reported to regional poison centers in the United States.

B. In 2004, > 11,000 deaths occurred as a result of poisoning.

C. Most events occur in the pediatric population; however, pediatric patients account for the fewest number of deaths.

III. Pathophysiology

A. Any substance can be poisonous depending on the dose and/or duration of exposure. Exposures can occur via oral, pulmonary, dermal, or ocular routes.

B. After exposure, factors such as absorption, distribution, and elimination are important determinants of toxicity. In the poisoned patient, the half-life of a substance might be much longer than reported by the pharmacologist, due to increased absorption times and enzyme saturation seen after toxic ingestions. **Toxicokinetics** assist in determining and predicting the onset of symptoms and duration of toxicity.

IV. Risk Factors

A. Risks to poisoning in children in the home include storage of poisons in unlocked cabinets close to the floor, pill bottles without child-proof caps, and storage of poisons in inappropriate containers (eg, storing hydrocarbons in soda cans or bottles).

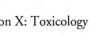

B. Taking multiple medications simultaneously may produce situations in which drug-drug interactions can occur. Examples include enzyme inhibition resulting in longer half-lives of certain drugs and multiple agents with similar pharmacology (eg, when several agents with pro-serotonergic activity result in serotonin syndrome).

V. Clinical Presentation

A. **History**
1. Obtaining history about location, occupation, pill bottles or chemicals from EMS, family, or friends may provide the necessary clues to determine the causative toxic agent.
2. **Time** of exposure is very helpful. This might be limited to when the patient was seen last in a "normal" condition.
3. **Amount** ingested in addition to whether the formulation was regular release or extended release.
4. **Chronicity** of exposure and symptoms (acute vs. chronic exposure).
5. **Symptoms** specific for different poisons provide valuable information (eg, vomiting after iron overdose or mushroom ingestion).
6. Previous suicide attempts, past medical history, pill counts, and the use of any recreational drugs may be helpful. Medication lists are essential and may require calling the pharmacy where the patient purchases medications.

B. **Physical Examination**
1. Use examination findings to appreciate specific **toxidromes** (Table 47–1).
2. **Vital signs** are important in evaluating hemodynamic abnormalities. Tachypnea or hyperpnea may indicate attempts to compensate for acidemia.
3. **Mental status** and neurologic examination are a priority. Delirium and CNS stimulation vs. obtundation or coma help determine the responsible toxin.
4. **Ocular examination.** Pupil size, evidence of nystagmus, or lacrimation.
5. **Bowel sounds.** Absent vs. active or hyperactive may differentiate anticholinergic from sympathomimetic toxicity, respectively.
6. **Skin.** Wet or dry, flushed or pale, burns, or ongoing dermal exposure that may require decontamination.

VI. Differential Diagnosis

A. AMS is frequently due to a toxicologic agent. Other entities that must be considered in such a patient include structural lesions (CNS bleeds, masses), metabolic abnormalities (hypo- or hyperglycemia, hyponatremia), infections (meningitis, urosepsis, pneumonia), and psychiatric conditions (paranoia, schizophrenia, mania).

B. The toxicologic agent involved is suggested based on the patient's vital signs, pupil size, presence of seizures, or skin changes (Tables 47–2 and 47–3).

VII. Diagnostic Findings

A. **Laboratory Studies**
1. **Electrolytes** are important to evaluate for evidence of an anion gap metabolic acidosis.
2. **ABG** (pH) may help to differentiate acid-base disorders.
3. **Co-oximetry** is used to evaluate for methemoglobinemia and elevated CO levels.

Table 47—1. Common toxidromes.

Toxidrome	Representative agent(s)	Most Common Findings	Additional Signs/Symptoms	Potential Interventions
Opioid	Heroin, morphine	CNS depression, miosis, respiratory depression	Hypothermia, bradycardia, respiratory arrest, acute lung injury	Ventilation or naloxone
Sympathomimetic	Cocaine, amphetamine	Psychomotor agitation, mydriasis, diaphoresis, tachycardia, hypertension, hyperthermia	Seizures, rhabdomyolysis, MI, cardiac arrest	Cooling, sedation with benzodiazepine, hydration
Cholinergic	Organophosphate insecticides, carbamate insecticides	Salivation, lacrimation, diaphoresis, nausea, vomiting, urination, defecation, muscle fasciculations, weakness, bronchorrhea	Bradycardia, seizures, respiratory failure	Airway protection and ventilation, atropine, pralidoxime
Anticholinergic	Scopolamine, atropine	AMS, mydriasis, dry/flushed skin, urinary retention, decreased bowel sounds, hyperthermia, dry mucous membranes	Seizures, dysrhythmias, rhabdomyolysis	Physostigmine (if applicable), sedation with benzodiazepine, cooling, supportive management
Salicylates	Aspirin, oil of wintergreen	AMS, respiratory alkalosis, metabolic acidosis, tinnitus, hyperpnea, tachycardia, diaphoresis, nausea, vomiting	Low-grade fever, ketonuria, acute lung injury	MDAC, alkalinization of the urine with K+ repletion, hemodialysis, hydration
Hypoglycemia	Sulfonylureas, insulin	AMS, diaphoresis, tachycardia, hypertension	Paralysis, slurring of speech, seizures	Glucose, octreotide, glucagon
Serotonin syndrome	Meperidine or dextromethorphan and MAOI; SSRI and TCA; SSRI/TCA/MAOI and amphetamines; SSRI alone	AMS, increased muscle tone, hyperreflexia, hyperthermia	Intermittent whole-body tremor	Cooling, sedation with benzodiazepine, supportive management

Table 47–2. MIOSIS: agents that affect pupil size.

Miosis (COPS)	Mydriasis (AAAS)
Cholinergics, clonidine	**A**ntihistamines
Opioids, organophosphates	**A**ntidepressants
Phenothiazine, pilocarpine	**A**tropine (anticholinergics)
Sedative-hypnotics	**S**ympathomimetics

4. **Serum lactate** (> 8–10 mmol/L) might indicate serious poisoning from a cellular poison-like cyanide.
5. **ECG** to evaluate for evidence of dysrhythmias, interval changes, or blocks in patients who may have ingested a cardiotoxic agent.
6. **Total CPK** and **renal function** to examine for rhabdomyolysis.
7. **Qualitative urine toxicology** screening rarely changes management, workup, or disposition of patients. In addition, false-positive results (eg, positive for PCP as a result of dextromethorphan use) and persistent positive results occurring much later than actual ingestion (positive opiates × 7 days after heroin use; positive cocaine × 3 days after cocaine use; positive cannabinoids x 30 days after marijuana use) render urine toxicology screens problematic.
8. **Quantitative blood levels** of acetaminophen, lithium, carbamazepine, valproic acid, lead, iron, and digoxin may provide useful information to guide treatment of the poisoned patient.

B. **Imaging Studies**
1. **Head CT scan** is important when AMS or neurologic abnormalities are present.

Table 47–3. OTIS CAMPBELL: agents that cause seizures.

OTIS CAMPBELL (town drunk on Andy Griffith show)
Organophosphates
Tricyclic antidepressants
Isoniazid, insulin
Sympathomimetics
Camphor, cocaine
Amphetamines, anticholinergics
Methylxanthines (theophylline, caffeine)
Phencyclidine (PCP)
Benzodiazepine withdrawal, botanicals (water hemlock), gamma-hydroxybutyrate
Ethanol withdrawal
Lithium, lindane
Lead, lidocaine

2. **CXR** in patients with hypoxia or history of inhalation of toxic fumes or aspiration (ingestion of hydrocarbons).
3. **Abdominal radiographs** are useful for products that are radio-opaque (eg, leaded paint chips, batteries, certain drug packets).

C. **Diagnostic Algorithm**

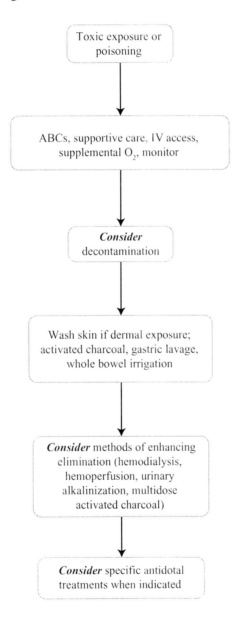

Toxic exposure or poisoning

↓

ABCs, supportive care, IV access, supplemental O_2, monitor

↓

Consider decontamination

↓

Wash skin if dermal exposure; activated charcoal, gastric lavage, whole bowel irrigation

↓

Consider methods of enhancing elimination (hemodialysis, hemoperfusion, urinary alkalinization, multidose activated charcoal)

↓

Consider specific antidotal treatments when indicated

VIII. Treatment

A. Supportive care is important for all poisoned patients. Specific antidotal therapy is listed in Table 47–4.

B. Treatment can be broken down into **ABCDE**.

1. **Airway.** Intubation must not be delayed if necessary, in pursuit of antidotal treatment.

2. **Breathing** and administration of supplemental O_2.

3. **Circulatory** issues such as hypotension must be addressed with fluid boluses initially, then vasopressors if necessary.

4. **Decontamination. Activated charcoal** (1 g/kg or a 10:1 ratio of charcoal to ingested drug) adsorbs poisons in order to prevent absorption. **Gastric lavage** is only considered early after ingestion (within 1 hr) of a potentially lethal toxin. Contraindications include hydrocarbon or other caustic ingestions. Complications from gastric lavage include increasing ICP, aspiration, and esophageal rupture. **Whole bowel irrigation** with polyethylene glycol (GoLYTELY) given at rate of 0.5 L/hr (pediatrics) to 2 L/hr functions to "flush" the gut of toxins that do not bind to charcoal (eg, leaded paint chips, drug packets). Contraindications to whole bowel irrigation include hemodynamic compromise (low BP = lack of gut perfusion) and decreased bowel

Table 47–4. Specific antidotes for toxicologic agents.

Poison	Antidote
Acetaminophen	N-acetylcysteine
Crotalidae bite	Antivenom Fab
Hydrofluoric acid, calcium channel antagonists	Calcium gluconate or calcium chloride
Cyanide	Sodium nitrite, thiosulfate
Iron	Deferoxamine
Digoxin	Digoxin Fab
Ethylene glycol, methanol	Ethanol 10% or fomepizole
Methanol, methotrexate	Folic acid/leucovorin
Calcium channel blocker, β blocker	Glucagon
Oxidizing chemicals (nitrites, benzocaine, sulfonamides)	Methylene blue
Refractory hypoglycemia after oral hypoglycemic	Octreotide
Opioid, clonidine	Naloxone
Anticholinergic (not TCA)	Physostigmine
Cholinergic	Pralidoxime (2-PAM)
Heparin	Protamine
Isoniazid	Pyridoxine
Anticoagulants	Vitamin K

sounds (poor gut motility). The most common adverse effect of gut decontamination is pulmonary aspiration. ***Patients must have an intact airway for these procedures to be pursued.***

5. **Enhanced elimination. Hemodialysis:** smaller size, small volumes of distribution (< 1 L/kg), and small amounts of protein-binding render agents amendable to hemodialysis. Examples of agents that can be successfully dialyzed include aspirin, toxic alcohols, or lithium. **Alkalinization of the urine** is common for weak acids such as aspirin and phenobarbital. The concept of trapping ions in the renal tubules after increasing the pH of the urine aids in the elimination of these agents. **Multiple doses of activated charcoal** (MDAC) are used in patients poisoned with theophylline, phenobarbital, carbamazepine, dapsone, or quinine in an attempt to utilize the gut wall as a dialysis membrane to drive the toxin into the gut, where it is then adsorbed to charcoal and eventually eliminated. MDAC can also be employed to further decontaminate the gut of agents that have erratic and persistent absorption (eg, salicylates, valproic acid).

IX. Disposition

A. **Admission.** Admit patients who have hemodynamic abnormalities, persistent mental status changes, metabolic or acid-base disruptions, ingested medications that require antidotal therapy, or have long-lasting or delayed effects (eg, sulfonylureas, extended-release calcium channel blockers, or β blockers). All suicidal patients require psychiatric consultation.

B. **Discharge.** Patients with accidental ingestions, no evidence of acute poisoning, and no chance that delayed effects would be detrimental can be discharged.

CASE PRESENTATION

A 28-year-old woman presents to the ED after ingesting her grandmother's medications. The grandmother noticed that the bottles were empty, and the patient was subsequently found in the garage with the automobile engine running. Her shirt is stained with a liquid that smells of gasoline. Vital signs on admission include a temperature of 35.5°C (96°F), BP 80/30 mm Hg, pulse 40 beats/min, RR 8, and O_2 saturation of 98%. Besides being obtunded, the physical examination is unremarkable.

1. *What other historical facts do you want to know?*

   - *Time of exposure (last seen in good health)? Amount of time spent in the garage (CO exposure duration)? What medications is the grandmother taking? Any antihypertensives (calcium channel blockers, β blockers, clonidine, digoxin)? Any chance of pregnancy?*

2. *What laboratory studies and diagnostic tests might you consider?*

   - *CXR, ECG, renal function, electrolytes, carboxyhemoglobin, pH, CT scan of head, urine pregnancy, and acetaminophen, salicylate, and digoxin levels.*

SUMMARY POINTS

- *Obtain a thorough history from the patient, friends, family, and EMS (time, chronicity, symptoms).*
- *Attempt to classify symptomatology into a "toxidrome." Vital signs are often important in categorizing the patient's toxidrome.*
- *Supportive care is most important in the initial management of poisoned patients.*
- *Consult your regional poison center (1-800-222-1222) or medical toxicologist colleague with questions pertaining to poisoned patients.*

CHAPTER 48
TOXIC ALCOHOLS

I. Defining Features

A. **Isopropanol, methanol,** and **ethylene glycol** are considered "toxic alcohols" that are capable of causing both generalized and specific toxic effects.

B. Time of ingestion is paramount when working up a patient with toxic alcohol ingestion and deciding on treatment modalities.

C. Toxic alcohols are ingested in suicide attempts or in patients trying to become intoxicated when ethanol is not readily available. Ethylene glycol's sweet flavor and methyl salicylate, which is commonly added to isopropanol, make both palatable. Each alcohol is capable of causing inebriation, with isopropanol being twice as intoxicating as ethanol.

II. Epidemiology

A. Toxic Exposure Surveillance System data reveal that over 15,000 exposures to the alcohols listed above were reported to United States poison centers in 2002, resulting in 33 deaths.

B. Isopropanol was associated with the most frequent toxic alcohol ingestion and the least number of deaths. In contrast, methanol was the least frequently reported ingestion, yet had the highest number of deaths reported.

III. Pathophysiology

A. While the parent compound results in inebriation, toxic metabolites are the reason for specific end-organ injury.

B. **Alcohol dehydrogenase** is responsible for the conversion of the alcohol to its dangerous metabolites.
   1. **Isopropanol** is converted to acetone (further CNS depression, hemorrhagic gastritis, hypotension).
   2. **Methanol** is converted to formic acid (acidemia, retinal toxicity).
   3. **Ethylene glycol** is converted to glycolic acid and oxalic acid (acidemia, renal insufficiency).

IV. Risk Factors

A. Individuals at risk for exposure to a toxic alcohol include those with depression or chronic alcohol abusers.

B. The amount ingested is a risk factor for poor outcome. Ingesting as little as 15 mL of a 40% solution of methanol has resulted in death.

V. Clinical Presentation

A. History

1. Merely obtaining the history that a toxic alcohol has been ingested can be challenging. Patients may be obtunded or not forthcoming with the ingestion history.
2. If an empty bottle is found, having someone from the scene read the ingredients on the label or bring the bottle into the ED is helpful.
3. Antifreeze contains ethylene glycol, and windshield-washing fluid contains methanol. Asking patients about ingesting these specific types of products is helpful. However, many products may contain different types of toxic alcohols (eg, antifreezes containing methanol).
4. **Time of ingestion.**

B. Physical Examination

1. **Neurologic examination** (mental status, cranial nerves, cerebellar findings, strength, and sensation) is important to document in any overdose patient.
2. **Ocular examination** may reveal blurred vision, decreased visual acuity, retinal edema, optic atrophy, or hyperemia of the optic disc in methanol poisoning.
3. **Abdominal and rectal examinations** looking for tenderness or blood is important because isopropanol toxicity causes hemorrhagic gastritis.

VI. Differential Diagnosis.
Ethanol, infection (eg, urosepsis, pneumonia, meningitis), CNS bleeds (eg, subdural/epidural hematoma, SAH), metabolic disruption (eg, hypo- and hyperglycemia, hypo- and hypernatremia), other ingestions (eg, aspirin, acetaminophen).

VII. Diagnostic Findings

A. Laboratory Studies

1. **Electrolytes.** The anion gap is calculated. The normal range is 8–14 mEq/L.
2. **ABG** to ascertain degree of acidemia.
3. **Serum ethanol level.**
4. **Serum osmolality** (measured).
5. **Calculated osmolality** is equal to 2 Na + glucose/18 + BUN/2.8 + ETOH/4.6.
6. **Osmolal gap** is the measured serum osmolality minus the calculated osmolality. The normal osmolal gap has a wide range, from -7 to +14. In toxic alcohol ingestion, the osmolal gap is elevated because the measured serum osmolality level detects the toxic alcohol, but the calculated osmolality does not. This is especially true early after ingestion before the toxic alcohols are metabolized. Later, as toxic metabolites build up and the parent compound decreases, an anion gap metabolic acidosis is the predominant finding and the osmolal gap is less significant (Figure 48–1). While ethylene glycol and methanol can result in a simultaneous anion gap metabolic acidosis and elevated osmolal gap, isopropanol usually only results in an elevated osmolal gap without an elevated anion gap.
7. **Serum toxic alcohol levels** are rarely available to aid in decision-making, but should be sent to a reference laboratory for STAT quantification.
8. **Serum acetone level** (isopropanol is converted rapidly to acetone).
9. The absence of **calcium oxalate crystal in the urine** or inability to fluoresce the urine of an ethylene glycol poisoned patient does not rule out exposure.

B. **Imaging studies. CT scan of the head** is important when mental status does not correlate with the exposure or trauma is a concern. In addition, methanol poisoning has resulted in basal ganglia hemorrhage or infarct.

C. **Diagnostic Algorithm**

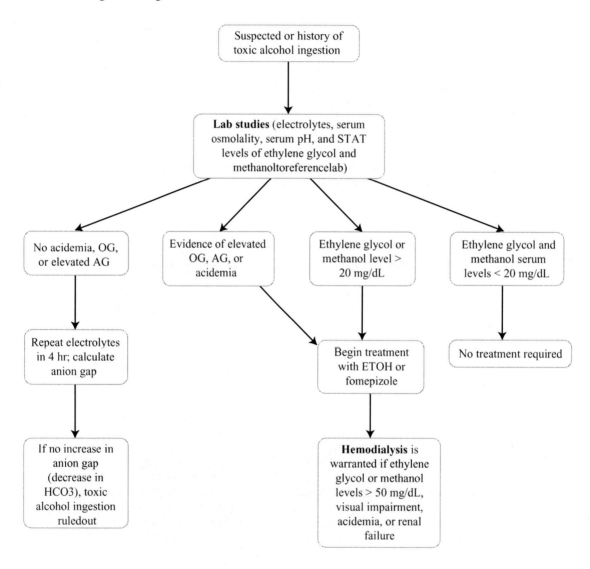

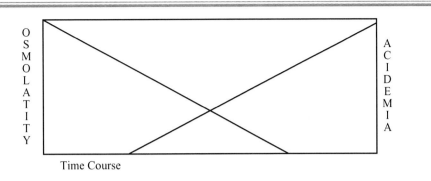

Figure 48–1. Relationship of degree of osmolality and acidemia during the course of methanol or ethylene glycol poisoning. "The Mountain"(tm) with permission from Mark B. Mycyk, MD.

VIII. Treatment

A. **Supportive care.** IV access, O_2, cardiac monitor. Isopropanol ingestions require good supportive care without alcohol dehydrogenase inhibition. Methanol and ethylene glycol require inhibition.

B. **Alcohol Dehydrogenase Inhibition** (2 methods)
   1. **Ethanol.** Goal is to achieve and maintain an ETOH level at 100–150 mg/dL. Load 10% ETOH in D5W at 10 mL/kg over a 30-minute period. Infusion of 10% ETOH in D5W at 1.5 mL/kg/hr.
   2. **Fomepizole** (Antizol, 4-MP). Load 15 mg/kg IV over a 30-minute period. Maintenance is 10 mg/kg IV q 12 hr x 4 doses (q 4 hr dosing during hemodialysis).
   3. Endpoint is ethylene glycol or methanol level < 20 mg/dL and no acidemia.

C. **Hemodialysis**
   1. Indications are renal failure, acidemia, visual impairment, ethylene glycol, or methanol levels > 50 mg/dL.
   2. Useful even when toxic alcohol levels are < 50 mg/dL and significant acidemia or other indications exist.

D. **Vitamin Therapy**
   1. **Folic acid** 50 mg IV q 4 hours may help convert formic acid to CO_2 and water.
   2. **Thiamine** 100 mg IV and **pyridoxine** 50 mg IV q 6 hours may help convert glyoxylic acid to non-toxic metabolites.

IX. Disposition

A. **Admission.** Any patient who is suicidal, requires treatment with hemodialysis, or requires alcohol dehydrogenase inhibition should be admitted to the hospital. Patients on ethanol drips usually require an ICU setting to appropriately follow ethanol levels, while patients receiving fomepizole may only require a regular hospital bed. All patients with abnormal vital signs, acidemia, or end-organ damage should be admitted to the ICU.

B. **Discharge** accidental ingestions with no evidence of acidemia or indication for treatment.

CASE PRESENTATION

A 30-year-old man presents to the ED with AMS. He was noted to vomit once en route per EMS, and he is well known to the department as a chronic alcoholic. He is awake, but slurring his speech. Laboratory studies indicate a normal ETOH level and an anion gap metabolic acidosis (anion gap = 26).

1. *What other historical facts and laboratory details do you want to know?*
   - *Time of ingestion? Agent ingested? Empty bottles at the scene?*
   - *Ethylene glycol and methanol levels (STAT), serum osmolality, pH, and urinalysis, checking for calcium oxalate crystals or fluorescence.*

2. *What is your next step in management?*
   - *Begin blockade with an alcohol dehydrogenase inhibitor (ETOH or fomepizole). Call a nephrologist to have the patient dialyzed for a suspected toxic alcohol (ethylene glycol, methanol) ingestion.*

SUMMARY POINTS

- *Consider the diagnosis of toxic alcohol ingestion when there is supporting history, an elevated osmolal gap, anion gap, or both.*
- *Block alcohol dehydrogenase in cases of ethylene glycol or methanol poisoning.*
- *Consult a nephrologist in all suspected cases, especially those that are acidemic.*

CHAPTER 49
ACETAMINOPHEN TOXICITY

I. Defining Features

A. Acetaminophen (APAP) is the most popular over-the-counter (OTC) analgesic used in the United States, and one of the most common exposures reported to regional poison centers.

B. The recommended maximum dosing is up to 4 g per day for adults and 60–90 mg/kg/day for children.

C. APAP is found in over 100 combination pharmaceuticals (cold, cough, and decongestant agents), in addition to being present in prescription opioid analgesics (eg, Vicodin®, Darvocet®).

D. Acute toxicity may result after an adult ingests 7 g or a child ingests 140 mg/kg.

II. Epidemiology.
According to the Toxic Exposure Surveillance System, in 2003, there were 127,171 toxic exposures to acetaminophen and 327 associated deaths.

III. Pathophysiology

A. Metabolism of APAP involves sulfonation and glucuronidation with renal excretion of non-toxic metabolites. Approximately 10% is metabolized via the cytochrome P450 system (CYP2E1, CYP1A2, CYP3A4) to a toxic reactive metabolite **N-acetyl-p-benzoquinone imine** (NAPQI).

B. Normally, endogenous hepatic glutathione is responsible for the detoxification of NAPQI. However, in an overdose, glutathione stores become depleted and NAPQI accumulates.

C. NAPQI then reacts directly with the hepatic macromolecules, causing liver injury. NAPQI production also occurs in the kidney, leading to potential renal insufficiency.

IV. Risk Factors

A. **Acute or chronic overdose.**

B. **Induced cytochrome P450 activity** (more NAPQI formed) anticonvulsants, antituberculosis agents, or alcoholism.

C. **Decreased glutathione stores** (less NAPQI detoxified) malnutrition, alcoholism, AIDS.

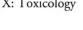

V. Clinical Presentation

A. History

1. **Time of ingestion,** especially if acute, is very important to ascertain.
2. **Amount ingested** influences the decision to treat.
3. **Number and frequency of doses** is used to categorize ingestion as acute or chronic.
4. **Symptoms** of GI upset, vomiting, AMS, or jaundice after chronic poisoning (or late presentation) increases the likelihood of a significant ingestion.
5. **Stages of APAP poisoning**
   a. *Stage 1: GI (0–24 hr).* Vomiting, abdominal pain, or asymptomatic.
   b. *Stage 2: latent (24–48 hr).* Resolution of nausea and vomiting, but rising transaminases and potential progression to significant toxicity.
   c. *Stage 3: hepatic (72–96 hr).* Severe hepatotoxicity (jaundice, hypoglycemia, vomiting, abdominal pain, coagulopathy, encephalopathy, acidemia, hyperbilirubinemia, significantly elevated transaminases).
   d. *Stage 4: recovery or death (4–14 days).* Resolution of toxicity or progressive deterioration beyond day 5 to renal failure, hyperammonemia, bleeding diatheses, and subsequent death.

B. Physical Examination

1. **Vital signs** are important to evaluate for hemodynamic abnormalities. Any signs of tachypnea or hyperpnea may indicate attempts to compensate for acidemia.
2. Examine the **skin and sclera** for any evidence of jaundice or icterus.
3. **Abdominal examination.** Diffuse abdominal tenderness is common after significant overdose. Hepatic enlargement and tenderness may be evident beginning in the latent stage.

VI. Differential Diagnosis. Other hepatotoxins (Amanita phalloides and Galleria autumnalis mushrooms, carbon tetrachloride, iron, isoniazid), viral hepatitis, biliary disease, ethanol.

VII. Diagnostic Findings

A. Laboratory Studies

1. **Serum APAP level.** Confirms presence after exposure and if acute ingestion has occurred, it can be used to plot the need for treatment on the Rumack-Matthew nomogram. Values above the treatment line indicate a greater potential for hepatotoxicity (Figure 49–1).
2. **Liver function studies** (AST, ALT) and **bilirubin levels** are important as baseline values in acute overdoses and essential in late presenters or chronic overdoses.
3. **Coagulation profile** (PT, PTT, INR). Elevations indicate significant hepatocyte injury.
4. **CBC** may be helpful in fulminant hepatic failure and bleeding diathesis.
5. **Electrolytes** may reveal a large anion gap in significant exposures.
6. **Renal function** is also of paramount importance, since NAPQI is also produced in the kidney.

B. Imaging Studies

1. **Head CT scan** is important when mental status does not correlate with an isolated ingestion.

2. Abdominal CT scan will not reveal any findings specific for APAP poisoning, but it should be considered if peritoneal findings are present.

C. **Diagnostic Algorithm**

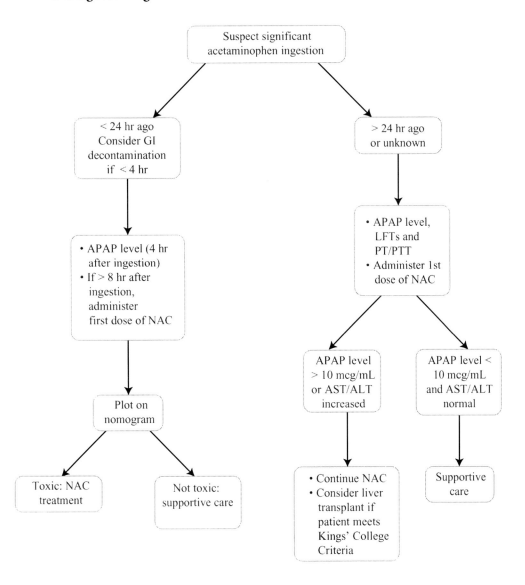

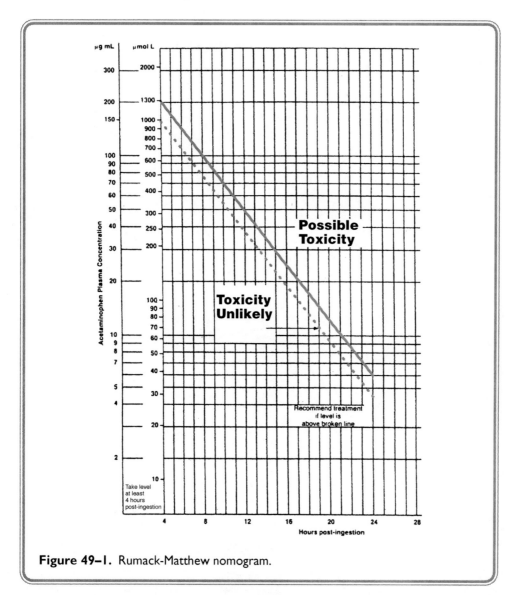

Figure 49–1. Rumack-Matthew nomogram.

VIII. Treatment

A. GI Decontamination

1. **Activated charcoal.** Charcoal readily absorbs APAP and it should be given, especially when the ingestion occurred within 4 hours of presentation. Dose is 1 g/kg, but more may be appropriate in significant ingestion. NAC is adsorbed by charcoal, but there is no evidence that there is less effectiveness when NAC and charcoal are given together orally.

2. **Gastric lavage** and/or **whole bowel irrigation** are not regularly utilized in light of the ability of APAP to adsorb to charcoal, and the availability of an effective antidote.

B. **N-acetylcysteine** (NAC, Mucomyst)

1. NAC can be given prior to knowing the serum APAP level.

2. **Indications**

a. Levels above the nomogram treatment line after acute ingestions (see Figure 49–1).

b. Evidence of significant ingestion over a period of time (or distant ingestion) with evidence of hepatotoxicity, regardless of the APAP level.

3. Oral dose is 140 mg/kg loading, followed by 70 mg/kg q 4 hour for 72 hours of treatment.

4. The oral formulation can be given IV through a 0.22 micron filter to prevent anaphylactoid reactions. Two protocols exist: **Rocky Mountain protocol** is 140 mg/kg load, 70 mg/kg q 4 hours for 48 hours of therapy. **Prescott protocol** is 150 mg/kg over 15 minutes to 1 hour, followed by 50 mg/kg over 4 hours, followed by 100 mg/kg over 16 hours.

5. Acetadote® is the trade name of an FDA-approved IV NAC formulation. Protocol is the same as the Prescott protocol. Advantages include reduced likelihood of anaphylactoid reactions and no need to filter. It is approved for patients with acute ingestions presenting < 8 hours after ingestion, and is utilized in pregnant patients or those with evidence of hepatotoxicity or intractable vomiting.

C. **Liver Transplantation**

1. Refer to a transplantation center if the following are evident (Kings' College Criteria): pH < 7.3 after resuscitation (or) PT > 100 (and) creatinine > 3.3 mg/dL (and) encephalopathy (grade 3 or 4).

2. Consider contacting a gastroenterologist who specializes in liver diseases prior to the patient developing these findings after significant overdose or hepatotoxicity.

IX. **Disposition**

A. **Admission.** Any patient who is suicidal, requires treatment with NAC, and/or has evidence of hepatotoxicity. All patients with abnormal vital signs, acidemia, or end-organ damage should be admitted to the ICU.

B. **Discharge.** Accidental ingestions with no evidence of acute poisoning and a non-toxic APAP level.

CASE PRESENTATION

A 20-year-old woman presents to the ED tearful because she recently broke up with her boyfriend. She states that she "took some pills," and was noted to vomit once en route per EMS. She is awake and has diffuse abdominal pain to palpation. EMS state that no medications other than OTC cold tablets were in her apartment. APAP level is pending.

1. *What other historical facts do you want to know?*

   · *Time of ingestion? Amount ingested? Agent(s) ingested? Chronicity of use? Any co-ingestion?*

2. *Laboratory studies indicate an APAP level of 250 mcg/mL and an undetectable salicylate level. The first dose of NAC is administered along with activated charcoal. ABG reveals a pH of 7.2. What is your next step in management?*

   · *Resuscitation with volume repletion.*

   · *Call for consultation with liver disease specialist or prepare for transfer to a tertiary care facility.*

SUMMARY POINTS

- *Obtain a thorough history from the patient (time, amount, acute or chronic).*
- *Remember that many OTC products, as well as prescription medications, contain APAP.*
- *When in doubt, administer NAC.*
- *Only utilize the Rumack-Matthew nomogram in acute ingestions presenting < 24 hours after exposure.*

CHAPTER 50
SALICYLATE TOXICITY

I. Defining Features

    A. In the United States, salicylate poisoning is most frequently attributed to ingestion of aspirin-containing products.

    B. Salicylates may be found in combination pharmaceuticals (combined with cold, cough, and decongestant agents), prescription analgesics (Fiorinal®, Soma Compound®, Percodan®), and methyl salicylate. One teaspoon of methyl salicylate contains > 7 g of salicylate, which is > twenty 325 mg tablets of aspirin.

    C. Overdose and poisoning must be approached, taking into account **acute, chronic,** and **acute on chronic** scenarios.

II. Epidemiology. According to the Toxic Exposure Surveillance System, in 2003, there were > 20,500 toxic exposures to salicylate and > 430 associated deaths.

III. Pathophysiology

    A. Absorption of aspirin can be very erratic, with peak levels potentially occurring > 20 hours after ingestion. Levels obtained 6 hours after ingestion reveal evidence of toxicity.

    B. Salicylate, the hydrolyzed byproduct of aspirin, is responsible for the therapeutic and toxic effects of aspirin.

    C. **Acid-base abnormalities.** Salicylates increase respiratory rate by *directly* stimulating the medullary respiratory center in the brainstem. This results in the early manifestation of respiratory alkalosis. Induction of lipolysis, uncoupling of oxidative phosphorylation, and the inhibition of Krebs cycle enzymes result in the accumulation of organic acids, which contributes to a metabolic acidosis. Significant volume depletion from vomiting may result in a metabolic alkalosis. The acid-base disturbance can be any or all of the above, yielding a mixed triple disorder (respiratory alkalosis, anion gap metabolic acidosis, and metabolic alkalosis).

    D. Other effects include CNS disturbance, disruption of glucose homeostasis (normo-, hyper-, or hypoglycemia), and pulmonary edema (non-cardiogenic).

    E. Using Michaelis-Menten kinetics, at levels > 30 mg/dL, salicylates are metabolized via zero-order elimination: a set amount is eliminated per unit time vs. a set fraction as in first-order elimination.

IV. Risk Factors

    A. Acute toxicity results after ingesting 150 mg/kg.

B. Chronic poisoning may occur with supratherapeutic administration (excessive dosing or frequent intervals).

V. Clinical Presentation

A. **History**
  1. **Time of ingestion** (especially if acute).
  2. **Amount ingested** will aid in predicting a potentially toxic dose.
  3. **Number and frequency of doses** helps to categorize a patient as acute or chronic.
  4. A history of tinnitus or hearing loss, vomiting, shortness of breath, or AMS may lead to the diagnosis.

B. **Physical Examination**
  1. **Vital signs** are important in evaluating hemodynamic abnormalities, and any signs of tachypnea or hyperpnea may indicate stimulation of the brainstem's breathing center or attempts to compensate for acidemia. Other potential abnormalities include tachycardia, fever, and low O_2 saturation (noncardiogenic pulmonary edema).
  2. **Skin examination** may reveal evidence of diaphoresis.
  3. **Abdominal examination** commonly reveals diffuse tenderness after acute overdose.
  4. Chronic salicylism should be considered in any patient with unexplained CNS dysfunction, unexplained noncardiogenic pulmonary edema, or seizures.

VI. Differential Diagnosis.
Other causes of an anion gap metabolic acidosis, sepsis (especially in the chronically poisoned patient), Reye's syndrome, DKA, alcoholic ketoacidosis, other poisonings (caffeine, theophylline, and heavy metals).

RULE OUT

Chronic poisoning mimics sepsis. A salicylate level should be obtained in all febrile elderly patients with AMS.

VII. Diagnostic Findings

A. **Laboratory Studies**
  1. **Serum salicylate level.** Being cognizant of your laboratory's *units* is of utmost importance. ***Therapeutic range is 15–25 mg/dL.*** Many references refer to levels of 100 mg/dL in acute exposures and 60 mg/dL in chronic exposures as significant enough to potentially warrant hemodialysis. However, *levels lower than this may cause severe illness and necessitate treatment with hemodialysis (eg, chronic poisoning, renal dysfunction, significant acidemia).*
  2. **Ferric chloride test** is a rapid bedside qualitative maneuver to determine the presence of salicylates. Adding 3 drops of ferric chloride to 1 mL of urine results in a purple coloration in the presence of salicylates.
  3. **Electrolytes** to appreciate any decrease in serum bicarbonate and an elevated anion gap.
  4. **Renal function** may dictate treatment choice.

B. **Imaging Studies**
  1. **Head CT scan** is important when mental status does not correlate with an isolated ingestion.
  2. Abdominal radiograph will likely *not* be able to visualize aspirin tablets.

C. **Diagnostic Algorithm**

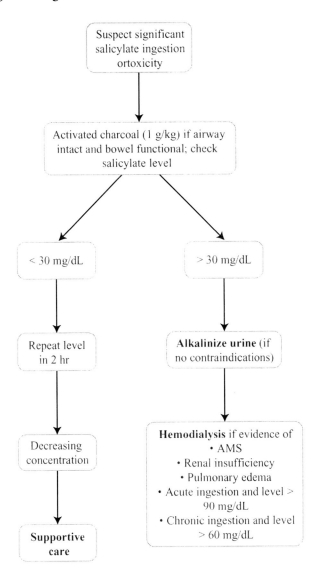

VIII. Treatment

    A. **Fluid resuscitation** should be aggressive, as patients are notably volume depleted from vomiting and insensible fluid losses.

    B. **Endotracheal intubation.** Patients who require intubation *must* have a higher than normal respiratory rate on the ventilator or be given the ability to hyperventilate. A normal rate will cause relative hypoventilation in the patient with salicylism, causing a respiratory acidosis, worsening the already present metabolic acidosis, and leading to death.

C. **GI Decontamination**

1. **Activated charcoal.** Salicylate is readily adsorbed to charcoal. The dose is 1 g/kg; however, more may be appropriate in significant exposure. The goal is 10:1 ratio of grams of charcoal per gram of salicylate. Repeat dosing is advantageous when subsequent levels indicate continual absorption from the GI tract.

2. **Gastric lavage** may be considered in a patient presenting early after a lethal overdose.

D. **Alkalinization of the Urine**

1. Enhances renal salicylate elimination via ion trapping of weak acids and probably through a mechanism of secretion into the renal tubules.

2. The main goal of alkalinization is shifting salicylate out of the CNS, which is most often the cause of death in these patients.

3. Add 3 amps of sodium bicarbonate to 1 L D5W and infuse at twice the maintenance rate. Goal is a urine pH of 7.5–8.0 to maximize elimination.

4. Serum potassium must be replaced for effective elimination. Low serum potassium yields acidic urine because of exchange of secreted hydrogen ion for reabsorbed potassium.

5. Contraindications include cardiopulmonary disease (eg, CHF, pulmonary edema), renal failure, AMS, or significant acidemia necessitating hemodialysis.

E. **Hemodialysis.** Consider if significant acidemia (pH < 7.1), renal insufficiency, pulmonary edema, AMS, or acute overdoses with levels > 90 mg/dL or chronic poisoning with levels > 60 mg/dL. Contact a nephrologist early in borderline cases.

IX. **Disposition**

A. **Admission** is indicated in any patient who is suicidal or requires treatment with a sodium bicarbonate infusion. All patients with abnormal vital signs, acidemia, AMS, or treatment with hemodialysis should be admitted to an ICU.

B. **Discharge.** Accidental ingestions with no evidence of acute poisoning or indication for treatment. Ensure subsequent levels are not increasing by checking a serum salicylate level every 2 hours until levels begin to decrease.

CASE PRESENTATION

A 30-year-old man presents to the ED with recent vomiting and abdominal pain. He has a hard time hearing your questions when you are taking his history. His roommate states that the man has been depressed lately. He also says that he saw an empty bottle of aspirin in the bathroom today. Physical examination reveals RR of 28 breaths/min and a temperature of 37.8°C (100.2°F). The patient also has shortness of breath. You notice that the pulse oximeter reads 92% saturation on room air.

1. *What other historical facts do you want to know?*

   · *Time of ingestion? Amount ingested? Agent(s) ingested? Chronicity of use? Any co-ingestion?*

2. *If his CXR reveals pulmonary edema or his pH is significant for profound acidemia, what is your next step in management?*

   · *Obtain a nephrology consult. This patient requires hemodialysis. He will likely not be able to tolerate a sodium bicarbonate infusion.*

SUMMARY POINTS

- *Obtain a thorough history from the patient (time, amount, acute or chronic).*
- *Consider chronic salicylism in all elderly patients with AMS or a sepsis-like presentation.*
- *Remember that many OTC products as well as prescription medications contain salicylate.*
- *Repeat dosing of activated charcoal is frequently helpful because of aspirin's characteristically erratic absorption and formation of concretions in the gut.*

CHAPTER 51
CARBON MONOXIDE POISONING

I. Defining Features

   A. Carbon monoxide (CO) is an odorless, colorless, tasteless, nonirritating gas.

   B. It is formed as a byproduct of the incomplete combustion of carbon-containing substances (coal, gasoline, fossil fuel).

   C. Other sources of CO include cigarette smoke, vehicle exhaust systems, and methylene chloride ingestion or inhalation (paint stripping solution, liquid in bubbling holiday lights). Methylene chloride is converted to CO by the liver, and may lead to poisoning on a delayed basis.

II. Epidemiology

   A. Historically, CO has consistently ranked as the number 1 cause of poisoning-related deaths.

   B. CO poisoning is more common during the winter months.

   C. According to the Toxic Exposure Surveillance System, 74 deaths and > 17,000 CO exposures occurred in 2004.

   D. CO poisoning can occur from fires or non-fire exposures. Between 1994 and 1998 in the United States, 11,000 patients were seen in EDs following non-fire exposures.

III. Pathophysiology

   A. CO poisoning results in tissue hypoxia via several mechanisms: CO binds to hemoglobin (Hb) with an affinity 240 times more than that of O_2. Reduced O_2 transport occurs because Hb-binding sites are occupied by CO. This results in impaired delivery of O_2 to tissues.

   B. In addition, the COHb molecule has a greater affinity for O_2, which does not allow delivery of O_2 to the tissues. This results in a left shift, and changing of the shape of the oxyhemoglobin-dissociation curve from sigmoidal to asymptotic. Both of these changes result in increased cellular hypoxia.

   C. At the cellular level, CO binds to cytochrome aa3, resulting in inhibition of electron transport and eventually halting ATP production from oxidative phosphorylation.

   D. Myoglobin (important for the uptake of O_2 by skeletal muscle) binds to CO with an affinity 40 times that of O_2. Myocardial myoglobin may also be affected, resulting in a reduction of contractility and cardiac output. This may lead to further reduction in tissue O_2 delivery.

IV. Risk Factors

A. Being in the close vicinity of a combusting engine (in a truck or automobile with a poor exhaust system; in a home with a faulty furnace; or behind speed boats or house boats). Other risks include using a gasoline-powered generator or motor or burning charcoal in a closed space (house, basement, or garage).

B. CO detectors in homes reduce the risk of significant poisoning and death.

V. Clinical Presentation

A. **History**
1. Headaches, vomiting, muscle aches, sleepiness, weakness, chest pain, shortness of breath, syncope, seizures, palpitations, or coma (Table 51–1).
2. Symptoms are very important in determining management. A patient who has had a syncopal event is managed much differently than a patient with a mild headache.
3. Pertinent historic features include the presence of sick or dead family members or animals in the home.
4. Time of exposure and chronicity of symptoms.

KEY COMPLAINT

Headache is a frequent complaint in patients with CO poisoning. The diagnosis of CO poisoning should be considered in patients with headache and other nonspecific symptoms, especially during the winter months.

B. **Physical Examination**
1. **Vital signs** are important in evaluating hemodynamic abnormalities, and any signs of tachypnea or hyperpnea may indicate attempts to compensate for

Table 51–1. Clinical findings in CO poisoning.

COHb Level (% of total Hb)	Symptoms
5	None or mild headache
10	Slight headache or dyspnea with extreme exertion
20	Headache, dyspnea with exertion
30	Severe headache, irritability, fatigue
40–50	Tachycardia, confusion, lethargy, syncope
60–70	Coma, convulsions
80	Rapidly fatal

acidemia. Other potential abnormalities in vital signs include tachycardia and hypotension. ***O₂ saturation is falsely recorded as high or normal in patients with CO poisoning.***

2. **Mental status** and **neurologic examinations** are a priority. A parkinsonian-like presentation after prolonged or remote exposure is possible.
3. **Cardiovascular examination** is paramount to examine for evidence of hemodynamic compromise, dysrhythmias, or murmurs that might suggest MI.
4. **Skin** rarely demonstrates bullous lesions.

VI. **Differential Diagnosis.** Other causes of an anion gap metabolic acidosis, influenza, acute gastroenteritis, common cold or viral syndrome, vasovagal syncope, migraine headache, CVA.

VII. **Diagnostic Findings**

A. **Laboratory Studies**
1. **COHb level** (venous or arterial) is obtained via CO-oximetry. This value quantifies a percent of Hb, which has CO bound. COHb levels are important in revealing exposure, yet many times do not correlate with degree of clinical toxicity. Symptomatology is as important, if not more than COHb levels.
2. **Electrolytes** are important to evaluate for any evidence of an anion gap. At high levels, CO poisoning will result in an anion gap metabolic acidosis.
3. **Arterial or venous pH** reveals evidence of acidemia.
4. **Serum lactate** (> 10 mmol/L) indicates serious poisoning or concomitant cyanide poisoning in victims of fires.
5. **ECG** and **cardiac enzymes** are used to evaluate for myocardial injury.
6. **Total CPK** and **renal function** to examine for rhabdomyolysis.
7. **Urine pregnancy test** should be obtained in females of childbearing age. Pregnancy is an indication for hyperbaric O₂, because HbF (fetal hemoglobin) avidly binds CO and may result in higher fetal levels than those of the mother.

B. **Imaging Studies**
1. **Head CT scan** is important when AMS or neurologic abnormalities are present. Globus pallidus densities have been reported in some patients.
2. **CXR** in patients with smoke inhalation or evidence of pulmonary edema or respiratory compromise.

C. **Diagnostic Algorithm (see page 305)**

VIII. **Treatment**

A. Treat concomitant injuries such as smoke inhalation, trauma, myocardial injury, or seizures.

B. **O₂.** CO has a half-life of 4–6 hours while breathing room air; 90 minutes with administration of 100% O₂; and approximately 23 minutes during hyperbaric O₂ delivery. Normobaric O₂ via a non-rebreather facemask should be administered until the CO level is < 5% and the patient is clinically stable. Hyperbaric O₂ therapy is indicated for those patients with significant exposures (Table 51–2). Most hospitals do not have hyperbaric chambers. Contacting the regional poison control center can be valuable in the management and disposition of these patients.

Diagnostic Algorithm

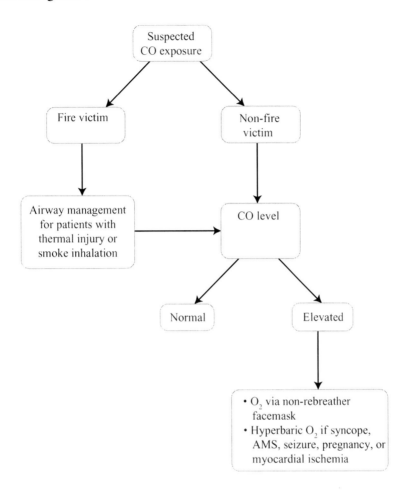

IX. Disposition

    A. **Admission.** Admit any patient who has AMS, neurologic manifestations, or any indication(s) for hyperbaric treatment. If the patient is otherwise well but poisoning was due to a suicide attempt, admission to a psychiatric hospital is warranted.

    B. **Discharge** is warranted when the exposure was accidental, the patient is clinically well, and the COHb level is < 5% after treatment with 100% O_2 via facemask. All discharged patients should be educated about CO poisoning and en-

Table 51–2. Indications for hyperbaric O_2 treatment in acute CO poisoning.

Definite Indication	Relative Indication
AMS and/or abnormal neurologic examination (if patient has normal evaluation while on supplemental O_2, temporarily take patient off O_2 and repeat evaluation) History of loss of consciousness or near-syncope History of seizure Coma History of hypotension during or shortly after exposure Myocardial ischemia History of prolonged exposure Pregnancy with COHb > 15%	Persisting neurologic symptoms including headache and dizziness after 4 h of 100% normobaric O_2 Persisting acidosis Concurrent thermal or chemical burns Pregnancy with history of carbon monoxide exposure regardless of COHb level

couraged to have their homes examined by the fire department or gas provider. Provide adequate follow-up for assessment of any delayed neurologic sequelae (parkinsonism, memory loss, lack of concentration).

CASE PRESENTATION

An 18-year-woman presents to the ED after being found unconscious in the garage with an automobile running. Her O_2 saturation is 98%, and she is unresponsive to verbal or noxious stimuli. A COHb level via CO-oximetry is 25%.

1. *What other historical facts do you want to know?*
   - *Time of exposure (last seen in good health)? Chronicity of exposure? Co-ingestion? Pregnancy?*
2. *What other laboratory studies and treatment might you consider?*
   - *Renal function. Electrolytes. pH. CXR. CT scan of head. Urine pregnancy.*
   - *Consultation with hyperbaric medicine specialist.*

SUMMARY POINTS

- *Consider CO poisoning in all patients with flu-like illness, headaches, AMS, or anion gap metabolic acidosis.*
- *Administer O_2 immediately to any patient with a presumptive diagnosis.*
- *Remember that pulse oximetry displays a falsely elevated value in patients with CO poisoning.*
- *Symptomatology is often more important than the COHb levels when it comes to making treatment and disposition decisions.*
- *Contact the poison control center and/or hyperbaric specialists for assistance in the management of these patients.*

SECTION XI
ENVIRONMENTAL EMERGENCIES

CHAPTER 52
HYPOTHERMIA

I. Defining Features

A. Hypothermia is defined as a core body temperature < 35°C (95°F).

B. Hypothermia is classified based on the core temperature: mild 35°–32°C (95°–89.6°F); moderate 32°–30°C (89.5°–86°F); and severe < 30°C (< 86°F).

II. Epidemiology

A. Although most common in cold climates, hypothermia may occur in temperate climates and may also occur during the summer.

B. In the United States, about 700 people die each year from hypothermia.

C. Over half of the deaths occur in patients > age 65.

D. Patients with an initial core temperature < 23°C (73.4°) usually do not survive.

III. Etiology

A. **Primary hypothermia** occurs when an otherwise healthy person is exposed to cold temperatures and is unable to compensate.

B. **Secondary hypothermia** occurs when a patient has a co-morbid medical illness that is disrupting their normal thermoregulatory mechanism (hypothyroidism, sepsis, intoxication).

C. **Anterior hypothalamus** normally controls body temperature; when the body is exposed to cold temperatures, the hypothalamus generates adaptive responses of heat production (shivering) and heat conservation (getting out of the cold; putting on warm clothing).

D. The body loses heat via 4 main mechanisms: **conduction, convection, evaporation,** and **radiation.** Prolonged exposure to a cold (radiation), wet (conduction, evaporation), and windy (convection) environment puts patients at risk for hypothermia.

IV. Risk Factors.
Psychiatric disorders, intoxication (alcohol and drugs), dehydration, extremes of age, infants/children (greater body surface area), medical illness (sepsis, hypothyroidism, hypoadrenalism, hypoglycemia, peripheral vascular disease).

V. Clinical Presentation

A. **History**

1. Patients with mild hypothermia attempt to increase heat production by shivering.

2. Patients with moderate hypothermia may experience a slowdown in their level of functioning and metabolism. Shivering ceases when body temperature is < 32°C.
3. Severe hypothermia may cause mild confusion, AMS, or coma.
4. Patients should be asked about co-morbid illnesses, medications, and intoxicants that may have precipitated or contributed to their hypothermia.

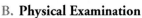

KEY COMPLAINTS

In the United States, most patients with hypothermia are intoxicated with alcohol or drugs or have a psychiatric illness or dementia.

B. **Physical Examination**
  1. **Assess patient's ABCs and vital signs** for possible unstable airway and presence or absence of pulses.
  2. An **accurate core body temperature** is imperative for the diagnosis. Most thermometers in the ED only read as low as 34.4°C (94°F). Rectal, bladder, or esophageal thermometers should be used to obtain an accurate temperature < 34.4°C.
  3. Completely undress the patient, removing all wet clothing.
  4. Focus examination looking for any signs of coexisting trauma, sepsis, hypothyroidism, hypoadrenalism, toxidromes, frostbite, or cardiac dysfunction.
  5. With decreasing temperatures, the patient's cardiac rhythm degenerates from sinus bradycardia to slow AF to VF.
  6. Perform a neurologic examination, evaluating LOC, pupils, and any focal deficits.

CLINICAL SKILLS TIP

In the severely hypothermic patient, pulses may be difficult to palpate. Use a handheld Doppler device when pulses are thready or difficult to palpate to confirm their presence.

VI. **Differential Diagnosis.** Primary hypothermia, hypoadrenalism, hypothyroidism, sepsis, hypoglycemia, drug overdose, hypothalamic dysfunction (CNS bleed), iatrogenic (exposure, fluids).

RULE OUT

Coexisting medical illnesses *that may be causing or exacerbating the hypothermia must be ruled out, especially sepsis in the elderly.*

VII. **Diagnostic Findings**
  A. **Laboratory Studies**
    1. Bedside glucose level should be obtained on all hypothermic patients because hypoglycemia may be present. More often, hyperglycemia is present from a cold-induced decrease in insulin secretion. This should not be treated with exogenous insulin because severe hypoglycemia may result upon rewarming.
    2. **Electrolytes** and **renal function** should be assessed. Hypothermia impairs renal concentrating ability and induces a diuresis exacerbating hypovolemia and dehydration.

3. Hypothermia impairs the coagulation cascade and platelet aggregation; therefore, patients are coagulopathic. However, laboratory measurement of PT and PTT will be normal because the blood is warmed prior to running the tests. Hypothermia also causes hemoconcentration, increasing the hematocrit by 2% for every 1°C drop in temperature.

B. **Imaging Studies**
   1. **Head CT scan** should be performed on all patients who have persistent AMS after rewarming.
   2. **ECG** should be performed on all patients with moderate or severe hypothermia to assess for pathologic rhythms. Bradycardia and QT prolongation are often found. Slow AF and VF are also found in more severe hypothermia. The **Osborn J wave** is a wide positive deflection at the end of the QRS complex. It is sensitive, but not a specific finding for moderate to severe hypothermia (Figure 52–1).

C. **Diagnostic Algorithm**

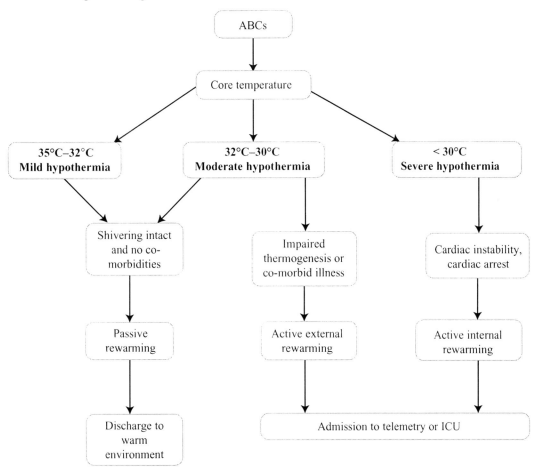

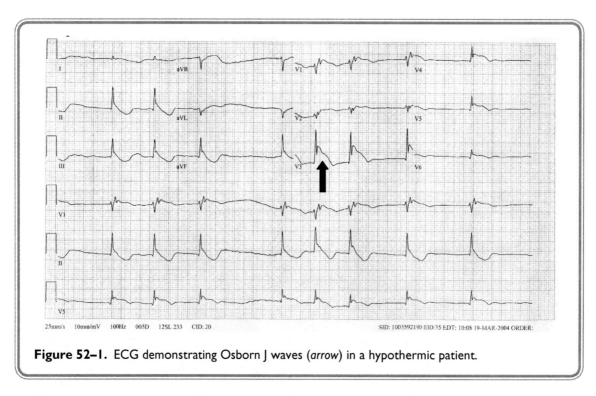

Figure 52–1. ECG demonstrating Osborn J waves (*arrow*) in a hypothermic patient.

VIII. Treatment

A. **Mild hypothermia. Passive rewarming** is usually effective. This technique uses the body's own heat production mechanisms for rewarming. Shivering response must be intact, and the patient should have sufficient energy stores (no severe co-morbidities or hypoglycemia). The patient should be undressed and placed in warm blankets. Rate of rewarming is usually < 1°C per hour.

B. **Moderate hypothermia.** Search for and treat co-morbid illnesses. If the patient has no serious co-morbidities and shivering is still present, **passive rewarming** may be adequate. For patients with serious underlying illness or impaired thermogenesis, **active external rewarming** should occur. This includes warmed IV fluids to 42°C, warmed humidified O_2 (up to 46°C), and forced-air rewarming blankets (Bair Hugger). These methods can rewarm at a rate of 3.5°C per hour.

C. **Severe hypothermia.** Patients with a strong pulse and no signs of cardiac instability are rewarmed with active external rewarming (see VIII B). Patients with cardiac arrest (or in cases of repeated cardiac instability) should have **active internal rewarming** methods employed, which consist of warmed saline (40°C) lavage of the stomach (only if intubated), bladder, and colon. Peritoneal irrigation and pleural irrigation may also be performed. Thoracotomy with internal cardiac massage and mediastinal irrigation is the most invasive procedure for active core rewarming, but has been used successfully in severe hypothermia with prolonged cardiac arrest. Patients with VF and temperatures < 30°C are often resistant to defibrillation. After the initial attempt at defibrillation, CPR should be started, and the patient should be rewarmed to 30°C. Defibrillation should again be attempted. ***A patient should not be pronounced dead until rewarmed to 32°C.***

IX. Disposition

A. **Admission.** Patients with moderate hypothermia who require active external rewarming or who have serious contributing co-morbid illnesses should be admitted to the hospital. Any patient with cardiac instability or cardiac arrest who undergoes active internal rewarming should be admitted to an ICU.

B. **Discharge.** Patients with mild to moderate hypothermia who undergo passive rewarming and have no serious co-morbid illnesses contributing to their hypothermia can be discharged as long as they have a warm environment to go to. Homeless patients will need a social worker to find them placement in a warming shelter, or they should be admitted.

CASE PRESENTATION

You are working in the ED on the first warm day of spring. EMS phones that they are bringing you an unresponsive person from the lakefront. They noted a bradycardic rhythm on the monitor. Upon arrival, you note a 22-year-old unresponsive male in wet swim trunks.

1. *What do you want to know next?*
   - *What was his blood glucose level? Does he have any serious medical problems? Did he ingest any intoxicating substances?*
2. *His friends arrive later and tell you he had been drinking alcohol all day and was one of the only people brave enough to swim in the cold waters of Lake Michigan. What else do you want to know?*
   - *An accurate core temperature, an alcohol level, and toxicology screen.*

SUMMARY POINTS

- *Most patients who present with hypothermia are intoxicated with either alcohol or drugs.*
- *Most ED thermometers will only accurately read temperatures as low as 34.4°C (94°F).*
- *Many patients have serious underlying illnesses that contribute to the development of hypothermia. It is imperative to search for and treat these illnesses.*
- *A patient should not be pronounced dead until core temperature is at least 32°C and defibrillation is still unsuccessful.*

CHAPTER 53
HEAT-RELATED ILLNESS

I. Defining Features

A. Heat exhaustion and heat stroke are on a continuum of disease severity. **Heat exhaustion** occurs when the body can no longer dissipate heat adequately, resulting in hyperthermia. **Heat stroke** is the result of complete thermoregulatory dysfunction.

B. **Classic heat injury** occurs in the elderly or ill with prolonged exposure to high environmental temperatures. Physical exertion is not required. Elevated temperatures and high humidity overwhelm the body's normal cooling mechanisms.

C. **Exertional heat injury** occurs in physically fit individuals who exert themselves during conditions with high heat and humidity. Heat gain from the environment combined with internal heat production overwhelms the body's normal cooling mechanisms.

II. Epidemiology

A. There are about 400 deaths from heat-related illness in the United States every year (the heat wave in July 1995 caused 465 deaths in Chicago alone).

B. The mortality rate in patients with heatstroke is between 10% and 70%.

III. Etiology

A. The body normally maintains its core temperature between 36°C (96.8°F) and 38°C (100.4°F).

B. In hyperthermia, there is an elevated body temperature without a resetting of the hypothalamic temperature center, as occurs with fever.

C. The body responds to heat stress through 3 main mechanisms: increased sweat production, decreased internal heat production, and removal from the hot environment.

D. Evaporation of sweat is the main mechanism through which the body dissipates heat. Radiation, conduction, and convection also allow the body to lose heat when the ambient temperature is lower than body temperature.

E. Evaporative mechanisms are impaired by high humidity, dehydration, obesity, and poor cardiac function.

IV. Risk Factors.
Chronic illness, extremes of age, alcoholism, decreased mobility, medications (eg, antipsychotics, anticholinergics, β blockers, diuretics), obesity, scleroderma.

V. Clinical Presentation

A. **Heat exhaustion.** Core temperature is usually normal but can be elevated to 40°C (104°F). Patients present with nonspecific symptoms and signs (weakness, dizziness, fatigue, nausea, vomiting, headache, myalgias, tachycardia, tachypnea, hypotension, and diaphoresis). Mental status is normal.

B. **Heat stroke.** Patients present with AMS ranging from mild confusion to coma. Body temperature is elevated above 40°C (104°F). They may or may not be sweating. Patients can exhibit a wide range of neurologic symptoms and signs, including ataxia, seizures, and hemiplegia. Multiorgan failure (hepatic, renal, cardiac) may also be present in severe cases.

VI. Differential Diagnosis. Meningitis, neuroleptic malignant syndrome (NMS), serotonin syndrome, sepsis, thyroid storm, drug intoxication (PCP, amphetamines, cocaine), cerebral hemorrhage, status epilepticus.

RULE OUT

NMS and *serotonin syndrome* should be considered in any patient taking psychiatric medications.

VII. Diagnostic Findings

A. **Laboratory Studies**
1. **Electrolytes** and **renal function.** Hypo- or hypernatremia and prerenal azotemia may be present.
2. Patients with severe cramping and pain should have **CPK** checked to rule out rhabdomyolysis.
3. Patients with heat stroke may have elevated **liver enzymes** (peaking at 24–72 hr), DIC (thrombocytopenia, low fibrinogen levels, elevated fibrin split products, elevated D-dimer), and coagulopathy (elevated PT/PTT).

B. **Imaging Studies**
1. **Non-contrast head CT scan** should be performed on patients presenting with AMS of unclear origin. In heat stroke, the CT is normal.
2. **ECG** should be performed on all patients with heat exhaustion and heat stroke, looking for ischemia or signs of electrolyte abnormalities.

C. **Diagnostic Algorithm (see page 316)**

VIII. Treatment

A. **Heat exhaustion.** Volume replacement (oral replacement for mild cases and IV for more severe cases). Electrolyte replacement (oral or IV, depending on severity of depletion). Rest and ambient cooling. Search for complications from co-morbid conditions.

B. **Heat stroke. IV volume** and **electrolyte replacement** (begin with 250–500 mL bolus NS and replenish other electrolytes based on laboratory values). Be careful not to fluid-overload older patients or those with cardiac problems. **Evaporative cooling** should begin as soon as life threats have been assessed and ABCs are secure. Completely expose the patient and mist them with tepid water, while a fan is blowing on them. This is the easiest and most practical method of cooling a patient in the ED. Stop this process when the body temperature reaches 40°C (104°F) to avoid overshoot hypothermia. Patients may

Diagnostic Algorithm

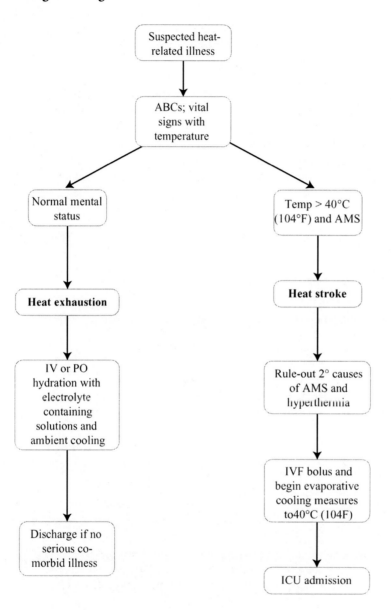

shiver during this process (which is counterproductive and produces heat). Treat shivering with low dose benzodiazepines (lorazepam 1 mg IV). **Search for complications** from heat stroke such as cardiac ischemia, hepatic and renal failure, DIC, and endocrine disorders. The number 1 factor that contributes to the morbidity and mortality of heat illness is the severity of underlying co-morbid illnesses, not the absolute height of the core temperature.

IX. Disposition

A. **Admission.** Patients with heat stroke should be admitted to an ICU. Patients with heat exhaustion and any serious co-morbidity should be admitted to the hospital, according to the complication.

B. **Discharge.** Patients with cases of heat exhaustion who improve in the ED may be discharged home.

CASE PRESENTATION

A 70-year-old man is brought to the ED by paramedics. They were called by the man's neighbor, who found the patient confused at home. The neighbor noted that the house was very warm, and it appeared that the air conditioning was not functioning.

1. *What else do you want to know?*
   - *When was the last time the neighbor saw the patient in his normal state?*
   - *What is the patient's past medical history?*
   - *Has he been ill recently?*
   - *What medications does he take?*
2. *His core temperature is 41.6° C (107° F). What is your differential diagnosis?*
   - *Heat stroke, sepsis, meningitis, drug toxicity, thyroid storm, intracerebral hemorrhage.*

SUMMARY POINTS

- *Always consider secondary causes of hyperthermia. Heat exhaustion and stroke should be diagnoses of exclusion.*
- *Do not fluid overload elderly patients while rehydrating them in the ED. Remember that their fluid and electrolyte deficits developed over days and they do not need to be fully repleted while in the ED.*
- *Begin cooling the severely hyperthermic patient as soon as other life threats and ABCs have been addressed. Delays in treatment can increase morbidity and mortality.*

SECTION XII
METABOLIC AND ENDOCRINE EMERGENCIES

CHAPTER 54
DIABETIC EMERGENCIES

I. Defining Features

  A. **Diabetes mellitus** is defined as fasting blood glucose > 126 mg/dL on 2 separate occasions or a random glucose > 200 mg/dL plus the classic symptoms of hyperglycemia (ie, polyuria, polydipsia).

  B. **Diabetic ketosis** is an intermediary metabolic state between hyperglycemia and ketoacidosis. Patients have an inadequate amount of insulin to provide the necessary energy substrates to the cell. As a result, lipolysis is stimulated to provide ketone bodies that can be used as substrates by the brain and other tissues. The ketone bodies include acetoacetate, acetone, and β-hydroxybutyrate.

  C. **DKA** is defined as blood glucose > 250 mg/dL, serum bicarbonate < 15 mEq/L, ketonemia, and an arterial pH < 7.3. When making the diagnosis of DKA, the physician should attempt to determine what has precipitated the illness. The most **common causes of DKA** are the **"3 I's"**-insulin lack, ischemia (cardiac), and infection.

  D. **Hyperosmolar hyperglycemic state** (HHS) occurs when a hyperglycemic osmotic diuresis causes extreme dehydration. Defining features include a serum glucose > 600 mg/dL, plasma osmolality > 320 mOsm/L, and the absence of ketoacidosis.

II. Epidemiology

  A. Diabetes mellitus is a common disorder, and is present in 6% of the population in the United States.

  B. DKA is present in 5–10% of hospitalized patients. It is the presenting illness of diabetes mellitus in 15–25% of patients. The mortality rate is approximately 5%, and most often is attributable to concomitant illness.

  C. Hyperosmolar hyperglycemic state is most common in elderly individuals. It results in < 1% of diabetes-related hospital admissions, but has a reported mortality rate of 20–60%.

III. Pathophysiology

  A. Hyperglycemia, even in the absence of DKA or HHS, has many deleterious effects. An osmotic diuresis occurs when an elevated glucose level overwhelms the kidneys and begins to pull electrolytes and water into the urine. In the healthy individual, serum glucose of 240 mg/dL is required before glucose is found in the urine. Additionally, hyperglycemia impairs leukocyte function and wound healing, making patients prone to infection. Chronic hyperglycemia causes renal failure, blindness, neuropathy, and atherosclerosis.

B. In DKA, reduced circulatory insulin levels do not allow glucose to reach the intracellular space. In response, the cell stimulates lipolysis, which provides the body with glycerol (substrate for gluconeogenesis) and free fatty acids. Free fatty acids are a precursor to the ketoacids acetoacetate, acetone, and β-hydroxybutyrate. The ketone bodies can be used as an energy source, but when they are present in excess, metabolic acidosis results.

C. The hyperosmolar hyperglycemic state occurs when a prolonged osmotic diuresis from hyperglycemia results in severe dehydration and an elevated serum osmolality.

IV. **Risk Factors.** Diabetes mellitus (history), medication noncompliance, elderly, medications (ie, steroids, diuretics), concomitant (precipitating) illnesses (ie, infection, ischemia, pancreatitis).

V. **Clinical Presentation**

A. **History**

1. **Hyperglycemia.** Patients report polydipsia and polyuria. They may also present with blurry vision due to changes in the shape of the lens, induced by osmotic movements of water. Recovery is spontaneous, but may take up to 1 month.

2. **DKA.** Nausea, vomiting, and abdominal pain may be present. Fatigue and generalized weakness are common. AMS also occurs in severe disease and is closely correlated with a high serum osmolality.

3. **HHS.** AMS is the most common presentation. Additional neurologic complaints include **seizures, hemiparesis, and coma.** Coma is present in only 10% of cases.

KEY COMPLAINTS

*Patients with DKA frequently present with **Kussmaul respirations** in an attempt to eliminate CO_2 and compensate for the underlying metabolic acidosis. These shallow, rapid respirations may be confused with respiratory illness initially until more information is gathered.*

B. **Physical Examination**

1. **Hyperglycemia.** Patients may exhibit evidence of mild dehydration.

2. **DKA.** Vital signs are often abnormal, with tachycardia and tachypnea predominating. If there is severe dehydration or sepsis, hypotension or hyperthermia may be present. Hypothermia is a poor prognostic sign. Fruity odor on the breath due to ketonemia may be present. Evidence of dehydration includes dry mucous membranes, decreased skin turgor, and tachycardia. Urine output may be maintained due to the ongoing osmotic diuresis.

3. **HHS.** Examination findings are similar to those of DKA. Patients usually show evidence of severe dehydration and diminished mental state. A focused neurologic examination is indicated in these patients to detect focal neurologic deficits.

VI. **Differential Diagnosis.** Alcoholic ketoacidosis, sepsis, gastroenteritis, appendicitis, pancreatitis, toxic ingestion (methanol, ethylene glycol, salicylates), renal failure, lactic acidosis, medications (iron, isoniazid).

Concomitant illness. In patients with DKA, the physician should consider and treat any precipitating factors that have caused the condition. The most common causes of DKA are the "3 I's"—insulin lack, ischemia (cardiac), and infection. Patients with hyperosmolar hyperglycemic state have a precipitating infection in 40–60% of cases.

VII. Diagnostic Findings

A. **Laboratory Studies**
1. **Bedside glucose** to rapidly establish the presence of hyperglycemia. The accuracy of these machines is known to decrease at extreme elevations and many will not read values > 600 mg/dL.
2. **Serum electrolytes, glucose, and renal function.** In DKA, the bicarbonate level will be low and there will be an elevated anion gap. The serum potassium level is frequently elevated due to acidemia, causing a shift of potassium into the extracellular space. As treatment is initiated, potassium is drawn back into the cells, exposing a total body potassium that is low. Sodium concentration is also frequently low, usually artificially, because water is drawn out of the intracellular space by the elevated glucose. To account for this, the sodium concentration is corrected by adding 1.6 mEq/L (correction factor) for every 100 mg/dL increase in the glucose. A correction factor of 2.4 mEq/L is more accurate for glucose levels > 400 mg/dL. In HHS, the measured (uncorrected) sodium concentration, glucose level, and BUN are used to calculate the serum osmolality:

$$\text{Serum osmolality (mOsm/L)} = 2(Na) + \text{glucose}/18 + BUN/2.8$$

3. **Urine ketones.** The nitroprusside test used for the detection of ketones on urinalysis identifies acetoacetate and acetone but does not detect β-hydroxybutyrate. In DKA, there is a predominance of β-hydroxybutyrate. Despite some earlier concerns that urine ketones could be falsely normal in DKA because of the predominance of β-hydroxybutyrate, this has not turned out to be the case in clinical practice. Urine ketones can be used as an accurate screen for the presence of serum ketones. However, it should be remembered that as treatment ensues, a shift to acetoacetate and acetone makes urine ketones more positive despite adequate treatment.
4. **ABG.** The pH of a venous blood gas is an accurate estimation of the arterial pH in DKA and can be used to guide management. To determine complex acid-base disorders, an ABG can be obtained, but this test rarely impacts treatment decisions.
5. **Urinalysis and blood cultures.** These tests are indicated when there is suspicion of an underlying infection.

B. **Imaging Studies**
1. **ECG** is obtained to evaluate for signs of hyperkalemia or cardiac ischemia.
2. **CXR** is indicated when clinical symptoms suggest pneumonia or another concomitant cardiopulmonary illness.
3. **Head CT scan** is indicated to rule out precipitating cranial pathology (ie, stroke, intracranial hemorrhage) if the patient has AMS.

C. **Diagnostic Algorithm**

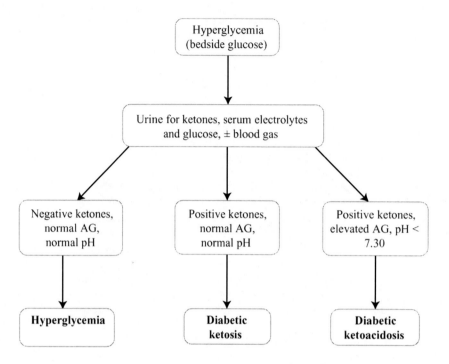

VIII. Treatment

A. **Hyperglycemia (uncomplicated).** Diabetic patients who are noncompliant or inadequately treated are frequently seen in the ED, and there is some controversy regarding the best treatment for these patients once it is determined that they do not have DKA or HHS. Treatment will depend on the degree of elevation of the glucose level and the presence of dehydration. Options include initiating or restarting an oral antihyperglycemic medication (ie, glipizide or metformin); administering IV or oral fluids and rechecking the glucose level; or administering insulin (usually regular insulin SQ) and rechecking the glucose level.

B. **DKA**

1. **IV fluids.** Initial liter over 30–60 minutes. Use 0.9 NS (1–2 L), then switch to 0.45 NS. Be careful to avoid fluid overload in patients with CHF.

2. **Insulin.** IV bolus (0.15 U/kg) is optional. IV infusion of 0.1 U/kg/hr regular insulin. Continue until pH is > 7.3 and anion gap has closed. Switch to D5 0.45 NS when glucose level is < 250 mg/dL.

3. **Potassium.** Treatment depends on the initial potassium level. **K > 5.5 mEq/L:** hold treatment; **K 3.5–5.5 mEq/L:** add 10–20 mEq to each liter of

IV fluids if renal function is normal; **K < 3.5 mEq/L:** add 40 mEq to each liter of IV fluids if renal function is normal.

   4. **Magnesium** repletion as needed.

C. **HHS**

   1. **IV fluids. Average fluid deficit is 9 L.** Give 0.9 NS for the initial resuscitation (1 L). Switch to 0.45 NS at a rate of 200–500 mL/hr. Goal of 3–4 L over the initial 4-hour period. The corrected serum sodium and the serum osmolarity should be gradually returned to normal.
   2. **Insulin.** IV infusion of 0.1 U/kg regular if the K > 3.3 mEq/L.
   3. **Potassium.** Replace in a similar manner to patients with DKA.
   4. **Magnesium** repletion as needed.

IX. Disposition

A. **Admission.** Indicated for patients with DKA and HHS. An ICU setting is appropriate for all patients with HHS. In DKA, AMS or pH < 7.0 generally necessitate ICU admission.

B. **Discharge.** Appropriate for patients with uncontrolled hyperglycemia once DKA and HHS have been excluded. Patients should be given instructions to obtain close follow-up.

CASE PRESENTATION

An 88-year-old woman with confusion is brought to the ED from a nursing home. Records indicate that she is diabetic. A bedside glucose by the triage nurse reads "HIGH."

1. What laboratory and imaging studies would be useful?

  · *Urinalysis for ketones would support a diagnosis of DKA, but can also be positive in HHS. Low pH or serum bicarbonate suggests DKA. High serum osmolality suggests HHS. Blood and urine cultures, leukocyte count. ECG, CXR, and CT scan of head.*

2. The basic metabolic panel reveals bicarbonate 22 mEq/L, glucose 900 mg/dL, BUN 80 mg/dL, creatinine 2.6 mg/dL, sodium 140 mEq/dL, and potassium 5.8 mEq/L. The urine ketone level is weakly positive. What is the diagnosis? How might you begin treatment?

  · *The patient meets the criteria for HHS. Her serum glucose is > 600 mg/dL and serum osmolality is > 320 mOsm/L. Her serum osmolality is 2(140) + 80/2.8 + 900/18 = 359 mOsm/L.*

  · *0.9 NS is the best initial fluid if the patient has a low BP and appears volume-depleted. After 1–2 L NS, switch to 0.45 NS, with a goal to replenish 3–4 L in the first 4 hours following the corrected serum sodium and osmolarity closely to assure appropriate correction.*

SUMMARY POINTS

· *Hyperglycemia causes an osmotic diuresis that may result in dehydration.*

· *Patients with DKA and HHS are treated with IV fluids and insulin. Potassium supplementation should begin as soon as the potassium level is in the normal range.*

· *Both DKA and HHS are often precipitated by another illness, frequently infection. An attempt should be made to search for and treat any precipitating illness.*

· *When treating patients with HHS, it is important to follow sodium and serum osmolality measurements to document return to normal values.*

CHAPTER 55
POTASSIUM DISORDERS

I. Defining Features

A. Potassium (K+) is involved in maintaining the resting cell membrane potential. Small shifts in potassium concentration result in problems with muscle and nerve conduction, leading to potentially life-threatening disorders of the cardiac and neuromuscular systems.

B. The normal plasma concentration of potassium is 3.5–5.5 mEq/L.

C. **Hyperkalemia** is defined as potassium level > 5.5 mEq/L. It can be classified as mild (5.6–6.0 mEq/L), moderate (6.1–7.0 mEq/L), and severe (> 7.0 mEq/L) forms.

D. **Hypokalemia** is defined as potassium level < 3.5 mEq/L. Mild hypokalemia is present when the serum potassium concentration is between 3.1 and 3.4 mEq/L. Moderate (2.5–3.0 mEq/L) and severe (< 2.5 mEq/L) hypokalemia is less common.

II. Epidemiology

A. Hyperkalemia is present in approximately 8% of hospitalized patients. If not treated promptly, two thirds of patients with severe hyperkalemia (> 7.0 mEq/L) will die.

B. Approximately 15% of ED patients are mildly hypokalemic. The percentage increases to 80% in patients taking diuretics.

III. Etiology

A. **Hyperkalemia**
   1. **Pseudohyperkalemia.** RBC hemolysis, extreme leukocytosis, or thrombocytosis.
   2. **Increased intake.**
   3. **Transcellular shifts.** Acidosis, insulin deficiency, medications (digoxin, succinylcholine), cell breakdown (crush injury, burns, tumor lysis).
   4. **Impaired excretion.** Renal failure, addisonian crisis, type 4 renal tubular acidosis, medications (ACE inhibitors, NSAIDs).

B. **Hypokalemia**
   1. **Decreased intake.**
   2. **Transcellular shifts.** β-2 adrenergic stimulation, thyrotoxicosis, insulin, respiratory or metabolic alkalosis, hypokalemic periodic paralysis.

3. **Excessive loss.** Renal loss (diuretics, hyperaldosteronism, Cushing's syndrome, type 1 renal tubular acidosis); GI loss (diarrhea).

IV. Risk Factors (see III)

V. Clinical Presentation

A. **History**
1. Symptoms of hyperkalemia and hypokalemia are vague and frequently include fatigue and generalized weakness.
2. Other features include paresthesias, nausea, vomiting, constipation, abdominal pain, psychosis, or depression.

KEY COMPLAINTS

Patients with abnormal K+ concentrations will have vague complaints, and disorders will not be detected unless the physician has a low threshold for ordering electrolyte levels.

B. **Physical examination.** Muscle weakness is a rare finding and may be recurrent in hyperkalemic or hypokalemic periodic paralysis.

VI. Differential Diagnosis (see III)

RULE OUT

*The most common cause of pseudohyperkalemia is RBC hemolysis. When **hemolysis** is suspected, the physician should obtain an ECG to rapidly assess for changes consistent with true hyperkalemia. Call the laboratory to confirm a hemolyzed sample, and test the K+ level again.*

VII. Diagnostic Findings

A. **Laboratory Studies**
1. **Electrolytes.** An electrolyte panel will detect abnormalities of potassium (turnaround time is approximately 30–40 min).
2. **ABG.** A potassium level can be obtained using many blood gas analyzers. Advantages include a more rapid turnaround time (2 min). However, blood gas analyzers are unable to detect a hemolyzed sample and therefore may overdiagnose hyperkalemia.
3. **Magnesium level.** A magnesium level should be obtained in patients with hypokalemia, because of the difficulty in correcting low potassium in the setting of low magnesium levels.

B. **Imaging Studies: ECG**
1. **Hyperkalemia.** Symmetrical T-wave peaking, P-wave flattening, QRS widening, or a sinusoidal pattern (Figure 55–1). Unfortunately, the ECG lacks sensitivity to detect elevated potassium levels. Only 50–60% of patients with potassium levels > 6.5 mEq/L have any of the above ECG findings.
2. **Hypokalemia.** U-waves, T-wave flattening, and ST segment depression. Dysrhythmias, including VF, may occur in patients with severe hypokalemia or in patients with moderate hypokalemia and a history of cardiac disease.

C. **Diagnostic Algorithm**

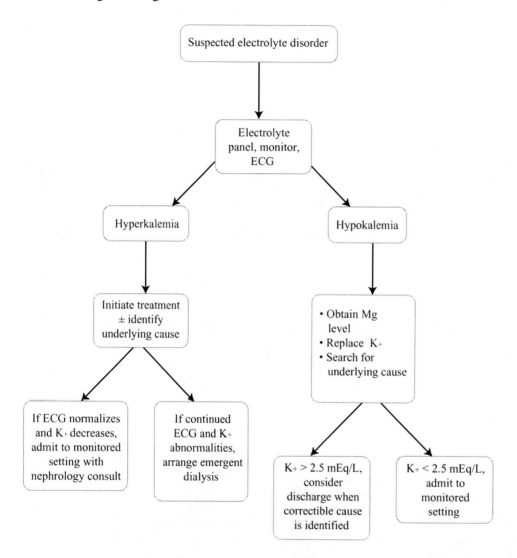

VIII. Treatment

A. **Hyperkalemia**

1. **Cardiac monitor.**

2. **Calcium** given as calcium gluconate 10% (less irritation to peripheral vein) or calcium chloride 10% (3x more calcium). Calcium should be administered whenever QRS widening or dysrhythmias are noted on the ECG. Calcium can be repeated every 5 minutes until the ECG normalizes. The duration of action is 30–60 minutes. Calcium is not indicated in the stable patient when the ECG shows only peaked T waves. ***Avoid giving calcium when treating***

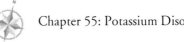

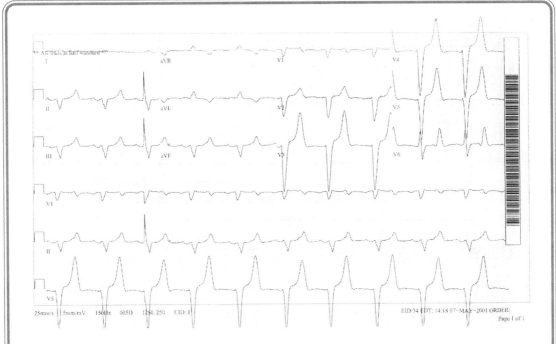

Figure 55–1. ECG obtained in a patient whose potassium level was 7.4 mEq/L. Note the significantly peaked T-waves and QRS complex widening, both of which resolved with treatment.

hyperkalemia with coexisting digoxin toxicity, because intracellular calcium is already elevated in digoxin toxicity. Further administration of calcium may cause asystole and death.

3. **Insulin** 0.1 U/kg IV is administered to shift potassium into the cell via an intracellular messenger. Within 30 minutes, insulin will reduce the potassium level by 0.5–1.0 mEq/L. In patients with normal glucose levels, administer 25–50 g (1/2–1 amp) of **dextrose** IV. An alternate method in stable patients is to add 10 U of regular insulin in 500 mL of D10W and administer this over a 1-hour period.

4. **Nebulized albuterol** shifts potassium back into cells. Albuterol 2.5 mg in 3 mL NS is given every 20 minutes.

5. **Sodium bicarbonate (NaHCO₃)** also shifts potassium back into cells and leads to increased potassium excretion by the kidneys. One amp (50 mEq) infused over a 5-minute period has an onset in 5–10 minutes and lasts 2 hours.

6. **Furosemide** 20–40 mg IV in patients not already taking the drug will reduce potassium levels. The onset is several hours, and the amount of decrease in the potassium level is variable.

7. **Cation exchange resins** like sodium polystyrene sulfonate (Kayexalate) remove up to 1 mEq potassium per gram. A standard dose is 30 g mixed with 50 mL of 20% sorbitol to induce diarrhea. It can be administered rectally (50 g with 200 mL 20% sorbitol), if necessary. Onset is 2–4 hours.

8. **Dialysis.** Consult nephrology early for patients in renal failure. Dialysis is also indicated in refractory cases.

9. Treat the underlying disorder (eg, steroids for addisonian crisis, Fab fragments for digoxin toxicity).

B. **Hypokalemia**

1. **Oral K+** replacement (40 mEq/day) is safe and generally recommended in patients with mild to moderate hypokalemia.

2. **IV K+** if cardiac dysrhythmias or severe hypokalemia are present. The rate of infusion should be no more than 20 mEq/hr, especially when the infusion is to run through a peripheral IV line. Pain and burning with peripheral IV potassium replacement can be treated by slowing down the infusion rate. Avoid IV potassium in patients in renal failure.

3. Treat concomitant hypomagnesemia.

IX. Disposition

A. **Hyperkalemia**

1. **Admission.** Because of the potential for life-threatening arrhythmias, all patients with moderate to severe hyperkalemia (K+ level > 6.0 mEq/L) should be admitted to a hospital bed with a cardiac monitor.

2. **Discharge.** Mild hyperkalemia (K+ level < 6.0 mEq/L) in patients who are asymptomatic and have an identifiable and correctable cause of their hyperkalemia.

B. **Hypokalemia**

1. **Admission.** To a monitored setting if severe hypokalemia (K+ level < 2.5 mEq/L).

2. **Discharge.** Mild to moderate hypokalemia (K+ 2.5–3.4 mEq/L) and no clinical effects of hypokalemia.

CASE PRESENTATION

An 82-year-old woman presents to the ED with a history of a nephrostomy tube. She states that the tube stopped draining 3 days ago and that she now feels weak and nauseous. Her vital signs are within normal limits.

1. *What should be done first?*

   · *Cardiac monitor and IV access. Obtain an ECG. Send blood for electrolyte levels.*

2. *The ECG shows peaked T-waves, small P-waves, and widened QRS complex, all changes compared to an ECG taken 1 month ago. What is the next step?*

   · *Administer treatment for hyperkalemia, including calcium, bicarbonate, insulin, glucose, albuterol, and Kayexalate.*

SUMMARY POINTS

· *Obtain an ECG early in patients with suspected hyperkalemia and never ignore a K+ > 6.0 mEq/L.*

· *Patients with ECG changes consistent with hyperkalemia require prompt treatment to avoid a life-threatening dysrhythmia.*

· *The most common cause of hypokalemia in patients in the ED is diuretic (loop or thiazide) use.*

· *Replacing K+ via the oral route is safe and is the preferred method for cases of mild-moderate hypokalemia.*

CHAPTER 56
THYROID EMERGENCIES

I. Defining Features

A. **Thyrotoxicosis** is a syndrome caused by excessive amounts of circulating thyroid hormone. It includes exogenous administration and endogenous overproduction.

B. **Hyperthyroidism** is defined as an overproduction of thyroid hormone by the thyroid gland. The most common cause of hyperthyroidism is Graves' disease.

C. **Thyroid storm** or **thyrotoxic crisis** represent the extreme manifestation of thyrotoxicosis. Unique findings include mental status changes, fever, and severe tachycardia. The distinction between thyroid storm and thyrotoxicosis is determined clinically. Thyroid storm usually occurs after a precipitating event such as infection or surgery.

D. **Hypothyroidism** is secondary to dysfunction of the thyroid gland in approximately 95% of cases. Secondary hypothyroidism, due to dysfunction of the hypothalamic-pituitary axis, is less common.

E. **Myxedema coma** is a severe manifestation of hypothyroidism that occurs most commonly in elderly patients. The principal clinical features are hypothermia and AMS. Myxedema refers to a dry, nonpitting edema due to the accumulation of mucopolysaccharides in the skin. The term "myxedema coma" is a misnomer because patients may not present with coma or myxedema.

II. Epidemiology

A. Hyperthyroidism affects 2% of women and 0.2% of men. Graves' disease accounts for 80% of cases and is 10 times more common in women.

B. Hypothyroidism is present in 0.5% of the population of the United States, but increases to 2–3% in the elderly population.

C. Thyroid emergencies, thyroid storm, and myxedema coma are uncommon, but will be missed if the physician does not consider the diagnoses.

III. Pathophysiology

A. Thyroid hormone is synthesized within the follicular cells of the thyroid gland. Production begins with the uptake of iodide into the follicular lumen.

B. Thyroglobulin, produced within the follicular cell, is bound to iodine and then coupled to produce the thyroid hormones thyroxine (T_4) and triiodothyronine (T_3).

331

C. Release of thyroid hormone is stimulated by the pituitary hormone, thyroid-stimulating hormone (TSH). High levels of T_4 and T_3 act to suppress production of TSH from the pituitary.

D. Thyroid hormone acts to stimulate cellular protein production, which promotes the function of the body's organs. The net effect is increased bone growth, CNS activity, basal metabolic rate, and O_2 consumption. Metabolic effects include increased glycogenolysis, gluconeogenesis, and lipolysis.

IV. **Risk Factors.** Female (hyperthyroidism) and elderly (hypothyroidism).

V. **Clinical Presentation**

A. **History**
1. **Thyrotoxicosis.** Patients report excessive sweating, heat intolerance, weight loss, palpitations, diarrhea, nervousness, and hair loss.
2. **Thyroid storm.** Patients are more likely to have AMS, seizures, and dyspnea from CHF.
3. **Hypothyroidism.** Patients with hypothyroidism report fatigue and lethargy, dry skin, memory impairment, constipation, cold intolerance, and weight gain.
4. **Myxedema coma.** New onset of AMS in a patient with a history of hypothyroidism should tip off the physician to this diagnosis.

KEY COMPLAINTS

Elderly patients with thyrotoxicosis may not present with the typical signs and symptoms of thyrotoxicosis. **Apathetic hyperthyroidism** *refers to an attenuated end-organ responsiveness that occurs in 10% of elderly patients. In these patients, cardiac manifestations and depressed mental status are more frequent.*

B. **Physical Examination**
1. **Thyrotoxicosis.** Patients usually have a goiter (Figure 56–1). Infiltrative ophthalmologic disease (proptosis) is clinically evident in 50% of patients with Graves' disease. Other findings include velvety skin, palmar erythema, tachycardia, systolic hypertension, and atrial fibrillation.
2. **Thyroid storm.** In addition to the findings of thyrotoxicosis, patients with thyroid storm are frequently febrile and tachycardic.
3. **Hypothyroidism.** Peripheral edema, hair loss, slowed speech, and skin pallor are frequent manifestations.
4. **Myxedema coma.** Hypothermia is universally present without a history of exposure to low ambient temperatures. The temperature is usually < 36°C (96°F), but may be as low as 27°C (80°F).

CLINICAL SKILLS TIP

Examination of the neck may reveal a goiter, thyroid nodule, or a mass that can be confused with a thyroid abnormality. Other masses found in the anterior neck include cervical lymphadenopathy, a thyroglossal duct cyst (midline above thyroid cartilage), and a branchial cleft cyst (lateral over sternocleidomastoid muscle).

VI. **Differential Diagnosis**

A. **Thyrotoxicosis.** Graves' disease (80%), toxic multinodular goiter (5–15%), exogenous administration of thyroid hormone, amiodarone (2% incidence), or thyroiditis (subacute, Hashimoto's, postpartum).

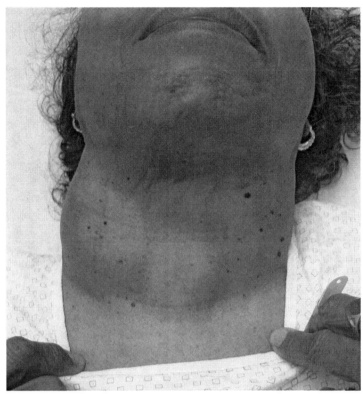

Figure 56–1. Photograph of a patient with a goiter.

B. **Hypothyroidism.** Hashimoto's thyroiditis, radioactive iodine ablation, lithium, or amiodarone (5–15% incidence).

RULE OUT

Both thyroid storm and myxedema coma are commonly due to an underlying precipitating illness/stress in patients with known thyroid disease. The physician must search for and treat precipitating events, especially infectious causes.

VII. Diagnostic Findings

A. **Laboratory Studies**

1. **Free T$_4$** and **TSH levels.** A normal TSH and a free T$_4$ make thyroid disease highly unlikely. A low TSH and high free T$_4$ accurately diagnose thyrotoxicosis. A high TSH and low free T$_4$ is consistent with primary hypothyroidism. It is important to remember that thyroid storm and myxedema coma are clinical diagnoses. No absolute level of TSH or free T$_4$ is diagnostic of thyroid storm or myxedema coma.

2. Other laboratory tests depend on the clinical situation but should include a CBC, electrolytes, renal function tests, urinalysis, and ECG.

B. **Imaging Studies**
   1. Imaging studies depend on the clinical presentation.
   2. ***CT scan with iodinated contrast should be avoided whenever possible*** in patients with thyrotoxicosis for 2 reasons. Rarely, thyroid storm has been precipitated in patients with untreated or poorly controlled thyrotoxicosis who receive iodinated contrast. In addition, iodinated contrast diminishes the effectiveness of nuclear thyroid imaging that is used for both diagnostic and treatment purposes. This effect persists for several weeks after an iodine load.

C. **Diagnostic Algorithm**

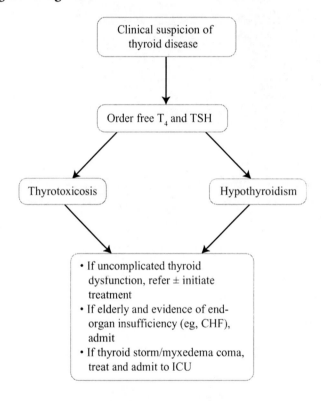

VIII. Treatment

A. **Thyrotoxicosis**
   1. **Thionamides.** These agents (propylthiouracil [PTU] and methimazole) inhibit the synthesis of thyroid hormone. Methimazole (Tapazole) is started at 15 mg BID, with maintenance doses of 5–10 mg/day. Alternatively, PTU is initiated at a dose of 100–150 mg TID, with maintenance doses of 50 mg TID. Up to 40% of patients receiving a thionamide will have remission within 6–18 months of therapy.
   2. **β-blocker therapy** is adjuvant treatment in patients with moderate to severe thyrotoxicosis. The most commonly used agent is oral propanolol 20–40 mg BID to TID.

B. **Thyroid Storm**
1. *Treat the underlying precipitating event.*
2. **PTU** 600–1000 mg PO/PR, then 250 mg q 4 hours.
3. **Inorganic iodine** (1 hr after PTU). Lugol's solution 8 drops PO/PR q 6 hours *or* saturated solution of potassium iodide (SSKI) 5 drops PO/PR q 6 hours. Inorganic iodine serves to block the release and reduce production of thyroid hormone. PTU is given prior to inorganic iodine to ensure that further substrate cannot be used for thyroid hormone production.
4. **Corticosteroids.** Dexamethasone 2 mg IV q 6 hours *or* hydrocortisone 300 mg IV, then 100 mg q 8 hours.
5. **β blocker** (if no evidence of decompensated CHF). Esmolol 250–500 μg/kg IV bolus, then 50–100 μg/kg/min infusion *or* propanolol 60–80 mg PO q 4 hours *or* propanolol 0.5–1 mg IV q 1 hour.
6. **Supportive care** (acetaminophen, cooling blankets, IV fluids).

C. **Hypothyroidism.** For uncomplicated hypothyroidism, replacement therapy with levothyroxine (Synthroid) can be initiated at 50–75 μg/day.

D. **Myxedema Coma**
1. Levothyroxine 200–500 μg IV followed by 75–100 μg/day IV/PO.
2. IV fluids, pressors, mechanical ventilation as needed.
3. Passive rewarming.
4. Hydrocortisone 100 mg IV or dexamethasone 6 mg IV.
5. Treat the underlying precipitating event (consider infection).

IX. **Disposition**

A. **Admission** for patients with concomitant illness such as CHF or dysrhythmia. An ICU setting is indicated for patients with thyroid storm or myxedema coma.

B. **Discharge** patients with uncomplicated thyrotoxicosis or hypothyroidism, with proper instructions, timely referral, and the initiation of treatment.

CASE PRESENTATION

An 86-year-old woman presents to the ED with confusion and is unable to give any history. The list of medications from the nursing home where she lives includes captopril and levothyroxine. Her temperature is 33°C (92°F). You suspect myxedema coma.

1. *What treatment should be provided?*
   - *Levothyroxine 200–500 μg IV. Dexamethasone 6 mg IV. Passive rewarming (active rewarming might precipitate hypotension due to peripheral vasodilation in a volume depleted patient). Fluids and pressors as needed.*

2. *What else is important to consider in this patient?*
   - *An underlying precipitating event such as infection.*

SUMMARY POINTS

- *In a critically ill patient with a goiter or history of hyperthyroidism, consider and treat thyroid storm early.*
- *Myxedema coma should be considered in elderly hypothyroid patients who present with hypothermia and confusion.*
- *Thyroid storm and myxedema coma are clinical diagnoses and do not depend on the absolute levels of TSH and free T_4.*

I. Defining Features

A. **Adrenal insufficiency** is failure of the adrenal cortex to produce adequate amounts of cortisol, aldosterone, or both.

B. **Primary adrenal insufficiency** (Addison's disease) refers to failure of the adrenal gland due to tissue destruction, most frequently from an autoimmune process.

C. **Secondary adrenal insufficiency** is due to inadequate production of adrenocorticotropic hormone (ACTH) from the pituitary gland. Cortisol production is decreased; however, aldosterone secretion is usually intact because its production is stimulated to a much greater extent by angiotensin.

D. **Acute adrenal insufficiency** (addisonian or adrenal crisis) is an emergent condition that occurs in a person who has underlying adrenal suppression and undergoes an acute stress or illness. Some patients have a history of chronic adrenal insufficiency; for others, adrenal crisis is the initial presentation.

E. **Cushing's syndrome** refers to a situation in which there is a symptomatic excess of glucocorticoids. The most common cause is prolonged exogenous steroid administration. **Cushing's disease** is present when Cushing's syndrome is due to excessive ACTH secretion from the pituitary gland.

II. Epidemiology

A. Primary adrenal insufficiency is uncommon, affecting 100 per 1 million persons. Autoimmune adrenalitis accounts for 70% of cases.

B. Secondary adrenal insufficiency due to suppression of the hypothalamic-pituitary-adrenal axis by exogenous steroid administration is the most common cause of adrenal insufficiency.

C. Exogenous administration of steroids is the most common cause of Cushing's syndrome. Endogenous Cushing's syndrome (Cushing's disease) is much less common, occurring in 13 per 1 million persons.

III. Pathophysiology

A. Cortisol secretion is regulated by ACTH, which, in turn, is regulated by corticotropin-releasing hormone (CRH) from the hypothalamus. Aldosterone secretion is regulated by the renin-angiotensin system.

B. Adrenal insufficiency due to exogenous steroid administration is based on the dose and duration of treatment. Administration of steroid for < 2 weeks or doses < 5 mg per day are unlikely to result in adrenal insufficiency.

C. HIV infection results in adrenal insufficiency at a much higher rate than in the general population. Up to 25% of patients with HIV have inadequate adrenal reserves. Contributing factors in HIV patients include the human immunodeficiency virus itself, opportunistic infections, and medications.

D. When not due to exogenous steroid administration, Cushing's syndrome is due to an ACTH-producing tumor of the pituitary (70%), adrenal gland (15%), or other (15%). Other tumors producing ACTH include pancreatic cancer, small cell lung carcinoma, and carcinoid tumors.

IV. Risk Factors

A. **Adrenal Insufficiency**
  1. **Primary (Addison's disease).** HIV infection, metastatic cancer (lung, breast, leukemia), infection (bacterial, fungal, viral, TB), sarcoidosis, or sepsis.
  2. **Secondary.** Steroid administration (withdrawal), pituitary tumors, or trauma.

B. **Cushing's Syndrome**
  1. **Exogenous.** Steroid administration (prolonged).
  2. **Endogenous (Cushing's disease).** Women aged 20–40 years or malignancy (lung, pancreatic).

V. Clinical Presentation

A. **History**
  1. **Adrenal insufficiency.** Patients report fatigue, nausea, vomiting, abdominal pain, lightheadedness, or diarrhea.
  2. **Cushing's syndrome.** Patients complain of fatigue and weakness. Proximal muscle weakness is present in 60% of cases. Menstrual irregularities and osteoporosis are also common.

KEY COMPLAINTS

Acute adrenal insufficiency should be considered in any patient who presents in shock.

B. **Physical Examination**
  1. **Adrenal insufficiency.** Patients with primary adrenal insufficiency will present with hyperpigmentation of the skin due to increased levels of circulating ACTH. This finding is present in 98% of these patients. Acute adrenal insufficiency is characterized by mental status changes, hypotension, and tachycardia. Hypothermia may be present, but fever can also be seen in the setting of a concurrent infection.
  2. **Cushing's syndrome.** Obesity (truncal), moon facies, buffalo hump, hypertension, hirsutism, and skin striae are common abnormalities.

VI. Differential Diagnosis

A. **Adrenal insufficiency.** Shock (cardiovascular, septic), dehydration, or influenza.

B. **Cushing's syndrome.** Polycystic ovary disease, depression, diabetes mellitus, or hypothyroidism.

RULE OUT

Acute adrenal insufficiency (addisonian crisis) is usually precipitated by an underlying illness (sepsis, myocardial ischemia, trauma). It is important to identify and treat both adrenal insufficiency and the underlying illness.

VII. Diagnostic Findings

A. **Laboratory Studies**

1. **Adrenal insufficiency**

   a. **Electrolytes.** Hyponatremia in 90%, hyperkalemia in 64%, and hypercalcemia in 6–33%. In secondary adrenal insufficiency, electrolyte levels are less likely to be abnormal because aldosterone production is not impaired.

   b. **CBC.** Anemia is present in 40%. An elevated WBC count suggests infection.

   c. **Glucose.** Hypoglycemia is present in two thirds of patients.

   d. **Cortisol and ACTH level.** A random serum cortisol level < 15 mcg/dL in an acutely ill patient will be diagnostic of adrenal insufficiency in most cases and can be performed in the ED. An ACTH level can be drawn, but the results are rarely available in the ED.

   e. **Cosyntropin (ACTH) stimulation test.** Used to test the responsiveness of the adrenal glands to ACTH 0.25 mg IV. In a patient with normal adrenal function, a repeat cortisol level at 30–60 minutes and 6 hours later should be twice the baseline level. In adrenal insufficiency, serum cortisol levels fail to increase after ACTH administration. This test is *infrequently* performed in the ED.

2. **Cushing's syndrome**

   a. Hyperglycemia due to insulin resistance is commonly present.

   b. A hypokalemic metabolic alkalosis is present in some patients with increased ACTH production.

   c. A random serum cortisol is not useful due to wide diurnal ranges.

B. **Imaging studies.** No imaging studies are routinely indicated for adrenal insufficiency or Cushing's syndrome, although a CXR, ECG, or head CT scan may be useful, depending on the clinical presentation (ie, AMS, suspected pneumonia).

C. **Diagnostic Algorithm (see page 339)**

VIII. Treatment

A. **Acute Adrenal Insufficiency**

1. **IV 0.9 NS** as needed for hypotension. Persistent hypotension may require vasopressors.

2. **Dextrose** is administered in the setting of hypoglycemia. An ampule of D50 is given initially and repeated as needed.

3. **Glucocorticoids.** Dexamethasone 4–6 mg IV q 6 hours or hydrocortisone 100 mg IV q 8 hours. Dexamethasone is preferred because, unlike hydrocortisone, it does not interfere with the cortisol response to ACTH or the cortisol assay. If hydrocortisone is given, the results of the ACTH (cosyntropin) stimulation test will be difficult to interpret.

Diagnostic Algorithm

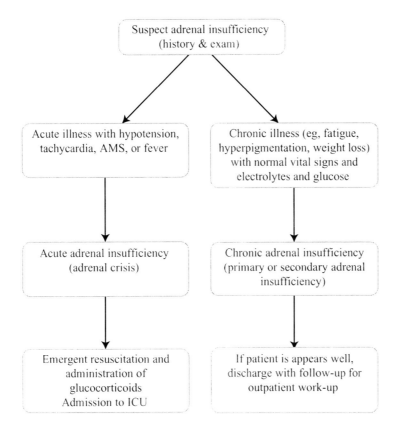

4. **Mineralocorticoids.** In primary adrenal insufficiency, administer fludrocortisone acetate (Florinef) 0.05–0.2 mg.
5. Correct electrolyte abnormalities.
6. Treat the underlying cause (eg, infection).

B. **Cushing's Syndrome**
1. The treatment depends on the underlying cause.
2. It is not the role of the emergency physician to make the definitive diagnosis of Cushing's syndrome but to suspect the condition and refer the patient for further testing and treatment.

IX. Disposition

A. **Admission.** All patients with acute adrenal insufficiency require hospital admission. Most patients will require an ICU setting.

B. **Discharge.** Patients with chronic symptoms of either adrenal insufficiency or Cushing's syndrome may be discharged with close follow-up with a primary physician and endocrinologist.

CASE PRESENTATION

A 37-year-old man presents to the ED with confusion. His girlfriend states that he has been feeling ill for the past 2 days with cough, but has no prior illnesses or medical problems. His BP is 70/40 mm Hg, HR is 130 beats/min, and temperature is 34°C (93°F). Bedside glucose is determined to be 34 mg/dL.

1. *What rapid interventions are required?*
   - *Establish IV access with large bore lines. Administer NS boluses (2 L initially). Administer 1 ampule D50.*
2. *The patient's vital signs improve with fluids, and his glucose level is corrected. What other clues might suggest adrenal insufficiency?*
   - *Hyperpigmentation of the skin, electrolyte abnormalities (hyponatremia, hyperkalemia), chronic steroid use, or history of HIV or HIV risk factors.*

SUMMARY POINTS

- *Adrenal crisis is a medical emergency and must be recognized and treated promptly.*
- *Administration of steroids, NS, and vasopressors agents (as needed) should be instituted when adrenal crisis is suspected.*
- *The preferred steroid for adrenal insufficiency is dexamethasone because it does not interfere with the cosyntropin stimulation test.*

SECTION XIII

HEMATOLOGIC AND ONCOLOGIC EMERGENCIES

CHAPTER 58
ONCOLOGIC EMERGENCIES

I. Defining Features

A. Oncologic emergencies occur in patients with recurrence of a previously diagnosed malignancy, complications of treatment, or signs and symptoms that may lead to a new diagnosis of cancer.

B. Emergency physicians must be aware of the common complications associated with malignancies and their available treatments.

II. Epidemiology

A. Improved cancer treatment has increased the number of survivors who may present to the ED with complications or recurrence.

B. The incidence of pulmonary embolus, superior vena cava (SVC) syndrome, infection, neutropenia, hypercalcemia, cauda equina syndrome, and tumor lysis syndrome are all increased in cancer patients.

C. Pain, vomiting, and dehydration are common presenting complaints of the cancer patient.

III. Etiology

A. Cancer patients have an underlying hypercoagulable state that predisposes them to **thromboembolism.** This is particularly common in patients with brain tumors, where the incidence is about 25%.

B. **Hypercalcemia** occurs in about 10–20% of patients with cancer. It occurs most commonly in cancers associated with bone (multiple myeloma), bony metastasis (breast, lung, prostate, renal), or cancers that secrete parathyroid-like substances (lung) or osteoclastic factors (lymphomas).

C. **Tumor lysis syndrome** is a metabolic complication occurring after treatment of neoplastic disorders. It is more common in cancers with high cell turnover (leukemia and lymphoma) as well as in patients with a high tumor burden. Patients develop acute renal failure, hyperuricemia, hyperphosphatemia, hyperkalemia, and hypocalcemia.

D. **SVC syndrome** results from obstruction (by tumor or thrombosis) of blood flow to the SVC, resulting in elevation of venous pressures in the lungs, neck, face, upper extremities, and brain.

E. **Neutropenia** occurs secondary to the cytotoxic effects of chemotherapy on the bone marrow. It should be suspected in any patient who has recently received chemotherapy.

IV. **Risk Factors.** Hypercalcemia (multiple myeloma, bony metastasis, lung cancer, lymphoma), SVC syndrome (lung cancer, lymphoma), tumor lysis syndrome (recent chemotherapy), and neutropenia (recent chemotherapy).

V. **Clinical Presentation**

A. **History**
1. Patients with a pulmonary embolus may present with shortness of breath, pleuritic chest pain, tachypnea, or signs of DVT.
2. Patients with SVC syndrome will often complain of headache, hoarseness, shortness of breath, dysphagia, facial and chest fullness, or facial swelling. Their symptoms are often exacerbated by bending over or lying down.
3. Patients with mildly elevated calcium levels are usually asymptomatic; however, with increasing levels, patients may complain of nausea, vomiting, constipation, hypertension, lethargy, or AMS.
4. Patients with tumor lysis syndrome most often present with symptoms associated with acute renal failure. They may have weakness, dizziness, nausea, or vomiting.
5. Neutropenic patients often present to the ED with weakness and dehydration. Associated fever is a medical emergency.

KEY COMPLAINTS

Patients with shortness of breath or hypoxia and a history of malignancy have a pulmonary embolus until proven otherwise.

B. **Physical Examination**
1. Patients with pulmonary embolus often exhibit hypoxia, tachypnea, and tachycardia.
2. Patients with SVC syndrome have edema and erythema of their upper chest and face. They also have dilated superficial veins (upper extremities, upper trunk, neck, and face), respiratory compromise, or AMS secondary to significant pulmonary or brain edema.
3. With very high calcium levels (> 14 mg/dL), patients may be lethargic or have AMS.
4. Patients with tumor lysis syndrome may have edema secondary to renal failure.
5. Chemotherapy patients with fever or infectious symptoms should have a thorough physical examination, looking for possible sources. Rectal temperature and examination should be avoided in patients who may be neutropenic.

VI. **Differential Diagnosis**

A. **Shortness of breath.** Airway obstruction by tumor, malignant pleural effusion, malignant pericardial effusion, pulmonary embolus, SVC syndrome.

B. **AMS.** Hypercalcemia, hyponatremia (SIADH), CNS malignancy, metastasis, infection, SVC syndrome.

C. **Acute renal failure.** Tumor lysis syndrome, obstructive uropathy from tumor.

D. **Fever.** Focal bacterial infection, sepsis, neutropenia.

VII. **Diagnostic Findings**
   A. **Laboratory Studies**
      1. **Chemistry** should be assessed on all patients with vague complaints, vomiting, or dehydration. Chemistry should also be ordered on those at risk for hypercalcemia (bony metastasis) and tumor lysis syndrome (recent cancer treatment). Patients with tumor lysis syndrome present with acute renal failure in the presence of hyperuricemia (> 15 mg/dL), hyperphosphatemia (> 8 mg/dL), hyperkalemia, and hypocalcemia.
      2. **CBC** should be obtained on all patients to assess for neutropenia (absolute neutrophil count < 500/mm^3), anemia, and thrombocytopenia. The absolute neutrophil count is determined by multiplying the total WBC count times the percentage of neutrophils plus bands.
   B. **Imaging Studies**
      1. **CXR** should be performed on all patients with shortness of breath or SVC syndrome.
      2. **ECG** should be performed on all patients with cardiopulmonary complaints and those with possible electrolyte abnormalities.
      3. **Chest CT angiogram** is indicated in patients with possible PE or SVC syndrome.
   C. **Diagnostic Algorithm (see page 346)**
VIII. **Treatment**
   A. **PE** should be treated with anticoagulation therapy (heparin or LMW heparin). The presence of CNS malignancy or metastasis is not an absolute contraindication to anticoagulation. An inferior vena cava filter may be an alternative.
   B. **Hypercalcemia** is treated in the ED with IV fluid administration. Levels > 13 mg/dL usually require treatment. An initial bolus of 1–2 L NS is initiated. Loop diuretics (furosemide) can also be given in a dose of 40–80 mg IV. Bisphosphonates may also be used, but their maximum effect does not occur for 2–4 days. Hemodialysis may be indicated in severe cases.
   C. **Tumor lysis syndrome** is treated with IV hydration (NS), loop diuretics, and allopurinol. Hemodialysis may be needed in patients with poor response to diuretics or with fluid overload.
   D. **SVC syndrome** is treated in the ED with IV steroids (dexamethasone 10 mg IV) and furosemide IV in an attempt to reduce venous pressures. Patients with cardiac or respiratory compromise or CNS dysfunction may require emergent endotracheal intubation or radiation therapy.
   E. **Neutropenic fever** is treated in the ED with ceftazidime 2 g IV. Vancomycin should be added for patients with sepsis, known methicillin-resistant *Staphylococcus aureus* (MRSA), or indwelling venous catheters.

Diagnostic Algorithm

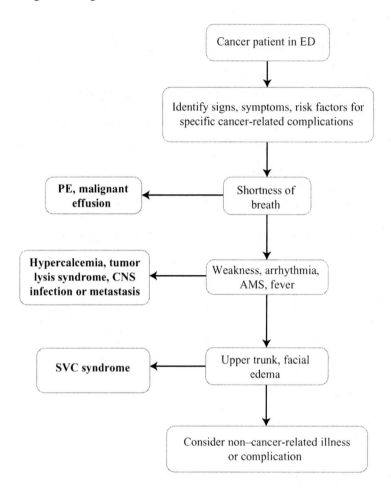

IX. Disposition

A. **Admission.** Neutropenic patients should be admitted to a reverse isolation room. Unlike an isolation room that has negative pressure and keeps infectious agents (eg, TB) from escaping, a reverse isolation room provides positive pressure (airflow) and keeps infectious agents from entering the room and further placing the immunocompromised patient at risk. Patients with severe electrolyte abnormalities or renal failure should be admitted to a monitored setting.

B. **Discharge.** Patients with correctable electrolyte abnormalities without renal failure can be safely discharged after follow-up has been arranged.

CASE PRESENTATION

A 50-year-old woman is brought to the ED by her family. She has been less responsive over the past few hours. The family notes that she had been doing well until 2 days ago when she received her first chemotherapy dose for lymphoma.

1. *After performing ABCs and a thorough history and physical examination, what tests do you want to order?*
   - *Electrolytes and renal function. CBC to assess for pancytopenia. ECG to assess for arrhythmia or electrolyte abnormality. Head CT scan to rule out mass or bleed.*
2. *Laboratory results reveal acute renal failure with elevated potassium and low calcium. What other tests and therapies would you initiate?*
   - *Obtain a phosphate and uric acid for suspected tumor lysis syndrome. Administer IV hydration and diuresis. Treat hyperkalemia and prepare for hemodialysis. ICU admission is indicated.*

SUMMARY POINTS

- *Pulmonary embolus should be considered in any patient presenting to the ED with hypoxia or shortness of breath and a history of malignancy.*
- *Electrolyte abnormalities should be considered in all patients with malignancy and nonspecific symptoms.*
- *Patients undergoing chemotherapy who present with fever should be considered neutropenic until proven otherwise.*

CHAPTER 59
SICKLE CELL EMERGENCIES

I. Defining Features

A. **Sickle cell anemia** is an inherited chronic disease characterized by abnormal hemoglobin synthesis and painful vaso-occlusive events (crises). It affects every organ system.

B. Patients present to the ED with symptoms of either acute vaso-occlusive events or complications and sequelae from vaso-occlusion. Some symptoms are potentially life threatening.

C. Patients with sickle cell disease must be adequately treated for pain. In addition, the emergency physician should diagnose and treat the precipitants of crises, life-threatening complications, and other coexistent diseases.

II. Epidemiology

A. **Sickle cell disease** is seen primarily in persons of African, Mediterranean, Middle Eastern, and Indian descent.

B. In the United States, **sickle cell trait** is diagnosed in approximately 8% of African Americans. Sickle cell disease is seen in approximately 0.3% of the population.

C. The life expectancy for men with sickle cell disease is 42 years and for women 48 years.

III. Pathophysiology

A. The basic defect is an abnormal hemoglobin (Hb) molecule. Normal Hb consists of 2 pairs of α and β globin. A single amino acid substitution (valine for glutamine) on the β-globin gene results in sickle hemoglobin (Hb S).

B. Individuals with 1 abnormal β-globin gene (heterozygous AS) have **sickle cell trait** and rarely have clinical manifestations of disease. Individuals with 2 abnormal β-globin genes (homozygous SS) have **sickle cell disease.** Other Hb abnormalities such as Hb C and thalassemia also occur in patients with Hb S.

C. Hb S polymerizes under biologic stress (ie, low O_2 state) and deforms the RBC, making it less able to pass through small blood vessels and ultimately resulting in vaso-occlusion, hemolysis, and end-organ damage. RBCs have a shorter half-life in sickle cell patients.

D. **Vaso-occlusion** is directly responsible for most acute manifestations of sickle cell disease.

1. **Acute pain crisis** (bone or joint pain).
2. **Infection.** Sickle cell patients are more prone to infection due to the loss of splenic function by age 6 months. Bone, pulmonary, and CNS infections are more common. Meningitis is 200 times more common in children with sickle cell disease. Causative organisms include *Streptococcus pneumoniae, Haemophilus influenzae, Staphylococcus aureus, Escherichia coli, and Salmonella.*
3. **Acute chest syndrome** is the most common cause of death in sickle cell patients, with a 2–14% mortality rate. It is more common in children but more severe in adults, and is characterized by fever, chest pain, respiratory symptoms, and an infiltrate seen on CXR.
4. **CVA** occurs in 11% of sickle cell patients by age 20, with the mean age of onset 6 years. There is a high recurrence rate, and seizures are commonly associated.
5. **Splenic sequestration.** Patients experience a rapid decrease in steady state Hb and have an enlarging spleen. This condition may be rapidly fatal, is most commonly seen in children, and has a mortality rate of 12%.
6. **Aplastic crisis.** The bone marrow stops producing RBCs in patients with folic acid deficiency or with Parvovirus B19 infection.
7. **Priapism** is painful failure of penile detumescence. Peaks occur in patients aged 5–13 and 21–29 years. When prolonged, impotence secondary to vascular damage may result.

IV. **Risk Factors.** Precipitants of crises include low O_2 states, dehydration, cold exposure, trauma, pregnancy, infection.

V. **Clinical Presentation**

A. **History**
1. Patients will generally present with pain that is usually moderate to severe and involves the extremities, back, chest, and abdomen. Ask the patient to characterize the pain as typical vs. atypical in relation to previous painful episodes.
2. Patients frequently have low-grade temperatures. Fever > 38.3°C (101°F) should prompt a search for an infectious precipitant.
3. Ask about prior episodes, possible precipitants, previous complications, analgesic regimen, and routine care.

KEY COMPLAINTS

Acute chest syndrome should be suspected in patients with shortness of breath, fever, and cough.

B. **Physical Examination**
1. Note the presence of abnormal vital signs, particularly fever, tachycardia, tachypnea, and hypotension. These signs may indicate complications of sickle cell or an additional independent acute process.
2. Determine hydration status.
3. Sickle cell patients are frequently mildly jaundiced due to rapid turnover of RBCs.

4. Chest auscultation to ascertain the presence of rales, rhonchi, or wheezing.
5. Abdominal examination, noting either splenomegaly or hepatomegaly.
6. Extremities for signs of infection, ulceration, or poor circulation.
7. Neurologic examination in patients with new neurologic complaints.

VI. **Differential Diagnosis.** Seizure, cholecystitis, pneumonia, PE, MI, cellulitis, osteomyelitis, septic arthritis

RULE OUT

Osteomyelitis and septic arthritis *may be mistaken for typical bone and joint pain. A thorough examination of the extremities should be performed in an undressed patient to rule out these infections.*

VII. **Diagnostic Findings**
  A. **Laboratory Studies**
    1. **CBC.** The Hb level is typically between 5 and 9 gm/dL. Compare to previous levels and note any acute decreases. Leukocytosis (12–20 K/mm^3) is common and not necessarily indicative of infection.
    2. **Reticulocyte count** is elevated during an acute pain crisis. Consider an aplastic crisis if the reticulocyte count is low.
    3. **Liver function tests** are indicated for patients with abdominal pain and/or jaundice.
    4. **Urinalysis** to assess for infection that may have precipitated the acute pain crisis.
    5. **Blood and urine cultures** if infection is suspected.
  B. **Imaging Studies**
    1. **CXR** when respiratory signs or symptoms are present or the patient has a fever.
    2. **Abdominal CT scan** in patients with significant abdominal pain.
    3. **Head CT scan** in patients with new neurologic symptoms to assess for possible CVA.
  C. **Procedures: Exchange Transfusion**
    1. This procedure may be useful during certain crises (priapism, CVA) when the hematocrit is > 35%. Removal of the abnormal Hb followed by replacement with a donor blood transfusion reduces vaso-occlusion.
    2. The procedure is simple to perform and involves removing blood (approximately 500 mL in an adult) through one IV line while administering saline in a second line. When the blood is removed, the patient is given the donor blood transfusion.
  D. **Diagnostic Algorithm (see page 351)**
VIII. **Treatment**
  A. Treat identifiable precipitants of pain.
  B. Begin analgesics promptly. Reassess frequently using pain scales. Opiates are first line therapy. Narcotic addiction does not result from treating pain.
    1. **Moderate to severe pain.** Morphine 0.1–0.15 mg/kg/dose IV, **or** hydromorphone 0.01–0.02 mg/kg/dose IV, **or** ketorolac 30 mg IV.
    2. **Mild pain.** Acetaminophen 1 g (peds: 15 mg/kg/dose) PO q 4 hr, **or** codeine 0.5–1 mg/kg/dose PO, **or** ibuprofen 800 mg (peds: 5–10 mg/kg/dose) PO q 8 hr.

Diagnostic Algorithm

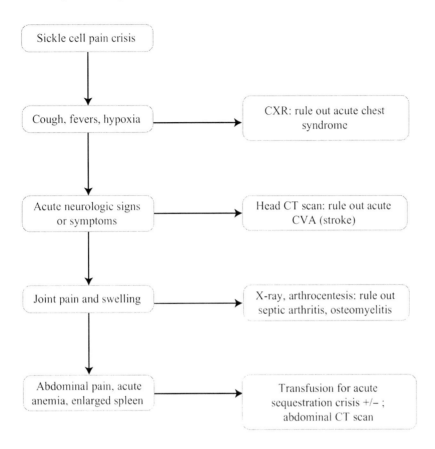

C. Use adjunctive agents such as hydroxyzine, prochlorperazine, or diphenhydramine for nausea or pruritus from morphine.

D. Replace fluids liberally; orally if possible. If the patient is hemodynamically stable and IV fluids are necessary, rehydrate with 0.45% NS.

E. Antibiotics are indicated only for patients with suspected infection (eg, osteomyelitis or acute chest syndrome).

F. Consider **simple blood transfusion** in patients with symptomatic anemia, sequestration crisis, hemolysis, or aplastic crisis. Consider **exchange transfusion** in acute chest syndrome, CVA, or priapism.

IX. Disposition

A. **Admission.** Refractory pain, acute chest syndrome, CVA or TIA, unexplained fever > 38.3°C (101°F) or focal infection, aplastic crisis, splenic sequestration, or refractory priapism.

B. **Discharge** when pain control is achieved and provide good outpatient follow-up.

CASE PRESENTATION

A 25-year-old man with a history of sickle cell anemia presents with a complaint of having had intermittent pain in his chest, back, arms, and legs for the past week. He has come to the ED twice over the past week, but says he is not feeling better. A nurse informs you that "he's always here." The patient states that he has taken Vicodin at home with no relief, and his chest pain is getting worse.

1. *What will you look for on physical examination?*
   - *Volume status, respiratory signs (rate, pulse oximetry, lung sounds), fever, abdominal or flank tenderness, or signs of infection.*

2. *His vital signs are BP 120/70 mm Hg, HR 120 beats/min, RR 24 breaths/min, temperature 37.9°C (100.2°F), and pulse oximeter 90%. He has rales in the right lung field, and the CXR shows an infiltrate. You make the diagnosis of acute chest syndrome. What is your next step?*
   - *O_2, hydration, pain control, antibiotics, and admission to ICU or monitored setting.*

SUMMARY POINTS

- *Control pain aggressively.*
- *Search for precipitants of painful events.*
- *Despite advances in treatment, patients with sickle cell anemia still have a decreased survival rate. Complications of the disease must be considered.*
- *Have a low threshold for admission when patients may have an occult infection.*

CHAPTER 60

ANTICOAGULANT THERAPY AND ITS COMPLICATIONS

I. Defining Features

  A. Anticoagulant therapies commonly used in the ED include **heparin, LMW heparin,** and **warfarin** (Coumadin).

  B. These agents are used frequently in patients with ACS, PE, venous thromboembolism, valve replacement, and AF.

  C. The risk of stroke in patients with AF is 5% a year. This risk is reduced by 70% with use of chronic warfarin therapy. Patients with AF without structural heart disease are at low risk for stroke and require only aspirin.

  D. When administered in the appropriate clinical setting, anticoagulant medications are lifesaving. Despite proper usage, bleeding complications are common.

  E. **Heparin-induced thrombocytopenia** (HIT) is due to IgG antibody that binds platelets and results in their activation, creating both thrombocytopenia and thrombosis. Onset of HIT is generally 5–12 days after onset of therapy.

II. Epidemiology

  A. In patients taking oral warfarin therapy, 15% will suffer a bleeding complication, 5% will develop a major bleeding complication, and approximately 1% will develop a fatal complication annually.

  B. The risk of a bleeding complication from heparin use is approximately 6%, and is no different than the risk of bleeding from LMW heparin.

  C. The incidence of HIT is 1–3% in patients treated with unfractionated heparin, but is much less common in patients taking LMW heparin.

III. Pathophysiology

  A. Heparin is a mixture of glycosaminoglycan chains of varying lengths that bind antithrombin III, resulting in inhibition of thrombin and coagulation factors IX and X.

  B. LMW heparin is prepared from unfractionated heparin and includes only short chains. LMW heparin binds to antithrombin III but inhibits only factor X. LMW heparin is advantageous because it has a more predictable dose response and greater bioavailability.

  C. Warfarin inhibits the cofactor of vitamin K, which normally allows for the production of anticoagulants (protein C and S) and coagulants (factors II, VII, IX, and X).

D. Because protein C has a half-life that is much shorter than the half-life of factors II, VII, IX, and X, a hypercoagulable state is seen first, necessitating the coadministration of unfractionated or LMW heparin until warfarin has reached its full anticoagulant potential after 5 days.

IV. Risk Factors

A. **Bleeding from warfarin.** INR > 4.0, > age 75, prior history of GI bleed, hypertension, cerebrovascular disease, renal insufficiency, alcoholism, known malignancy.

B. **Bleeding from heparin.** Increasing dose, degree of elevation of PTT, recent surgery or trauma, renal failure, use of another anticoagulant (aspirin, glycoprotein inhibitor), > age 70.

V. Clinical Presentation

A. **History**

1. Consider why the patient is taking the anticoagulant. Patients who have had a recent PE or a prosthetic heart valve have a greater need for anticoagulation than a patient with isolated AF. This information is frequently useful when there is a severe bleeding complication that requires reversal of anticoagulation.

2. GI bleeding is a common complication and may not be noticed by the patient. Inquire about blood in the stool or melena.

3. Any history of trauma, especially head trauma, should be taken very seriously in the patient on anticoagulant medications. Intracranial bleeding is much more likely in these patients after minor trauma.

4. Administration of additional medications to patients already taking warfarin will either increase or decrease the anticoagulant effects. Medications that increase the INR include antibiotics, NSAIDs, prednisone, cimetidine, amiodarone, and propanolol. A decrease in INR is induced by carbamazepine, haloperidol, and ranitidine.

KEY COMPLAINTS

Any patient taking warfarin who suffers minor head trauma with or without a headache should have a head CT scan to rule out intracranial hemorrhage.

B. **Physical Examination**

1. **Vital signs.** Abnormalities that suggest hypovolemia and shock should be addressed immediately in any patient with a bleeding complication.

2. **HEENT.** Look for any evidence of head trauma. Also, sublingual or neck hematomas are airway emergencies, especially if they are expanding.

3. **Cardiovascular examination.** Listen for murmurs or an irregular heart rhythm that suggests AF.

4. **Abdominal examination.** Tenderness may suggest intraperitoneal hemorrhage. Rectal examination is indicated to diagnose GI bleeding.

5. **Skin.** Patients recently started on warfarin may develop coumadin skin necrosis due to capillary thrombosis in the subcutaneous tissues. Patients with HIT may also develop similar skin lesions. Ecchymosis and hematomas should be noted.

VI. Differential Diagnosis

A. **Bleeding.** Intracranial, sublingual, pericardial, GI, splenic or liver, or retroperitoneal.

B. **Skin lesion.** Heparin-induced thrombocytopenia, Coumadin skin necrosis.

VII. Diagnostic Findings

A. **Laboratory Studies**

1. **CBC** is used to detect anemia and thrombocytopenia.

2. Pro-time (PT), INR, PTT.

B. **Imaging studies.** Lower the threshold to obtain an imaging study to detect bleeding in patients on anticoagulant medications.

C. **Diagnostic Algorithm**

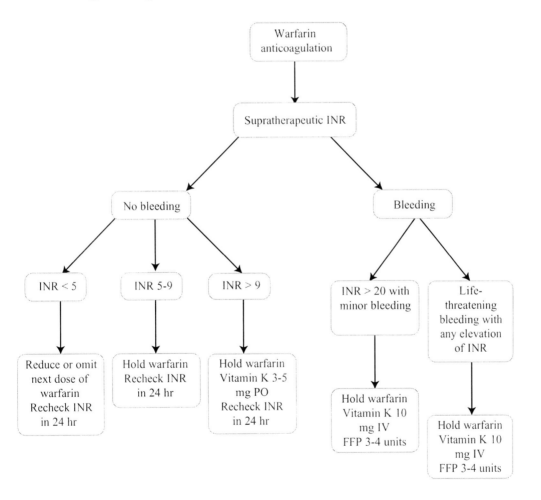

VIII. Treatment

A. Heparin

1. **Therapy.** An 80 IU/kg bolus followed by continuous infusion of 18 IU/kg/hr. For patients receiving fibrinolytic therapy or a glycoprotein inhibitor, the dose is reduced (60 IU/kg bolus, 12 IU/kg/hr infusion). PTT is measured 6 hours after initiation of the bolus, with a goal of 1.5 to 2.5 times normal.

2. **Bleeding complication.** When clinically significant bleeding is present, stop the heparin infusion. Anticoagulation lasts up to 3 hours after the infusion is stopped. If major bleeding occurs, administer protamine (1 mg/100 IU heparin) IV, given slowly over 1–3 minutes to a maximum dose of 50 mg.

B. LMW Heparin

1. **Therapy.** Enoxaparin (Lovenox) 1.0 mg/kg SC q 12 hours. Dosing in morbidly obese patients or those in renal failure may vary.

2. **Bleeding complication.** Protamine (1 mg/1 mg enoxaparin) can be administered, but reversal is not as effective as with unfractionated heparin.

C. Warfarin

1. **Therapy.** Initiate doses of 5 mg daily. Lower doses are usually required in the elderly, in patients with liver disease, or those with poor nutrition. The therapeutic range for the INR depends on the indication. Patients with mechanical valves are considered therapeutic at INR levels of 2.5–3.5, while other patients (eg, with AF) are therapeutic at INR levels of 2–3.

2. **Bleeding complication or supratherapeutic INR** (see Diagnostic Algorithm). IV administration of **vitamin K** is most rapid, with onset within 1–2 hours (compared with 6–10 hr for oral dosing) but carries a small risk of anaphylaxis. High doses of vitamin K (10 mg) may result in warfarin resistance (up to 1 week) when it is time to restart anticoagulation therapy. **FFP** is used as the first-line agent for reversal of bleeding due to warfarin. The initial dose is 2–4 units.

IX. Disposition

A. **Admission.** A patient requiring anticoagulation therapy is usually admitted to the hospital for heparin coadministration with warfarin. This is to prevent the hypercoagulable state that occurs in the early phase of warfarin treatment. Patients with a supratherapeutic INR and bleeding require admission. Patients with a supratherapeutic INR who have a poor social situation or are at risk of falling should also be admitted.

B. **Discharge.** A patient with no other admission indications who requires anticoagulation may be discharged with warfarin and a 5-day course of LMW heparin injections. Close follow-up should be arranged, and the patient must be knowledgeable about self-injecting. Patients with supratherapeutic INR without bleeding are frequently safe to discharge if they are not at increased risk of falling.

CASE PRESENTATION

A 75-year-old man presents to the ED after falling in his home. He states that he struck his head but did not lose consciousness. He denies any vomiting, but states that he has a mild headache. Review of his medications reveals that he takes warfarin for AF. Physical examination reveals a small abrasion to the forehead.

1. *How do you want to proceed with the work-up for this patient?*
   - *PT/INR and head CT scan without contrast.*
2. *The patient's INR returns, at 3.0. Head CT scan reveals an intracranial hemorrhage. How do you want to proceed now?*
   - *Administer vitamin K 10 mg IV slowly and FFP 4 units.*
   - *Consult neurosurgery.*

SUMMARY POINTS

- *In the anticoagulated patient, have a low threshold to obtain imaging studies following trauma.*
- *When initiating warfarin therapy, co-administration with heparin (5 days) is necessary to avoid a paradoxical hypercoagulable state.*
- *When the INR is supratherapeutic in a patient who is not bleeding, a cautious approach to vitamin K administration is important. Administering excess vitamin K may over-correct the INR, leaving the patient refractory to further anticoagulation.*

SECTION XIV
HEENT EMERGENCIES

CHAPTER 61
SLIT LAMP EXAMINATION

I. **Indications.** Slit lamp examination is indicated for examination of the anterior eye. It is the definitive tool for diagnosing corneal abrasions, foreign bodies, iritis, and anterior chamber hemorrhage and inflammation.

II. **Contraindications.** The patient must be awake and alert when the examination is performed.

III. **Equipment**

    A. The slit lamp consists of 3 components: mechanical assembly, binocular microscope, and light source (Figure 61–1).

    B. **Mechanical assembly.** The patient should be comfortably seated with the forehead pressed against the forehead brace and the chin in the chin rest. Align the patient's eye level with the mark on the headrest support rods by adjusting the chin support.

    C. **Binocular microscope.** Low power is most useful, either 10x or 16x. Focus the eyepieces first by moving the entire instrument forward and backward until the patient's cornea is in focus. Then adjust each eyepiece individually to produce an equally sharp image.

    D. **Light source.** The light is mounted on a swinging arm. Knobs and switches allow the examiner to vary the width and height of the beam as well as place white and blue filters in front of the beam. Vertical white light is best for most of the examination. The entire apparatus is moved with a joystick in front of the examiner. To raise or lower the apparatus, twist the joystick. To make subtle changes in the focal point, move the joystick forward or backward.

IV. **Procedure**

    A. **Overall screening.** For examination of the right eye, the light source is placed at a 45° angle to the left of the examiner, with the microscope directly in front of the eye. Using white light, the beam is set to maximum height and minimum width. Using the joystick, the examiner first focuses on the conjunctiva and cornea and scans side to side. Then the examiner pushes forward to scan across the iris. The light source should not be moved during the examination. The reverse set-up is used for the left eye.

    B. **Corneal foreign bodies.** If a foreign body is encountered during the screening examination, the examiner can remove the foreign body with a small (27–29 gauge)

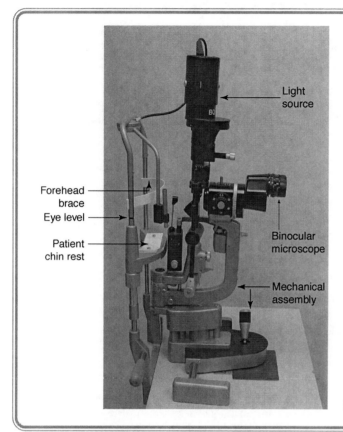

Figure 61–1. Slit lamp.

needle after anesthetizing the cornea with tetracaine. The needle is moved toward the object, parallel to the surface of the cornea. The tip of the needle is then used to pull the object off the cornea, while causing as little injury to the cornea as possible.

C. **Corneal abrasions.** Tetracaine is used to anesthetize the eye. The patient's eye is then stained with fluorescein. Before application of fluorescein, make sure the patient is not wearing contact lenses because the fluorescein will stain the lens. The cobalt blue filter is moved in front of the light, and the width of the beam is widened to 3–4 mm. *Be careful not to confuse the cobalt blue light with the green light.* Using the joystick, the apparatus is moved back and forth to focus the microscope. The cobalt blue light is then moved across the eye to scan for fluorescein uptake representing a corneal abrasion (Figure 61–2). Fluorescein seen percolating from the site of injury suggests a full-thickness injury to the cornea with aqueous leakage (**Seidel's sign**).

D. **Cell and flare.** The height of the beam is shortened to 3–4 mm, and the width is made as narrow as possible. The light source is switched to high power. The beam is focused initially on the cornea and then moved forward until it is focused on the center of the lens. Next, the joystick is pulled back so the focal point is posi-

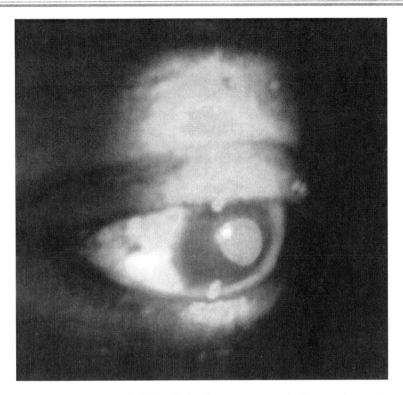

Figure 61–2. Using the cobalt blue light, fluorescein uptake is seen in a patient with a large corneal abrasion.

tioned between the cornea and the lens. The beam will now be focused on the anterior chamber. Particles noted floating in the light, like "dust motes in a sunbeam," are cells. Flare is when the beam lights up the chamber like a "flashlight through fog," which is caused by protein present in the anterior chamber.

V. Complications. Avoid placing pressure on the eye when the possibility of a globe rupture exists. Excessive pressure may cause the intra-ocular contents to be extruded.

CHAPTER 62
RED EYE

I. Defining Features

A. **Conjunctivitis** is present in patients who have a complaint of a red eye associated with a gritty foreign body sensation and discharge. The cause of conjunctivitis can be bacterial, viral, or allergic. The hallmark is a red eye without a change in vision or pain. When associated with a corneal ulcer, visual impairment and pain are present and permanent visual loss can occur unless treated promptly.

B. **Subconjunctival hemorrhage** is blood between the conjunctiva and the sclera. It may be alarming to the patient, but it is usually a benign process. The hemorrhage is most commonly seen after trauma, but can be spontaneous or related to systemic illness.

C. **Corneal abrasions** are characterized by pain, foreign body sensation, tearing, and photophobia. Abrasions are usually the result of trauma; the patient may not remember the event, however. If the abrasion is large enough, the patient may note blurry vision.

D. **Acute uveitis** is defined as inflammation of the uveal tract (iris, ciliary body, and choroid). Acute anterior uveitis (iritis) is most common and involves the iris and ciliary body. It is characterized by severe photophobia. In extreme cases, the patient may complain of blurry vision.

II. Epidemiology

A. Eye complaints account for 3% of all ED visits.

B. Conjunctivitis is one of the most common eye complaints in the ED. About 15% of persons will develop allergic conjunctivitis at some point during their lifetime.

C. **HSV** is the most common cause of a corneal ulcer.

D. Corneal abrasions represent 10% of all ED visits for eye complaints.

E. Uveitis occurs in 15/100,000 persons.

III. Etiology

A. **Conjunctivitis** is bacterial, viral, or allergic. Viruses are the most frequent cause of conjunctivitis, especially adenovirus. HSV and varicella zoster virus are 2 other important causes that have significant associated morbidity if not promptly treated. The most common bacterial cause is *Staphylococcus aureus*.

However, in neonates and sexually active adults, consider *Neisseria gonorrhea* and *Chlamydia trachomatis*. Allergic conjunctivitis is due to recurrent seasonal inflammation from allergen exposure.

B. **Subconjunctival hemorrhage** is a result of a conjunctival vessel rupture, frequently due to a sudden increase in pressure from sneezing, coughing, straining, or vomiting. If atraumatic, the etiology is usually hypertension or an idiopathic spontaneous rupture.

C. **Corneal abrasions** occur secondary to trauma or foreign body. If the history is of a slow, progressive worsening of symptoms, consider abrasion secondary to contact lens use.

D. **Acute anterior uveitis** is secondary to a variety of causes. Commonly, uveitis is due to trauma, and patients usually present 1 to 4 days after the traumatic event. Systemic causes of acute uveitis include ankylosing spondylitis, Reiter's syndrome, inflammatory bowel disease, and chronic granulomatous conditions such as TB or sarcoidosis. Corneal ulcerations due to infectious processes can cause acute anterior uveitis.

IV. Risk Factors (see III)

V. Clinical Presentation

A. **History**

1. **Bacterial conjunctivitis** presents with redness, gritty foreign body sensation, and **mucopurulent discharge,** which may result in the eyelids being stuck together, especially in the morning. Viral conjunctivitis presents as redness, itching, and a **watery discharge.** Often it begins unilaterally and then spreads through autoinoculation. Constitutional symptoms (fever, rhinorrhea, myalgias) are common with a systemic viral infection. Allergic conjunctivitis is associated with more intense itching, a burning photophobia, and a seasonal history.

2. **Subconjunctival hemorrhage** may be preceded by direct trauma or indirect injury such as sneezing or coughing.

3. **Corneal abrasion** is associated with pain, foreign body sensation, tearing, and photophobia. The patient may also complain of visual loss and blurring if the abrasion is central or very large. It is important to elicit the events leading up to the abrasion in order to determine the likelihood of a foreign body.

4. **Acute anterior uveitis** presents with a gradual onset of a painful red eye with severe photophobia. The patient will often be sitting in a dark room with eyes closed or a hand over the eyes. They may complain of associated blurring of their vision, which is frequently secondary to tearing. Often a prior history of similar symptoms can be elicited. Be sure to inquire about recent trauma and systemic signs and symptoms.

KEY COMPLAINTS

Patients with a corneal abrasion will have relief of symptoms after use of a topical anesthetic agent, whereas patients with anterior uveitis have ongoing pain.

KEY COMPLAINTS

B. **Physical Examination**

1. The physical examination should always follow the same pattern: visual acuity, lids and lashes, conjunctiva, sclera, cornea, pupil, and anterior chamber (Table 62–1).

2. **Conjunctivitis.** Eyelids demonstrate bilateral cobblestone papillae with allergic conjunctivitis. In patients with herpes zoster ophthalmicus (HZO), a rash is usually present on the forehead and nose in the distribution of the first branch of the trigeminal nerve. **Hutchinson's sign** is present when there are lesions on the tip of the nose, indicating involvement of the nasociliary branch of the trigeminal nerve (V_1). Although the presence of Hutchinson's sign makes ocular involvement twice as likely, one third of patients without the sign will still have ocular involvement. Conjunctiva will have diffuse injection. **Chemosis** (the appearance of fluid in the conjunctiva) is common (Figure 62–1). The sclera is typically clear, but may have white ulcers at the limbus (junction between the cornea and sclera) resulting from allergic reaction or staphylococcus toxin. The cornea will have no fluorescein uptake; however, ulceration and perforation can occur. In HSV infection, a branching **dendritic ulcer** is characteristic, while in varicella zoster virus infection, a thin wavy lesion similar to tangled spaghetti is seen. Gonorrhea may cause corneal ulceration.

3. **Subconjunctival hemorrhage.** Clinical diagnosis is based on an area of bright red blood on the sclera.

4. **Corneal abrasions.** Visual acuity is unaffected unless there is central involvement or a very large abrasion. Lids and lashes are unaffected; however, it is important to evert lids to look for a foreign body. Pain is relieved by a topical

Table 62–1. Physical examination findings in patients with red eye.

Examination	Conjunctivitis	Subconjunctival Hemorrhage	Corneal Abrasion	Acute Anterior Uveitis
Visual acuity	Normal	Normal	Decreased when central	Decreased due to pain, tearing
Lids	Edema, erythema	Normal	Normal	Normal
Conjunctiva	Injection	Normal	Injection	Normal
Sclera	Normal	Erythema	Normal	Ciliary flush
Cornea (fluorescein uptake)	None, unless associated corneal ulcer	None	YES	None
Pupil	Normal	Normal	Normal	Constricted
Anterior chamber (cell and flare)	None	None	None	Yes

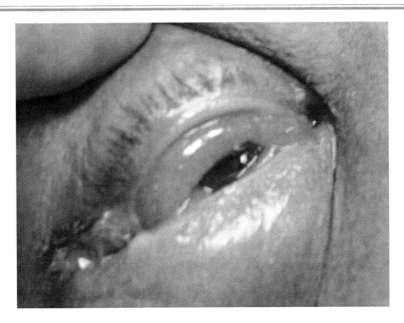

Figure 62–1. Chemosis.

anesthetic agent (tetracaine). The cornea will have fluorescein uptake in the affected area, which is seen with a cobalt blue light from the slit lamp. The fluorescein will light up as bright green where it pools in the abrasion. If multiple lines are seen, check for a foreign body under the eyelid that is scratching the cornea every time the patient blinks. If a branching pattern is seen, consider a viral herpetic infection.

5. **Acute anterior uveitis.** Visual acuity is often decreased secondary to pain and tearing. Sclera may demonstrate **ciliary flush** (redness at the limbus). The cornea demonstrates no fluorescein uptake, and pain is *unrelieved* by a topical anesthetic agent (tetracaine). Pupils are often constricted and irregular. Consensual photophobia, pain produced by shining light in the unaffected eye, is frequently present. The anterior chamber will demonstrate **"cell and flare."** Cells and protein floating through a light projected through the anterior chamber will flash and shine like dust motes in a sunbeam. This finding is diagnostic. When cellular debris is significant, it can layer out at the bottom of the anterior chamber between the cornea and iris. This finding is called a hypopyon (Figure 62–2).

VI. Differential Diagnosis (see I)

RULE OUT

Foreign body. *When examining the eye in patients with a corneal abrasion, always evert the eyelid to rule out a foreign body.*

VII. Diagnostic Findings

A. **Laboratory and imaging studies.** None are routinely indicated.

B. **Diagnostic Algorithm**

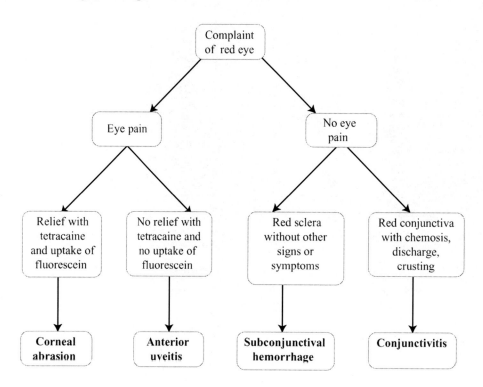

VIII. Treatment

A. **Conjunctivitis**

1. **Uncomplicated conjunctivitis.** Frequent hand washing to limit spread. For symptomatic relief, patients can use cool compresses and artificial tears. If a bacterial cause is suspected, treat with topical antibiotic drops or ointment (eg, sulfacetamide, quinolones, aminoglycoside, trimethoprim, and polymyxin) for 5–7 days.

2. **HZO.** Oral acyclovir within 72 hours of onset of symptoms reduces the likelihood of eye involvement from 50% to 25%, and is the treatment of choice when the eye is involved. IV acyclovir is indicated for immunocompromised patients. Ophthalmology consultation is indicated.

3. **HSV.** Treatment of HSV requires topical antiviral drops (Viroptic) and consultation with an ophthalmologist.

4. **Contact lens.** Patients with conjunctivitis associated with contact lens use must discontinue use of the lens and be given an aminoglycoside or quinolone to treat pseudomonas.

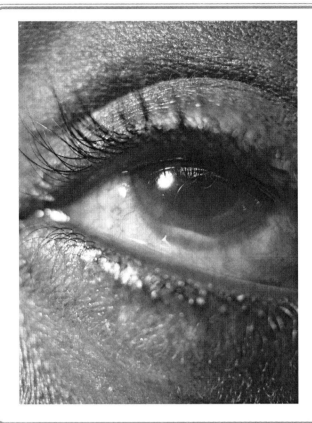

Figure 62–2. Hypopyon.

5. **Corneal ulcer.** An immediate ophthalmology consultation is required. The first-line regimen usually consists of a topical aminoglycoside and a first-generation cephalosporin every 15–30 minutes.

6. *C. trachomatis* **or** *N. gonorrhea* **infection.** Both require systemic and topical antibiotics. Patients with suspected gonorrhea (Gram stain showing gram-negative intracellular diplococci) must have an immediate ophthalmologic consult and may require hospital admission.

B. **Subconjunctival hemorrhage.** Requires no specific treatment. Reassure the patient that the condition usually resolves within 2 weeks. If recurrent, the patient may need coagulation studies and a further work-up to rule out a bleeding disorder.

C. **Corneal abrasion.** Pain relief and infection prophylaxis. Patients benefit from a cycloplegic to relieve ciliary spasm and reduce pain, using either cyclopentolate or homatropine. They will often also require narcotic analgesia. To prevent secondary infection, prescribe a topical antibiotic (10% sulfacetamide). If the patient wears contact lenses, use an aminoglycoside or quinolone to cover pseudomonas. Do not use an eye patch, as it is associated with corneal ulceration and pseudomonas infection. Tetanus prophylaxis should be updated.

D. **Acute anterior uveitis.** *Treatment should be instituted only in consultation with an ophthalmologist,* as continual monitoring and treatment is required. To eliminate ciliary spasm, use a long-acting cycloplegic such as homatropine 5%. To relieve inflammation, prescribe a topical steroid such as prednisolone acetate 1%.

IX. Disposition

A. **Admission.** Patients with bacterial conjunctivitis secondary to gonorrhea should be admitted for IV antibiotic therapy. Consider admission of patients with corneal ulcers if the patient is unable to self-administer antibiotics; there is a high likelihood of non-compliance or a large ulcer is present.

B. **Discharge.** Patients with corneal abrasion and acute anterior uveitis should be discharged with ophthalmology follow-up within 24–48 hours. Patients with conjunctivitis and subconjunctival hemorrhage can be discharged to follow up with their primary physicians. Patients with herpetic keratitis should follow up with an ophthalmologist within 24 hours.

CASE PRESENTATION

A 32-year-old man is sitting in a dark exam room with his eyes closed and a hat pulled down over them. The patient states that he gradually developed redness and pain in his right eye, and it is much worse when the lights are on. He reports a decrease in vision associated with the pain and no discharge or foreign body sensation. He denies any other medical problems.

1. *What will you look for on physical examination?*

   • *Visual acuity: the vital sign of the eye. Lids and lashes: foreign bodies, styes? Conjunctiva: redness and discharge? Sclera: redness, ciliary flush? Cornea: relief with topical anesthetic, fluorescein uptake? Pupil: constricted, irregular, consensual photophobia? Anterior chamber: cell and flare?*

2. *The patient has decreased visual acuity in the right eye compared to the left. Lids and lashes are normal, and conjunctiva are normal. A ciliary flush is noted in the sclera. No relief is gained with the application of a topical anesthetic, and there is no fluorescein uptake. You elicit severe pain when shining light in both pupils. The anterior chamber is positive for cell and flare. You make the diagnosis of acute iritis. How will you proceed?*

   • *Apply and prescribe a long-acting cycloplegic to eliminate ciliary spasm. Call ophthalmology for consideration of a topical steroid to relieve inflammation and arrange follow-up within 24 hours.*

SUMMARY POINTS

• *Always begin with visual acuity, the vital sign of the eye.*

• *Follow a systematic approach to the physical examination: visual acuity, lids and lashes, conjunctiva, sclera, cornea, pupil examination, and anterior chamber.*

• *Never prescribe topical steroids without consulting with an ophthalmologist.*

CHAPTER 63
ACUTE VISUAL LOSS

I. Defining Features

A. The most important first step in addressing the patient with acute visual loss is to determine if the loss of vision is associated with pain.

B. **Painless loss of vision** is secondary to the following:
   1. **Central retinal artery occlusion** (CRAO) is a sudden monocular loss of vision due to obstruction of the central retinal artery.
   2. **Central retinal vein occlusion** (CRVO) is a sudden painless monocular *decrease* in vision due to retinal vein obstruction.
   3. **Retinal detachment** refers to separation of the inner layers of the retina from the underlying retinal pigment epithelium.

C. **Painful loss of vision** is secondary to the following:
   1. **Optic neuritis** is a painful rapid reduction of central vision secondary to an inflammatory process of the optic nerve.
   2. **Temporal (giant cell) arteritis** is a vasculitis that results in monocular loss of vision associated with a unilateral temporal headache.
   3. **Acute angle-closure glaucoma** is a sudden painful monocular loss of vision secondary to increased pressure in the anterior chamber.
   4. **Corneal abrasions and ulcerations** may cause decreased vision if they are central and large (see Chapter 62).

II. Epidemiology

A. CRAO and CRVO occur most frequently in elderly patients. About 90% of cases of CRVO occur in patients > age 50.

B. Optic neuritis occurs more commonly in women aged 15 to 45.

C. Retinal detachment is most prevalent in advanced age and in patients with significant myopia. The prevalence in the United States is 0.3%.

D. Temporal arteritis occurs most commonly in woman > 50. Caucasians are more frequently affected than are other races.

E. Acute angle-closure glaucoma represents < 10% of all cases of glaucoma in the United States. It is more common in women, and is also more common in African American and Asian populations.

371

III. Etiology

A. CRAO is a result of a thrombotic plaque or more commonly an embolus of the central retinal artery, whereas central retinal vein occlusion is caused by thrombosis of the retinal vein.

B. Optic neuritis is secondary to an inflammatory process of the optic nerve.

C. Retinal detachment results from traction of the vitreous humor on the retina. This causes a tear in the retina and a separation of the inner neuronal retina from the outer retinal pigment epithelial layer.

D. Temporal arteritis is a vasculitis of medium and large arteries and can lead to optic nerve infarction and blindness.

E. Acute angle-closure glaucoma occurs in patients with shallow (narrow) anterior chamber angles. As the pupil dilates, the iris leaflet touches the lens. This impedes the flow of aqueous humor from the posterior to the anterior chamber with a subsequent increase in hydrostatic pressure.

IV. Risk Factors

A. **CRAO.** Risk factors are similar to other vascular disease entities. Hypertension, carotid artery disease; diabetes mellitus; cardiac disease, especially AF and valvular disease; vasculitis; temporal arteritis; and sickle cell disease.

B. **CRVO.** Risk relates to likelihood of thrombosis. The physician should have increased suspicion in patients with diabetes mellitus, hypertension, arteriosclerosis, chronic glaucoma, and vasculitis.

C. **Optic neuritis.** In patients without a previous diagnosis, 25–65% will develop MS.

D. **Retinal detachment.** Risk is related most closely to severe myopia. Other risk factors include trauma, previous cataract surgery, family history, Marfan's syndrome (or other inherited connective tissue disorder), and diabetes mellitus.

E. **Temporal arteritis.** Polymyalgia rheumatica, female, Northern European, and > age 50.

F. **Acute angle-closure glaucoma.** Farsighted (hyperopic) persons are at risk secondary to the shape of their anterior chamber; female and elderly.

V. Clinical Presentation

A. **History**

1. **CRAO.** Sudden, painless, complete, monocular loss of vision without other associated factors.

2. **CRVO.** The presentation of central retinal vein occlusion is more insidious than retinal artery occlusion. The patient will have a sudden painless monocular *decrease* in vision that is most commonly noted upon awakening. Patients may also describe a sudden decrease, acutely imposed on a chronic gradual worsening over a longer period of time (eg, 1 week).

3. **Optic neuritis.** Patients with optic neuritis will present with rapidly progressive reduction or blurring of their vision. Ocular pain worsens with eye movement.

4. **Retinal detachment.** Patients with retinal detachment present with painless loss of vision often described as a sensation of a curtain moving across the visual field. Flashing lights, "spider webs," or "coal dust" in the visual field may precede visual loss.

5. **Temporal arteritis.** Temporal arteritis presents as a sudden monocular loss of vision associated with a unilateral temporal headache. Eye pain usually is not present.
6. **Acute angle-closure glaucoma.** Acute angle-closure glaucoma presents as cloudy vision associated with halos around lights. In addition, the patient will complain of eye pain or headache along with nausea and vomiting and possibly abdominal pain. Often patients will have no previous history of glaucoma.

KEY COMPLAINTS

A patient with a retinal detachment frequently will describe loss of vision as a shade being pulled down over the eye.

B. **Physical Examination**
1. **CRAO. Visual acuity** is markedly decreased, with the patient often only able to perceive shadows or count fingers. Initial **pupil examination** may be normal; however, after 1–2 hours the pupil may dilate. The pupil is poorly reactive to direct light but has a greater consensual response to light shown in the opposite eye (afferent pupillary defect). On **funduscopic examination,** the physician may see a pale retina with a cherry-red spot in the macular area, which represents the fovea (Figure 63–1).
2. **CRVO. Visual acuity** is variable but the deficit is usually less severe than retinal artery occlusion. On **pupil examination,** the pupil will react sluggishly to light. On **funduscopic examination,** there may be retinal hemorrhage, tortuous retinal veins, and disc edema, referred to as "blood and thunder" (Figure 63–2).
3. **Optic neuritis. Visual acuity** varies from mildly reduced to no light perception. Often the visual deficit will be limited to the central visual field, and the patient will complain more of a defect with color vision rather than sight.

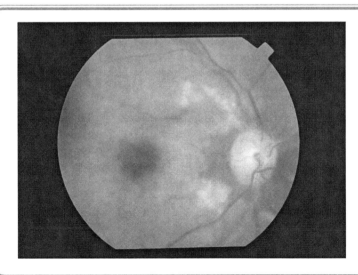

Figure 63–1. Central retinal artery occlusion.

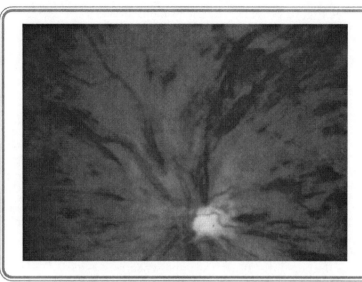

Figure 63–2. Central retinal vein occlusion.

This can be evaluated using the red desaturation test. Have the patient look at a dark red object with one eye and then test the other eye to see if the object looks the same color. The affected eye will often see the object as lighter or pink. An afferent pupillary defect will often be present on **pupil examination.** If the fundus is normal on **funduscopic examination,** the patient has retrobulbar optic neuritis. However, if the fundus is swollen or hyperemic, the patient has papillitis.

4. **Retinal detachment. Visual acuity:** the extent of the loss of vision is dependent on the degree of detachment. Visual field defects will be noted on confrontation. **Pupil examination** is unremarkable. **Funduscopic examination** reveals an undulating, dull grey, detached retina.

5. **Temporal arteritis.** Palpation of the temples may reveal tender, tortuous and sometimes pulseless temporal arteries. The degree of loss of vision depends on when the diagnosis is made. If diagnosed late, visual acuity will be markedly decreased. An afferent pupillary defect may be present on **pupil examination.** On **funduscopic examination,** a pale, swollen optic disc will be present.

6. **Acute angle-closure glaucoma. Visual acuity** is markedly decreased. The patient's sclera will be red due to ciliary injection. The cornea will be cloudy. On gentle palpation, the eye may have a rock hard consistency. **Pupil examination** shows fixed, mid-dilated, and non-reactive pupils. **Funduscopic examination** is difficult to perform in the face of a cloudy cornea, but is otherwise unremarkable.

CLINICAL SKILLS TIP

Funduscopic examination: allow the patient to sit in a dark room for several minutes before attempting the examination. When the eye is sufficiently dilated, ask the patient to focus on an object on the wall and ignore the examiner. Focus the ophthalmoscope on the eye and gradually approach the eye from a

lateral position. The optic disc is noted medially. If only vessels are seen, the optic disc can be located by knowing that the blood vessel's branches "point" to the direction of the disc.

VI. Differential Diagnosis (see I)

RULE OUT

Central retinal artery occlusion must be considered and treated early because irreversible visual loss occurs after 90 minutes.

VII. Diagnostic Findings

A. **Laboratory studies.** ESR > 50 mm/hr is almost universally present in patients with temporal arteritis. Normal ESR for males is age/2; females (age + 10)/2.

B. **Imaging studies.** Diagnosis in patients with acute visual loss hinges on the patient's history and physical examination; imaging studies have little role.

C. **Procedures**

1. **Intra-ocular pressures.** To diagnose acute angle-closure glaucoma, intraocular pressure is measured with a Schiötz tonometer or Tono-Pen (Figures 63–3 and 63–4). Normal pressure is < 20 mm Hg. A pressure > 40 mm Hg is diagnostic.

2. **Temporal artery biopsy** performed by a surgeon is used to confirm the diagnosis of temporal arteritis.

D. **Diagnostic Algorithm (see page 376)**

VIII. Treatment

A. **CRAO.** Treatment of CRAO must begin as soon as the diagnosis is suspected because permanent visual loss typically occurs after 90 minutes. The goal of treatment is to restore retinal artery blood flow by dislodging the clot. This is

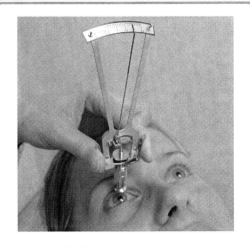

Figure 63–3. Schiötz tonometer.

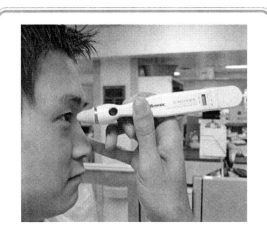

Figure 63–4. Tono-Pen.

Diagnostic Algorithm

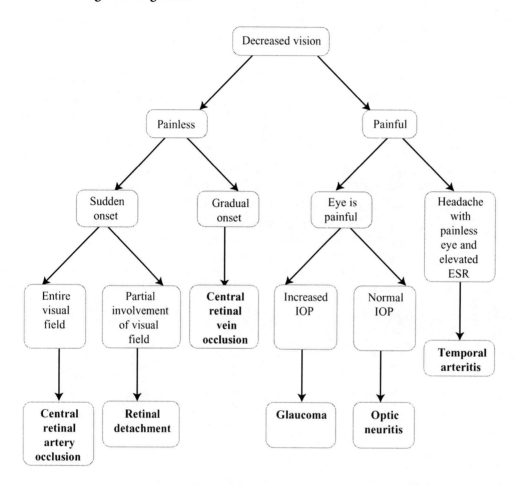

accomplished by dilating the artery and reducing intraocular BP through the following modalities: **intermittent digital massage** of the globe (5 sec on, 5 sec off) for 5–15 minutes; **hyperventilation** into a paper bag 10 minutes of every hour; **acetazolamide** 500 mg IV and a **β blocker** (timolol 0.5% drops intraocular). Immediate ophthalmology consultation is paramount for paracentesis (aspiration of aqueous fluid) of the anterior chamber.

B. **CRVO** is not as emergent as CRAO because no immediate treatment is effective. Patients should be referred to ophthalmology for confirmation of the diagnosis and monitoring of disease progression.

C. **Retinal detachment.** Immediate ophthalmology consultation is indicated to evaluate for retinal reattachment surgery. The patient should be instructed to avoid activity and remain on bed rest until seen by an ophthalmologist.

D. **Optic neuritis.** A short course of high-dose IV methylprednisolone followed by a rapid oral taper of prednisone provides a rapid recovery of symptoms in the acute phase. This treatment may also delay the short-term development of MS.

E. **Temporal arteritis.** Treatment with oral prednisone (80 mg/day) should begin in the ED when the diagnosis is suspected. Follow-up with an ophthalmologist for evaluation; temporal artery biopsy should be arranged.

F. **Acute angle-closure glaucoma.** Treatment of acute angle-closure glaucoma consists of the sequential administration of several agents to decrease intraocular pressure: **β blocker** (Timoptic 0.5%) 1 drop; **α agonist**(Iopidine 0.1%) 1 drop; **acetazolamide** 500 mg orally or IV; **steroid** (pred forte 1%) 1 drop; **mannitol** 1–2 g/kg IV; and **pilocarpine** 1–2% is administered to constrict the pupil and pull the iris back, helping to prevent a recurrence. The unaffected eye should be treated prophylactically. Consult ophthalmology immediately, since the definitive treatment is bilateral laser iridectomy.

IX. **Disposition**

A. **Admission.** Optic neuritis is frequently managed as an inpatient for treatment and an expedited work-up, including MRI. CRAO, retinal detachment, and acute angle-closure glaucoma require immediate ophthalmology consultation. Admission is required when definitive treatment cannot be accomplished in the ED.

B. **Discharge.** Temporal arteritis can be managed on an outpatient basis after the initiation of steroids if the patient has appropriate follow-up. CRVO is managed on an outpatient basis with ophthalmology referral.

CASE PRESENTATION

A 62-year-old woman presents with the complaint of sudden monocular loss of vision. She had been at lunch with a friend and suddenly could not see out of her left eye.

1. *What other information do you want to know?*

   • *Does she have pain in the eye? Associated symptoms: headache, abdominal pain, nausea, vomiting? Is vision loss central? Did she notice a sensation of a "curtain dropping"? What are her other medical problems? Hypertension, diabetes mellitus, AF?*

   • *Examination. Visual acuity: Can she see the Snellen visual acuity eye chart or just shadows or fingers? Is there red desaturation? Sclera: Is it red or cloudy? Is there a ciliary flush? Pupil: Is it fixed and mid dilated? Is there an afferent papillary defect? Fundus: Is there hemorrhage? Is it pale or swollen? Cherry red spot? Is her intraocular pressure elevated?*

2. *The patient denies having any pain in her eye, headache or nausea or vomiting. She has a history of HTN and AF and has not been taking her warfarin (Coumadin) because she ran out 3 weeks ago. On examination, you note complete loss of vision in the left eye and 20/40 in the right. Normal sclera and pupil are present, but a pale fundus with a cherry red spot is seen. Intraocular pressure is normal. You make the diagnosis of central retinal artery occlusion. What is your next step?*

   • *You have 90 minutes before visual loss is permanent. Call for immediate ophthalmology referral for paracentesis of the anterior chamber. Next, initiate intermittent digital massage of the globe (5 sec on, 5 sec off) for 5–15 minutes, hyperventilation into paper bag 10 minutes of every hour, acetazolamide 500mg IV, and topical β blocker (timolol 0.5%).*

SUMMARY POINTS

- *History and physical examination alone will lead to the diagnosis in most patients presenting with acute visual loss.*
- *Begin with visual acuity, the vital sign of the eye, and then proceed with pupillary and funduscopic examination. If indicated, measure intraocular pressure.*
- *An ophthalmologist should be consulted immediately when CRAO or acute angle-closure glaucoma are diagnosed in the ED.*

CHAPTER 64
EPISTAXIS

I. Defining Features

A. Epistaxis, like all hemorrhage, needs prompt evaluation and treatment.

B. The primary goal of diagnosis is to determine the location of bleeding: anterior versus posterior.

C. Once the site of bleeding is identified, bleeding is stopped using various techniques ranging from chemical cautery (silver nitrate) to nasal packing.

II. Epidemiology

A. Epistaxis occurs in 1 of every 7 persons in the United States.

B. The incidence is highest in persons aged 2 to 10 and 50 to 80 years.

III. Etiology

A. **Vascular anatomy.** The lower half of the nose is supplied by the sphenopalatine and greater palatine arteries. Both are distal branches of the external carotid artery. The anteroinferior nasal septum is the location of **Kiesselbach's plexus,** the most common source of anterior bleeds. The posteroinferior turbinate is the location of Woodruff's plexus, the most common **venous** source of posterior bleeds.

B. **Anterior epistaxis** accounts for 90% of nosebleeds. Most commonly, the bleeding is **venous** from Kiesselbach's plexus.

C. **Posterior epistaxis** represents 10% of nosebleeds. Posterior bleeds are more commonly **arterial,** from the sphenopalatine artery.

IV. Risk Factors

A. **Anterior epistaxis.** Trauma, dry air leading to dry mucous membranes (during winter months), or foreign body (eg, finger). Other causes include allergies, nasal irritants such as cocaine or nasal spray, pregnancy, rapid changes in atmospheric pressure, infection, and Osler-Weber-Rendu syndrome.

B. **Posterior epistaxis.** Elderly debilitated patients with co-morbid diseases such as a coagulopathy, atherosclerosis, neoplasm, or hypertension.

V. Clinical Presentation

A. **History**

1. Ask about onset and duration to assess severity of blood loss.

2. Ask about co-morbidities and medications, especially blood thinners and anti-platelet drugs.

B. **Physical Examination**
1. To appropriately evaluate the origin of the blood, first have the patient clear clot from the nose by blowing the nose.
2. Next, look inside the nares to see if a site of bleeding can be identified. If the site of bleeding cannot be identified, have the patient hold pressure over the nares, and then look in the patient's oropharynx.
3. If blood is seen trickling down the oropharynx while the patient is holding anterior pressure, consider a posterior bleed.

CLINICAL SKILLS TIP

Blood that continues to drain down the posterior pharynx while the anterior portion of the nose is being squeezed suggests a posterior source of epistaxis.

VI. Differential Diagnosis (see IV)

RULE OUT

Posterior epistaxis. *Bleeding from the posterior portion of the nose is less common (10%), but because it is frequently due to an arterial source, bleeding can be severe and result in significant morbidity. When the diagnosis is unclear, clues to the presence of a posterior nosebleed include significant bleeding in the posterior pharynx with a properly placed anterior pack.*

VII. Diagnostic Findings
A. **Laboratory Studies**
1. **CBC.** This test is not routinely indicated but may be useful to identify patients with thrombocytopenia or anemia.
2. **Coagulation studies.** PT/INR/PTT is indicated in patients taking anticoagulant warfarin or in cirrhosis.
B. **Imaging studies. Angiography** is rarely indicated but can be used to diagnose and treat refractory posterior bleeding from the sphenopalatine and greater palatine arteries.
C. **Diagnostic Algorithm (see page 381)**

VIII. Treatment

A. If bleeding is significant, insert an IV and place the patient on a cardiac monitor. Intubation is occasionally necessary when bleeding is severe and is compromising the airway.

B. **Anterior Bleed**
1. If an anterior bleed is suspected, have the patient hold pressure over the soft cartilaginous portion of the nose for 10 minutes.
2. Assemble equipment: nasal speculum, headlight, suction, vasoconstrictor, and anterior packing (Figure 64–1).
3. After 10 minutes, re-examine the nose.
a. ***Bleeding stopped.*** Apply bacitracin to anterior nares and discharge with follow-up.

Diagnostic Algorithm

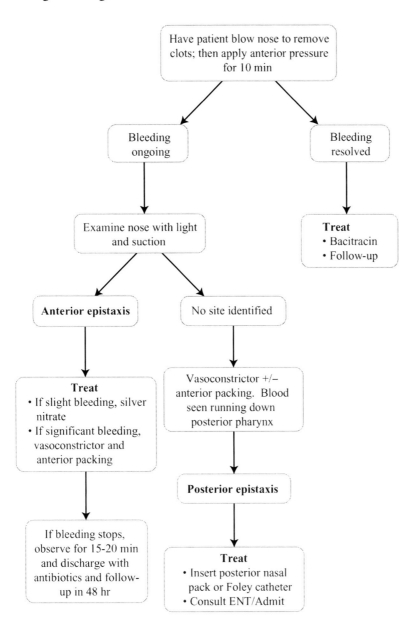

Have patient blow nose to remove clots; then apply anterior pressure for 10 min

Bleeding ongoing

Bleeding resolved

Treat
• Bacitracin
• Follow-up

Examine nose with light and suction

Anterior epistaxis

No site identified

Treat
• If slight bleeding, silver nitrate
• If significant bleeding, vasoconstrictor and anterior packing

Vasoconstrictor +/− anterior packing. Blood seen running down posterior pharynx

Posterior epistaxis

If bleeding stops, observe for 15-20 min and discharge with antibiotics and follow-up in 48 hr

Treat
• Insert posterior nasal pack or Foley catheter
• Consult ENT/Admit

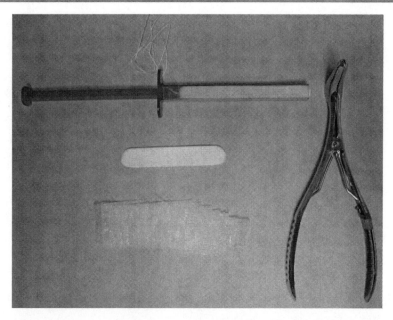

Figure 64–1. Left, from top to bottom, anterior packs include the Rhino Rocket, Merocel, and petroleum gauze. Right, nasal speculum.

    b. ***Bleeding mild.*** Consider chemical cautery with silver nitrate sticks. Roll the stick over the area until a grey eschar is formed. Never hold the stick in one place > 5 seconds and never use silver nitrate bilaterally.

    c. ***Bleeding significant.*** If bleeding has not stopped, insert pledgets with an anesthetic-vasoconstrictor combination such as 4% cocaine or 4% lidocaine and 1% phenylephrine in a 1:1 dilution. Then hold pressure for 10 minutes and check again. If the bleeding still has not stopped, pack the nare with petroleum gauze, a compressed sponge (Merocel or Rhino Rocket), or an anterior epistaxis balloon. When using a compressed sponge, remember to lubricate the sponge before putting it into the nose, and use at least 10 mL saline to expand the sponge once it is in the nostril. Hemostatic material (Surgicel, Gelfoam, topical thrombin) may also be useful in controlling hemorrhage.

  4. If the patient's nose requires packing, then prescribe prophylactic antibiotics (amoxicillin 500 mg TID) against staphylococci to prevent TSS, sinusitis, and otitis media.

  5. Have the patient follow-up with ENT or with their primary care physician in 2–3 days.

C. Posterior Bleed

  1. Posterior bleeds are an emergency because it is difficult to tamponade the bleeding site. In addition, bleeding is often arterial, and patients frequently have significant co-morbidities.

  2. Attempt tamponade using a balloon device or a Foley catheter (Figure 64–2).

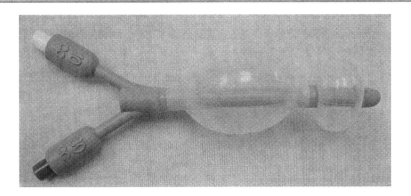

Figure 64–2. Epistat nasal catheter® for posterior epistaxis. The 30-mL balloon tamponades the anterior nares, and the 10-mL balloon is used to provide posterior tamponade of bleeding.

3. **Balloon device method.** Insert catheter into the nose until the tip is seen in the oropharynx. Inflate the posterior balloon with 4–8 mL of air; then pull the device anteriorly to tamponade the bleeding. Inflate the anterior balloon with 10–25 mL of air. Assess the posterior oropharynx to assure cessation of bleeding.

4. **Foley catheter method.** Obtain a 14 F Foley with 30 mL balloon. Cut the tip of the catheter just *distal* to the balloon. Suction, anesthetize, and vasoconstrict the nose. Insert the catheter into the nose until the tip is seen in the oropharynx. Inflate the balloon with 10–15 mL air. Pull back on the catheter until bleeding has stopped. Place an anterior pack. Use gauze to secure the catheter and prevent pressure necrosis on the nasal tip.

5. Consult ENT.

6. Place the patient on prophylactic antibiotics (amoxicillin 500 mg TID) to prevent TSS, sinusitis, and otitis media.

IX. Disposition

A. Admission to a monitored setting is indicated for patients with posterior epistaxis, even if hemorrhage is controlled. Severe bleeding and fatal airway obstruction secondary to dislodgment of the packing can occur. Although rare, patients may develop a nasopulmonary reflex, manifested by hypoxia, hypercarbia, dysrhythmias, or coronary ischemia secondary to packing placement.

B. Discharge can be arranged for patients with anterior epistaxis once bleeding is controlled. Remember to prescribe antibiotics to patients who have had their nose packed. Follow-up should be arranged in 2 days to have the packing removed.

CASE PRESENTATION

A 76-year-old man presents to the ED because he has had a severe nosebleed for the past 3 hours. He is upright on the stretcher and holding a basin on his lap into which he is continually spitting bright red blood.

CASE
PRESENTATION

1. *He tells you that he has a history of a mitral valve replacement 2 months ago and since then he has been on warfarin. What will you look for on physical examination?*
   * *Are you able to easily identify the site of bleeding? After evacuating clot, does the bleeding stop with anterior pressure or does it continue down the oropharynx?*

2. *After blowing out large amounts of clot, you apply pressure to the patient's nose and look inside the oropharynx, where you continue to see a trickle of blood. Now that you have made the clinical diagnosis of posterior nose bleed, what is your next step?*
   * *Attempt tamponade using a balloon device or a Foley catheter. Consult ENT emergently. Check a hemoglobin and INR. Place patient on prophylactic antibiotics. Admit to a monitored setting.*

SUMMARY POINTS

* *Anterior epistaxis is more common than posterior epistaxis.*
* *Anterior epistaxis generally stops with pressure, but may require nasal packing.*
* *Posterior epistaxis is an emergency and requires emergent ENT consultation and admission.*
* *Any patient who requires nasal packing must be given antibiotics to prevent TSS or sinusitis.*

CHAPTER 65
DENTAL EMERGENCIES

I. Defining Features

A. Dental Trauma
1. **Tooth fractures** are managed differently, depending on the patient's age and the extent of the fracture.
2. **Avulsed tooth** management depends on whether the avulsed tooth is a permanent or a deciduous tooth. Preservation of the periodontal ligament and limiting the length of time out of the socket relates directly to subsequent tooth viability. A *subluxed* tooth refers to a tooth that is "loose" due to trauma.
3. **Mandible fractures** occur at the symphysis (16%), body (28%), angle (25%), ramus (4%), condyle (26%), and coronoid process (1%). Fractures are multiple in half of cases because of the ring shape of the mandible.

B. Odontogenic Infections
1. **Mandibular infections** can arise in the sublingual, submental, or submandibular spaces. **Ludwig's angina** is an infection of the floor of the mouth involving all 3 spaces bilaterally. Its name originates from the sensation of choking and suffocation that a patient with this infection experiences. *Ludwig's angina is an emergency because the massive swelling can result in airway obstruction.*
2. **Other abscesses. Masticator space abscess** is bound by the muscles of mastication. Patients with infection in this space present with trismus. The origin of infection is most frequently the 3rd molar. **Buccal space abscess** presents with swelling in the cheek and is due to infection of a premolar or molar tooth (Figure 65–1). **Canine space abscess** presents with swelling in the anterior face and is due to an infection of a maxillary canine (Figure 65–2). When severe, infection may spread to the cavernous sinus.

II. Epidemiology

A. Dental Trauma
1. Approximately 80% of traumatized teeth are maxillary teeth.
2. Tooth avulsion occurs with a prevalence of up to 15% of cases.
3. Mandible fractures are the 2nd most common fracture of the facial bones, with nasal bone fractures being the most common.

B. Odontogenic infections. Dental caries and abscesses are commonly seen in the ED. Fortunately, deep space abscesses and Ludwig's angina are rare.

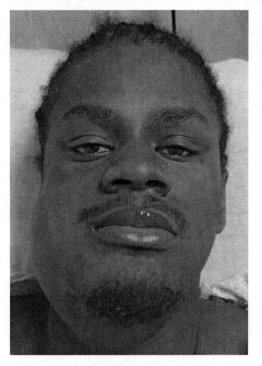

Figure 65–1. Buccal space infection.

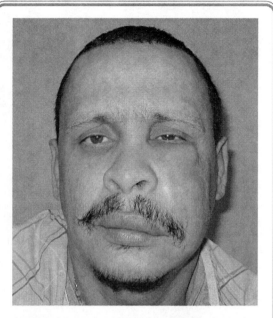

Figure 65–2. Canine space infection.

III. Etiology

A. **Dental Trauma**
1. **Tooth fractures** are based on the Ellis classification. Ellis I fractures involve only the enamel. Ellis II fractures include the dentin, and Ellis III fractures are present when both the dentin and pulp are exposed (Figure 65–3).
2. **Tooth avulsion** is a result of disruption of the tooth's attachment apparatus. The periodontal ligament is the primary source of attachment of the tooth to the alveolar bone, and is of primary concern to the emergency physician.
3. **Mandible fractures** are most common after blunt trauma to the jaw from either an altercation or an MVC.

B. **Odontogenic Infections**
1. Due to periodontal disease, traumatic injury, or postsurgical infections. A typical odontogenic infection originates from caries, which decay the protective enamel.
2. Once the enamel is dissolved, bacteria travel through the microporous dentin to the pulp, tracking to the root apex, soft tissues, and finally into the deeper fascial planes.

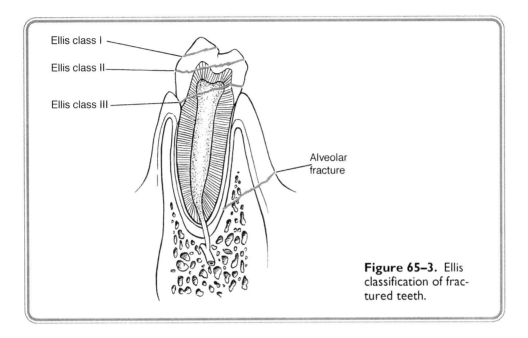

Ellis class I

Ellis class II

Ellis class III

Alveolar fracture

Figure 65–3. Ellis classification of fractured teeth.

3. Ludwig's angina occurs secondary to an abscess of the posterior mandibular molars in 75% of cases. If the infection continues to spread, the potential exists for adjacent retropharyngeal and mediastinal infection. Ludwig's angina is most commonly due to anaerobic (Bacteroides) and aerobic (Streptococcus, Staphylococcus) oral flora in an immunocompromised patient who is often elderly, diabetic, or an alcoholic.

IV. Risk Factors

A. **Dental trauma.** Male, MVC, sports activity, or assault.

B. **Odontogenic infection.** Dental caries, alcoholic, elderly, or diabetes mellitus.

V. Clinical Presentation

A. **History**

1. **Dental trauma**

   a. *Ellis fractures.* Ellis I fractures are painless, and the patient may only note a jagged edge to the tooth. Ellis II fractures present with the primary complaint of hot and cold sensitivity as the exposed dentin is quite sensitive. Patients with Ellis III fractures present with severe pain, although pain may be absent if there is neurovascular compromise (see Figure 65–3).

   b. *Tooth avulsion.* The time the tooth spends out of the socket is one of the most important pieces of information to obtain. If the tooth is out for < 20 minutes, prognosis is good. If > 60 minutes has elapsed, a successful re-implant is much more difficult.

   c. *Mandible fracture.* Patients report jaw pain, inability to open the mouth, and possible malocclusion of the teeth. Numbness of the lower lip suggests an injury to the inferior alveolar nerve.

2. **Odontogenic infection.** When evaluating for an abscess, elicit a history of fever, trismus, drooling, inability to handle secretions, and recent dental infection or trauma. Ludwig's angina presents with dysphagia, odynophagia, dysphonia, trismus, and drooling. The patient may also complain of severe neck and sublingual pain. Patients with a masticator space abscess will present with pain, fever, trismus, and marked lateral facial swelling on examination.

Trismus is the inability to fully open the jaw due to tonic spasm of the muscles of mastication (lockjaw). In the absence of trauma, a patient with facial swelling and trismus has a masticator space infection until proven otherwise.

B. **Physical Examination**
   1. **Dental trauma**
      a. *Ellis fractures.* The dentin is visualized on examination as a creamy yellow color present in the center of the broken tooth. The pulp is seen as a pink tinge or drop of blood within the exposed dentin.
      b. *Tooth avulsion.* Evaluate the socket and surrounding soft tissue for lacerations, ecchymosis, or foreign bodies. When examining the tooth, do not touch the root.
      c. *Mandible fracture.* Malocclusion may be noted. An intra-oral laceration may represent an open fracture. Ecchymosis under the tongue is highly suggestive of a mandible fracture.
   2. **Odontogenic infection**
      a. **Submental space infection** is characterized by a firm midline swelling beneath the chin. This abscess is due to infection from the mandibular incisors.
      b. **Sublingual space infection** is indicated by swelling of the floor of the mouth and pain and dysphagia. It is due to an anterior mandibular tooth infection.
      c. **Submandibular space infection** is identified by swelling around the angle of the jaw. Mild trismus is frequently present. These abscesses are caused by an infection of the mandibular molar.
      d. **Ludwig's angina** presents with massive swelling on the floor of the mouth and is painful to palpation. The swelling may produce an elevation of the tongue, which can occlude the oropharynx. The patient's anterior neck may be brawny in character secondary to edema.
      e. **Buccal space infection** presents with cheek swelling (see Figure 65–1).
      f. **Canine space infection** is characterized by anterior facial swelling and loss of the nasolabial fold. This infection can extend into the infraorbital region and be confused with ocular pathology (see Figure 65–2).
      g. **Masticator space infections** present with trismus.

Tongue blade test is used to clinically exclude a mandible fracture. The patient is asked to bite on a tongue blade. If the examiner is able to break the blade by turning it while the patient bites down, then a mandible fracture is unlikely. The sensitivity of this test is 95%.

VI. Differential Diagnosis (see I)

VII. Diagnostic Findings
   A. **Laboratory Studies**
      1. No laboratory test is essential for the diagnoses of dental trauma or odontogenic infections.
      2. **CBC** may reveal a leukocytosis in a patient with a dental abscess.
   B. **Imaging Studies**
      1. **Panorex radiograph** is useful to diagnose a mandible fracture, and allows for the visualization of the entire mandible with 1 radiograph (Figure 65–4).
      2. **Soft-tissue lateral neck radiograph** can be used to visualize the retropharyngeal space and exclude other diagnoses.
      3. **CT scan** can be used to diagnose mandible fractures and to localize odontogenic infections. In patients with potential airway compromise, evaluation and treatment should not be delayed while waiting for imaging studies.
   C. **Diagnostic Algorithm (see page 390)**

VIII. Treatment
   A. **Dental Trauma**
      1. **Ellis fractures.** Ellis I fractures require no immediate treatment; patients should be referred to a dentist. For Ellis II fractures, place a calcium hydroxide paste, cement, or moist gauze over the dentin, then cover the tooth with aluminum foil to decrease contamination of the pulp. Patients will require urgent follow-up with a dentist within 24 hours. Ellis III fractures should be covered with calcium hydroxide, cement, or moist gauze and then covered with foil. These patients require immediate dental referral to avoid pulpal necrosis and loss of the tooth.

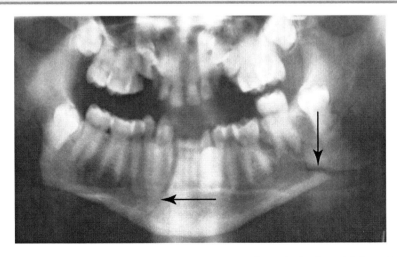

Figure 65–4. Panorex demonstrating fractures to the right body and left angle of the mandible.

Diagnostic Algorithm

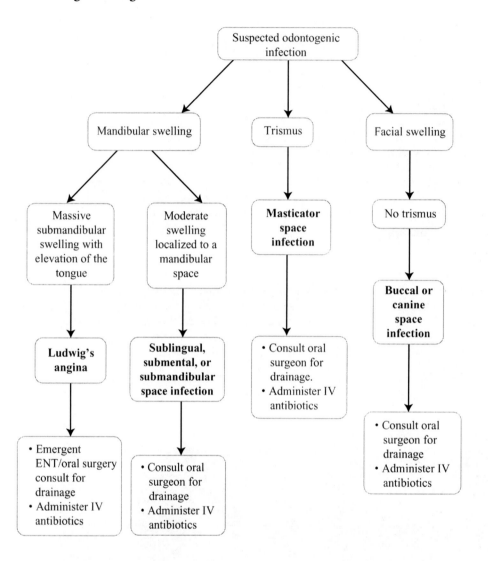

2. **Avulsed tooth.** If it is a permanent tooth, care should be taken to hold the tooth by the crown, carefully avoiding the periodontal ligament. If the ligament is damaged, the success of re-implantation may be compromised. In the ED, the tooth should be rinsed gently with saline; do not "brush" the tooth clean, as this will disrupt the periodontal ligament. The socket is rinsed with NS to remove blood clot. Then re-implant the tooth in its socket with a firm pressure into the socket. Have the patient bite on gauze to maintain the tooth in the socket. If unable to replace the tooth, place it in Hank's solution,

which preserves the ligament for 4–6 hours. Milk is an acceptable alternative if Hank's solution is not available. Patients require prophylactic antibiotics, tetanus immunization, and an immediate dental referral for tooth stabilization.

3. **Mandible fracture.** Narcotic pain control and antibiotics (penicillin G 2–4 million U IV or clindamycin 900 mg IV) are indicated for open fractures. Oral surgery consultation for operative repair is indicated, with the exception of isolated nondisplaced condylar fractures, which can be managed non-operatively.

B. **Odontogenic Infection**

1. **Ludwig's angina.** Primary concern is maintenance of the patient's airway. Maintain the patient in a seated position and place airway equipment at the bedside. The patient should be given parenteral antibiotics, such as penicillin plus metronidazole, cefoxitin, or clindamycin. ENT should be consulted immediately and arrangements made for transfer to the OR.

2. **Masticator space abscess.** Administer IV antibiotics. Penicillin G 2–4 million U IV or clindamycin 900 mg IV. Consult ENT or oral surgery for surgical drainage.

IX. Disposition

A. **Admission.** Patients with an open mandible fracture require admission for IV antibiotics and operative repair. Patients with odontogenic deep space infections and Ludwig's angina require drainage of the abscesses in a controlled setting. These patients require admission.

B. **Discharge.** Most patients with dental trauma can be discharged to follow up with a dentist. Patients with minor odontogenic abscesses can be discharged after I&D by a consulting oral surgeon. These patients will require oral antibiotics and follow-up.

CASE PRESENTATION

A 47-year-old man with the odor of alcohol on his breath presents to the ED complaining of pain under his tongue, difficulty swallowing and opening his mouth, and drooling. He states that the problem began 2 days ago after he broke a tooth in the back of his mouth. Since then it has gotten significantly worse.

1. *What will you look for on physical examination?*

   · *Does the patient have any swelling on the floor of the mouth that is painful to palpation? Is there any elevation of his tongue? Does he have any systemic signs such as fever?*

2. *His triage vital signs demonstrate a tachycardia and a fever. The patient has noted elevation of his tongue, and it is quite tender to palpation on the floor of his mouth. Now that you have made the clinical diagnosis of Ludwig's angina, what is your next step?*

   · *Definitive airway equipment at bedside. Immediate ENT consultation for operative drainage. Administer antibiotics: penicillin + metronidazole, cefoxitin, or clindamycin.*

SUMMARY POINTS

· *Tooth fractures are categorized and treated according to the Ellis classification.*

· *Clean avulsed teeth with care to avoid dislodging the periodontal ligament.*

· *Ludwig's angina is a surgical emergency that requires prompt drainage.*

SECTION XV
NEUROLOGIC EMERGENCIES

CHAPTER 66
ALTERED MENTAL STATUS

I. Defining Features

A. Altered mental status (AMS) may have an organic (ie, structural, biochemical, pharmacologic) or functional (ie, psychiatric) cause.

B. Consciousness has 2 main components: arousal and cognition. Arousal is controlled by the **ascending reticular activating system** (ARAS) in the brainstem. Cognition is controlled by the **cerebral cortex.**

C. Lethargy, stupor, obtundation, and coma are imprecise terms used to describe alterations of arousal. A description of the patient's arousal level (eg, opens eyes to voice) is preferable.

D. **Delirium** is an alteration of both arousal and cognition. Patients exhibit restlessness, agitation, and disorientation. **Dementia** is an alteration of cognition, not arousal.

II. Epidemiology

A. AMS accounts for 5% of ED visits.

B. About 80% of patients with AMS have a systemic or metabolic cause, and about 15% have a structural lesion.

III. Pathophysiology

A. ARAS is a complex system of nuclei in the brainstem. It may be impaired by small structural lesions in the brainstem such as ischemic or hemorrhagic stroke, shear forces from head trauma, or external compression from brain herniation. Severe toxic and/or metabolic derangements (eg, hypoxia, hypothermia, drugs) can also cause impairment.

B. Bilateral cerebral cortex dysfunction must occur to cause decreased levels of arousal or profound AMS. This is usually caused by toxic/metabolic derangements, infection, seizures, SAH, or increased ICP. Unilateral lesions such as stroke do not by themselves cause profound AMS.

IV. Risk Factors

A. **Elderly** are more prone to infection, have co-morbid illnesses, and take multiple medications.

B. **Substance abuse.** Heroin, cocaine, alcohol withdrawal, and liver failure.

C. **Psychiatric patients** may be on mood stabilizing drugs, which, when taken in excess, have toxic effects that cause abnormal arousal or cognition.

V. Clinical Presentation

A. **History**
1. AMS represents a spectrum of disease presentations from profoundly depressed arousal requiring emergent intubation to severe agitation and confusion requiring restraint and sedation. ***Initial stabilizing measures are often needed before a complete history and physical examination can be performed.***
2. If the patient is unable to give a coherent history, alternate sources of history should be sought. Pre-hospital providers should be questioned about the patient's condition in the field, therapies given and the response, and the condition of the home environment (pill bottles, suicide note). Family members should be contacted to ascertain past history of similar episodes, medical history, trauma, substance abuse, and the last time the patient was seen in a normal state.
3. The patient's belongings should be searched for medical identification bracelets, pill bottles, phone numbers, or other potential sources of information.

B. **Physical Examination**
1. Vital signs, ABCs, pulse oximetry, and bedside glucose should be assessed, looking for immediate life threats and treatable causes of AMS (hypoglycemia, hypoxia or abnormal respiratory pattern, hyper- or hypotension, hyper- or hypothermia). Naloxone (Narcan), glucose, and thiamine should be administered, as dictated by history and examination.
2. A "head-to-toe" examination should follow, looking for systemic causes of AMS and focal neurologic deficits.
3. **HEENT examination.** The head should be examined for any signs of trauma. Pupil size, symmetry, and reactivity should be assessed. Pinpoint pupils are a sign of opiate overdose or pontine hemorrhage. An asymmetrically dilated "blown" pupil is a sign of uncal herniation. Fundi should be assessed for presence of papilledema or subhyaloid hemorrhage associated with SAH.
4. **Neck** stiffness indicates meningeal inflammation caused by either SAH or infection.
5. **Heart examination.** Assess for dysrhythmias (AF), murmurs (endocarditis), or rubs (pericarditis).
6. **Lung examination.** Assess for symmetric breath sounds, respiratory rate, wheezes, rhonchi, and rales.
7. **Abdominal examination.** Assess for masses and organomegaly (alcoholic liver disease, splenic sequestration in sickle cell disease).
8. **Skin examination.** Assess for color, turgor (dehydration), rashes (petechiae, purpura suggesting TTP or meningococcemia), and infection (cellulitis, fasciitis).
9. **Neurologic examination.** If you cannot perform a complete examination due to the patient's mental status, document what you are able to do and how the patient appears. Mental status: AVPU (alert, responds to voice, responds to pain, unresponsive). If the patient responds to voice, is the response coherent and appropriate? Cranial nerves, motor, and sensory examinations.

CLINICAL SKILLS TIP

The Glasgow Coma Scale (GCS) was developed to stratify patients with head injuries, but has evolved into a way to categorize patients with decreased LOC. Scores range from 3 to 15. Intubation for airway protection is usually considered for scores < 8 (see Chapter 72).

VI. **Differential Diagnosis.** The mnemonic AEIOU-TIPS is useful for remembering the treatable causes of AMS (Table 66–1).

VII. **Diagnostic Findings**

A. **Laboratory Studies**

1. Multiple laboratory tests are obtained in an attempt to gain more information, although a cause can usually be ascertained from a thorough history and physical examination.

2. Initial laboratory tests should include CBC (leukocytosis, anemia, thrombocytopenia); chemistry (electrolyte abnormalities, acidosis, renal failure); urine (pregnancy test, toxicology screen, infection); coagulation and liver studies (liver failure, coagulopathy); blood cultures (if infection suspected); ABG (hypoxia, hypercarbia, acidosis, lactate); alcohol level; and serum toxicology screen.

B. **Imaging Studies**

1. **Head CT scan** to assess for mass lesion, hydrocephalus, and intracerebral or subarachnoid bleed.

2. **CXR** if hypoxia, abnormal respirations, or evidence of pulmonary infection is present.

3. **ECG** should be performed on all patients, looking for ischemia, QT or QRS prolongation, or changes consistent with electrolyte abnormalities.

Table 66–1. AEIOU TIPS: differential diagnosis of patients with AMS.

A - Alcohol
E - Epilepsy, **E**lectrolytes, **E**ncephalopathy (HTN and hepatic)
I - Insulin (hypo- and hyperglycemia), **I**ntussusception (peds)
O - Opiates, **O**verdose
U - Uremia
T - Trauma, **T**emperature (hypo- and hyperthermia)
I - Infection, **I**ntracerebral hemorrhage
P - Psychiatric, **P**oison
S - Shock

C. **Diagnostic Algorithm**

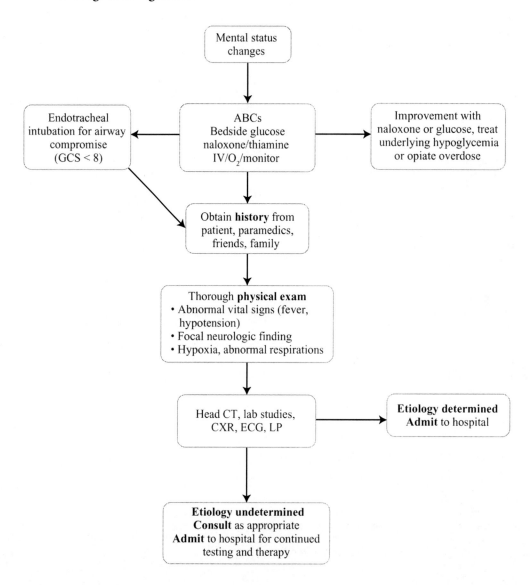

VIII. Treatment

    A. **ABCs,** IV access, cardiac monitor, and pulse oximetry.

    B. **Hypoglycemia. Adults:** 1 amp D50 (50% glucose solution). **Pediatrics:** 2–4 mL/kg D25 (25% glucose solution).

    C. **Narcotic overdose.** Treat based on history and pupillary examination. **Adults:** naloxone 2–4 mg IV given in 0.2–0.4 mg increments to avoid precipitating opiate withdrawal in chronic abusers. In a non-emergent setting, administer naloxone 2–4 mg in a nebulizer with 3 mL saline. **Pediatrics:** naloxone 0.01–0.1 mg/kg IV.

D. **Hypoxia.** Administer 100% O_2, mechanical ventilation as needed, and search and treat potential causes (pneumonia, CHF, pneumothorax, or PE).

E. **Seizures.** Lorazepam 0.1 mg/kg IV.

F. **Infection.** IV fluids and broad-spectrum antibiotic coverage.

G. **Encephalopathy.** Reduce MAP by 25% within 30 minutes in patients with hypertensive encephalopathy. Administer lactulose in patients with hepatic encephalopathy.

H. **Trauma** (see Chapter 72).

I. **Toxicologic overdose** (see Chapters 47–51).

IX. Disposition

A. **Admission.** Most patients with AMS who are not immediately treatable require admission to the hospital for further work-up, therapies, and observation. The level of admission (observation unit, floor, telemetry, ICU) should be guided by the patient's vital signs, reassessments in mental status, and co-morbid illnesses.

B. **Discharge.** Patients with hypoglycemia caused by insulin, who are able to eat and remain normoglycemic after a period of observation, may be safely discharged. *If on long-acting oral hypoglycemics, admit for observation.* For patients with narcotic overdose, discharge is appropriate if the patient improves with naloxone and remains stable after the duration of action of naloxone has elapsed (ie, 1–4 hours). Patients with AMS due to a seizure may be discharged if the seizure is typical in a patient with history of seizures. Antiepileptic medications (eg, phenytoin) should be loaded prior to discharge.

CASE PRESENTATION

A 32-year-old man is transported by EMS to the ED. He was found in an alley by a pedestrian. He is minimally responsive to painful stimuli. Physical examination reveals RR of 8 and pinpoint pupils.

1. *What will you do first?*
   - *ABCs, O_2, naloxone, bedside glucose.*
2. *If the patient responds to the naloxone, what will you do next?*
   - *Speak with the paramedics about the scene, contact family, speak with the patient, and perform a complete physical examination.*

SUMMARY POINTS

- *Do not delay bedside glucose determination, administration of glucose, and naloxone, if indicated. This can prevent the need for endotracheal intubation.*
- *Talk to the paramedics and family; they can often identify the cause of AMS.*
- *Identify level of AMS, systemic conditions, and any focal deficits with the physical examination.*
- *Re-examine your patients frequently and note any changes in condition and response to therapy.*

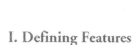

CHAPTER 67
HEADACHE

I. Defining Features

A. Headache is the presenting complaint in 3–5% of all visits to the ED.

B. Headaches are classically divided into **primary headache syndromes** (migraine, tension, cluster) and **secondary causes,** which can range from **benign** (sinusitis) to **emergent** (SAH, meningitis, tumor with increased ICP).

C. In clinical practice, the emergency physician attempts to classify a patient's headache as **emergent** (cannot miss diagnosis that is life or organ threatening) or **benign** (treat the pain and discharge home).

II. Epidemiology

A. The majority of headaches in patients presenting to the ED have a benign etiology; however, there are still 5–10% of patients who may have a serious or potentially life-threatening cause for their headache (Table 67–1).

B. Although SAH represents < 1% of headaches in patients who present to the ED, SAH occurs in approximately 12% of patients with a severe sudden headache and a normal neurologic examination.

C. About 55% of patients with an intracerebral hemorrhage have a headache, compared with 17% of ischemic stroke patients.

III. Etiology

A. Brain tissue is insensate. In benign headache syndromes, pain originates from blood vessels, venous sinuses, the dura, cranial nerves, or extra-cranial sources (muscle tension). In emergent headaches, pain may arise from mass effect (tumor or subdural hematoma), inflammation of the meninges (meningitis and SAH), vascular inflammation (temporal arteritis), vascular dissection (carotid and vertebral artery dissection) or extra-cranial sources (dental caries, otitis media, sinusitis).

B. **Emergent Headaches**

1. **SAH.** Rupture of an aneurysm is the most common cause. Median age of patient is 50. Sudden onset of a severe headache in the occipital region. Pain may resolve spontaneously in ED. Over 50% of patients have a normal neurologic examination.

2. **Meningitis.** Classic triad of headache, fever, and meningismus is often *not present.* More difficult to diagnose at extremes of age. Immunosuppression can cause atypical subacute presentations.

Table 67–1. Headache classification by incidence.

Type of Headache	Incidence (%)
Tension	50
Unknown cause	30
Migraine	10
Serious secondary cause	3–8
Life threatening	1

    3. **Intracranial bleed. Subdural** bleed can occur with minimal or unrecognized trauma (warfarin use, elderly). **Epidural** bleed usually occurs with significant trauma. **Intracerebral** bleed is often associated with severe hypertension.

    4. **Temporal arteritis.** Occurs in patients > age 50, and is more frequent in women. Caused by a systemic panarteritis involving arterial walls. Patients present with frontotemporal throbbing headache, jaw claudication, and a non-pulsatile or tender temporal artery. It can cause visual loss from ischemic optic neuritis.

    5. **Carotid and vertebral artery dissection.** Acute unilateral headache and neck pain. Associated with or without trauma. Median age of patient is 40. May present with hemiparesis.

    6. **Pseudotumor cerebri.** Benign intracranial hypertension of unclear cause. Often occurs in young, obese females with chronic headaches. Papilledema is usually the only abnormal examination finding.

    7. **Other.** Stroke, tumor, acute angle-closure glaucoma, hypertensive encephalopathy, pheochromocytoma, CO poisoning, venous sinus thrombosis.

C. **Benign Headaches**

    1. **Migraine.** Abnormal vascular activity is causal. More common in females, with onset usually in teen years, and less commonly begins > age 40. Unilateral pulsating headache that may have associated aura. Usually follows a typical pattern for individual patients. Improves during pregnancy (estrogen excess). Associated nausea and vomiting or photophobia and phonophobia.

    2. **Tension.** Most common primary headache. Bitemporal non-pulsating. No associated nausea, vomiting, photophobia, or phonophobia.

    3. **Cluster.** Uncommon headache overall, but more common in men. Acute, severe, unilateral retro-orbital pain. Associated lacrimation, eye injection, and rhinorrhea. Occur in "clusters" over days to weeks and resolves spontaneously.

IV. **Risk Factors.** **"Red flags"** in the history should cause consideration of an emergent secondary cause of headache, including acute onset, worst or first ever, trauma, progressive nature, fever, focal neurologic deficit, AMS, immunocompromise (eg, HIV), malignancy, coagulopathy (eg, warfarin), or uncontrolled hypertension.

V. Clinical Presentation

A. **History**

1. **Onset.** Sudden and severe suggests a more serious vascular cause such as SAH.

2. **Pattern.** Different from previous, worst ever (SAH), first ever, progressive, mornings (tumor or mass lesion), better supine, worse standing (post-LP headache).

3. **Location.** Usually nonspecific. However, migraines are typically unilateral, tension headaches are bilateral, and SAH is usually occipital or nuchal. Neck pain with or without neurologic deficits may represent a carotid or vertebral artery dissection.

4. **Character.** Migraines pulsate, tension headaches squeeze, cluster and SAH headaches are acute and sharp.

5. **Associated symptoms.** Syncope, AMS, neck pain or stiffness, seizure, fever, cough or cold, hypertension.

6. **Family history.** Migraines and SAH are both more common if a first-degree relative is affected. Consider CO poisoning when many family members are affected during the fall and winter.

B. **Physical Examination**

1. **Vital signs.** Fever (meningitis), severe hypertension (hypertensive encephalopathy or intracerebral bleed).

2. **HEENT examination.** Sinus tenderness, dental caries, otitis media, temporal artery tenderness, eye examination including visual acuity, pupil reactivity (angle-closure glaucoma), and funduscopy (papilledema from increased ICP).

3. **Neck examination.** Meningismus, pulses, and bruits.

4. **Neurologic examination.** Mental status, cranial nerves, strength, sensation, reflexes, cerebellar, and gait.

CLINICAL SKILLS TIP

A thorough neurologic examination should be documented on the chart of any patient complaining of a headache.

VI. Differential Diagnosis (see III)

VII. Diagnostic Findings

A. **Laboratory studies.** General laboratory studies (CBC, chemistry panel, urinalysis) add little to the diagnosis of emergent headaches. Elevated WBC count may point to an infection; elevated ESR is present in cases of temporal arteritis.

B. **Imaging studies.** Non-contrast **head CT scan** is the test of choice when working up possible emergent causes of headache. It can assess for acute SAH (sensitivity 98% within 12 hours, 93% within 24 hours), intracerebral, acute subdural and epidural hematomas, and lesions causing mass effect. **IV contrast** is added in patients with HIV, possible subacute or chronic subdural, or with suspected CNS infections.

C. **Procedures**

1. **LP** to rule out meningitis, or SAH if the head CT scan is non-diagnostic. It can also be performed to check the opening pressure (normal < 20 cm H_2O) in patients with suspected pseudotumor cerebri. LP can be safely performed

without previous head CT scan in alert immunocompetent patients, < age 60, with a non-focal neurologic examination and no papilledema or other signs of increased ICP and no seizure activity.

   2. CSF findings in acute meningitis and SAH (Table 67–2).

D. Diagnostic Algorithm

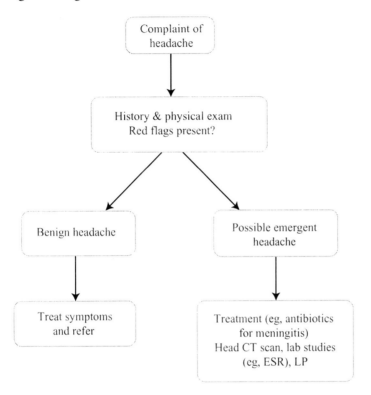

Table 67–2. CSF findings in meningitis and SAH.

CSF	Normal	Bacterial	Viral	SAH
Cells	< 5 WBC	200–5000 PMN	< 1000 monocytes	100's–million RBC
CSF/serum glucose ratio	0.6	Low	Normal	Normal
Protein	15–45 mg/dL	High	High	Normal to increased
Gram stain	Negative	Positive	Negative	Negative
Xanthochromia	Negative	Negative	Negative	Positive

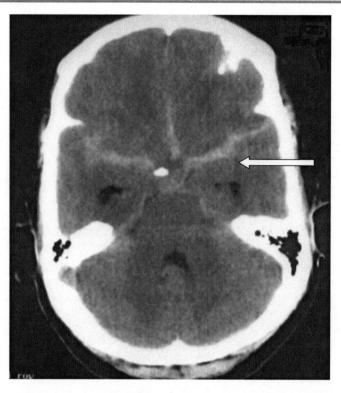

Figure 67–1. Non-contrast head CT scan showing SAH. Note the blood (*white areas*) in the basal cisterns and interhemispheric fissure. This is referred to as the "star sign." (arrow)

CLINICAL SKILLS TIP

Interpreting CSF results in the face of a traumatic LP can be difficult. A decrease in RBCs to near zero from tubes 1 to 4 suggests that the blood in tube 1 was from LP-induced trauma, not SAH. Xanthochromia, when present, is indicative of SAH. In general, there will be 1 WBC in the CSF for every 700 RBCs when from a traumatic LP. More WBCs suggests meningitis or SAH.

VIII. Treatment

A. **Benign headache** (typical migraine, tension, cluster). Oral pain medications for mild pain. For more severe pain (migraine and cluster), IV antiemetics (prochlorperazine 5–10 mg IV). Decrease sensory stimuli (dark quiet room). IV morphine for continued pain.

B. **Emergent Headache**
   1. **Subarachnoid hemorrhage.** Emergent neurosurgical consult for aneurysm clipping or coiling. Nimodipine 60 mg PO to reduce subsequent vasospasm.
   2. **Meningitis.** Do not delay antibiotics for CT scan or LP (ceftriaxone + vancomycin). Perform CT scan before LP if patient has AMS, focal neurologic findings, HIV, seizures, signs of increased ICP, or is > age 60.

3. **Intracranial bleed.** Emergent neurosurgical consultation for evacuation of subdural or epidural bleed. FFP if patient is coagulopathic. BP control for intracerebral bleed (reduce MAP by 25%).

4. **Temporal arteritis.** Administer oral prednisone 80 mg. Patient should be discharged home on prednisone 40 mg daily. Close follow-up for biopsy and definitive diagnosis.

5. **Pseudotumor cerebri.** CT scan followed by LP to assess opening pressure. An opening pressure > 25 cm H_2O suggests the diagnosis (normal 10–20 cm H_2O). Remove 20 mL of CSF. Give acetazolamide and steroids after consulting with a neurologist.

6. **Carotid or vertebral artery dissection.** CT scan is often normal, with focal neurologic findings. MRA or duplex ultrasound is needed to determine diagnosis.

IX. Disposition

A. **Admission.** All patients with an emergent secondary headache should be admitted to the hospital. Patients with SAH, intracranial hemorrhage, or mass effect with signs of increased ICP should be admitted to an ICU.

B. **Discharge.** Patients with benign headache syndromes whose pain is well controlled can be discharged home. Patients with headaches that are not life or organ threatening (brain tumor without mass effect, temporal arteritis, pseudotumor cerebri) can be discharged home after close follow-up is arranged. These patients should be given very specific instructions to return if headache worsens or they experience any new or different symptoms, including focal weakness, numbness, speech or visual problems, or vomiting.

CASE PRESENTATION

A 23-year-old woman presents to the ED with complaints of headache for the past 3 months. The headache has been constant, frontal, and is worse with exertion. She denies a previous history of headache. She is obese and papilledema is present. A non-contrast head CT scan shows no mass lesion.

1. *What is your next step?*

   · *Perform an LP to assess the opening pressure. To obtain an accurate opening pressure, the patient should be in the lateral decubitus position (not sitting up).*

2. *The opening pressure is 45 cm H_2O. You diagnose pseudotumor cerebri. What should be done to treat the patient?*

   · *Remove approximately 20 mL of CSF. Consult neurology. Give acetazolamide. Steroids are considered when there is visual loss.*

SUMMARY POINTS

· *Consider emergent causes of headache first.*

· *Have a low threshold to perform a CT scan on patients with "red flags" in their history and physical examination.*

· *Never delay administering antibiotics while waiting for a CT scan or LP when considering the diagnosis of meningitis.*

· *When SAH is suspected, follow a normal CT scan with LP*

CHAPTER 68
DIZZINESS

I. Defining Features

  A. **Dizziness** is a word commonly used by the patient to describe symptoms, but it can mean many different things. The term must be further clarified into 1 of 4 general categories: vertigo, presyncope, disequilibrium, or lightheadedness.

  B. **Vertigo.** Feeling, sensation, or illusion of movement.

  C. **Presyncope.** Patient feels as though they may "pass out."

  D. **Disequilibrium.** Patient feels a sense of imbalance without vertigo.

  E. **Lightheadedness.** Vague, poorly defined symptoms that do not fall into the above categories.

II. Epidemiology

  A. About 25% of patients presenting to the ED have dizziness as some component of their complaint.

  B. Dizziness is the number 1 complaint in patients > age 75.

III. Pathophysiology

  A. **Vertigo.** Causes of vertigo can be divided into **central** and **peripheral** processes. Central vertigo implies pathology within the cerebellum, whereas peripheral vertigo occurs when there is an abnormality of the semicircular canals or labyrinth of the inner ear.

  B. **Benign paroxysmal positional vertigo** (BPPV) is the most common cause of peripheral vertigo. It is due to the accumulation of floating calcium carbonate particles in the semicircular canals. This stimulates the labyrinth, causing asymmetric input from the semicircular canals and the sensation of movement.

  C. **Ménière's disease** is a disorder in which there is an increase in volume and pressure of the endolymph of the inner ear, which eventually leads to damage of the endolymphatic system.

  D. **Labyrinthitis and vestibular neuronitis.** The pathophysiology of labyrinthitis is not completely understood, although many cases are associated with systemic or viral illnesses. Viral infection of the vestibular nerve is believed to be the most common cause of vestibular neuronitis.

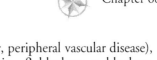

IV. Risk Factors. Elderly (cardiovascular, cerebrovascular, peripheral vascular disease), medications (anticonvulsants, aminoglycosides, diuretics, β blockers, α blockers, calcium channel blockers, tranquilizers), peripheral neuropathy, decreased visual acuity, head trauma, or tympanic membrane rupture.

V. Clinical Presentation

A. **History**

1. The cause of "dizziness" can be elicited by history alone in more than half of all cases.

2. **Vertigo.** Patients complain of a sensation of movement, or "the room spinning" around them, with associated nausea and vomiting. **BPPV** usually has an abrupt onset, lasts < 1 minute, and is provoked by head movement. VBI, TIA, and cerebellar hemorrhage may also have an acute onset. **Ménière's disease** is associated with hearing loss and tinnitus, and the vertigo usually lasts for hours. **Labyrinthitis** and **vestibular neuronitis** usually last for a few days. In contradistinction, the symptoms of central vertigo are usually less acute, more persistent, and may have associated neurologic symptoms (Table 68–1).

3. **Presyncope.** Patients complain of feeling as though they are going to pass out. This may be associated with a stressful event (vaso-vagal episode), exertion (aortic stenosis), sudden change in posture (hypovolemia), or palpitations (dysrhythmia).

4. **Disequilibrium.** Patients are usually elderly. They complain that their symptoms are worse at night (limited visual acuity is further impaired) and later in the day (more fatigued).

5. **Lightheadedness.** Patients usually have vague complaints. They may have a medical or psychiatric cause for their symptoms. Medications should be assessed as a possible cause.

Table 68–1. Differentiating peripheral vertigo from central vertigo.

Symptoms	Peripheral Vertigo	Central Vertigo
Onset	Acute	Insidious
Nausea and vomiting	Usually present	Usually absent
Nystagmus	• Horizontal or rotatory • Fatigable • Suppressed with fixation • Unidirectional	• Vertical or any direction • Not fatigable or suppressible • May change directions with gaze
Head movement	Exacerbates	Minimal effect
Ataxia	Minimal	Moderate to severe
Neurologic deficits	None	May be present

B. **Physical Examination**

1. A complete physical examination should be performed, paying special attention to a few key areas.

2. **Vital signs.** Hypotension suggests causes related to decreased cerebral perfusion, whereas hypertension may point to VBI, stroke, or hemorrhage. Bradycardia or tachycardia may cause presyncope from impaired cardiac output.

3. **HEENT examination.** Ears should be carefully examined for presence of ruptured tympanic membrane, decreased hearing, infection, cerumen impaction, and foreign bodies.

4. **Cardiovascular examination.** Assess for signs of vascular insufficiency (carotid bruits, decreased peripheral pulses). Auscultate for any arrhythmia or the systolic murmur of aortic stenosis.

5. **Neurologic examination.** Assess for presence and type of nystagmus. Pay special attention to CN VII, VIII, and IX. Associated cranial neuropathies suggest brainstem involvement and a central cause of vertigo. Patients with peripheral vertigo should be able to ambulate, although they may veer to one side. Patients with cerebellar infarction or hemorrhage usually cannot ambulate.

CLINICAL SKILLS TIP

A Romberg test can be used to differentiate cerebellar from spinal cord (posterior column) dysfunction. Have the patient stand, with feet together, and then have them close their eyes. Excessive swaying or imbalance is a positive test and is seen in patients with significant proprioceptive loss from posterior column dysfunction.

VI. **Differential Diagnosis**

A. **Vertigo. Peripheral:** BPPV, Ménière's disease, vestibular neuritis, or labyrinthitis. **Central:** vertebrobasilar insufficiency, ischemic stroke, cerebellar hemorrhage, or cerebellopontine angle tumor.

B. **Presyncope and lightheadedness.** Vasovagal, cardiac (arrhythmia, valvular disease), hypovolemia, anemia, medications, or electrolyte abnormalities.

C. **Dysequilibrium.** Decreased vision or peripheral neuropathy.

RULE OUT

Cerebellar hemorrhage should be ruled out in patients with central vertigo. Because of the limited space in the posterior fossa, hemorrhage can cause herniation and death in a relatively short period of time.

VII. **Diagnostic Findings**

A. **Laboratory studies.** No specific laboratory test can aid in the diagnosis of vertigo. However, older patients on multiple medications with non-specific symptoms should have **hemoglobin, electrolytes,** and **renal function** evaluated. **ECG** should be performed in patients suspected of having a cardiac cause for their symptoms.

B. **Imaging studies. Head CT scan** is indicated in patients with a suspected central cause for their symptoms (focal neurologic findings, AMS, severe headache), or significant cerebrovascular disease risk factors (Figure 68–1).

C. **Diagnostic procedures. Dix-Hallpike** maneuver can be used to elicit BPPV and differentiate it from a central cause for vertigo. The procedure involves rapidly moving the patient from a seated to supine position with the head rotated 45° to the right with the eyes open. If no symptoms are elicited, the procedure should be repeated with the head rotated to the left. The latency, duration, and direction of nystagmus and presence of vertigo should be noted. With BPPV or peripheral vertigo, the nystagmus is horizontal or rotatory, has a latency period (up to 60 seconds), is fatigable, and suppresses with fixation (Figure 68–2).

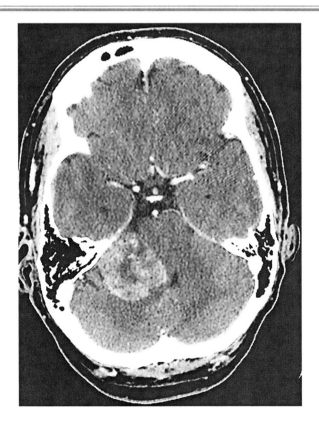

Figure 68–1. CT scan showing cerebellopontine angle tumor (acoustic neuroma).

D. **Diagnostic Algorithm**

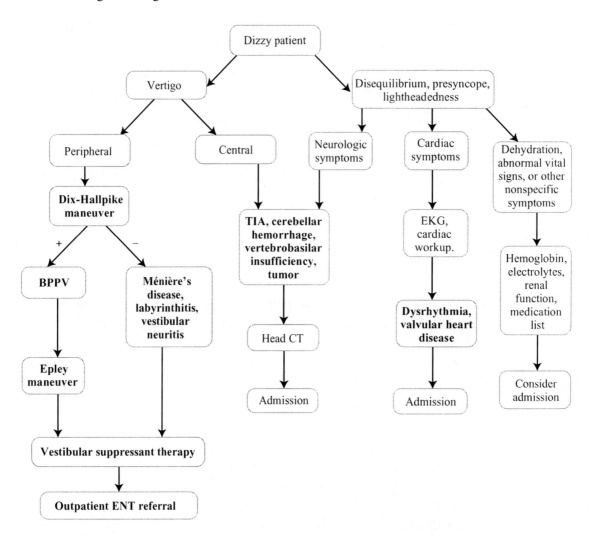

VIII. Treatment

A. **Peripheral Vertigo**

1. **BPPV.** The Epley maneuver is used to reposition the particulate debris from the semicircular canal to the utricle (Figure 68–3). Once the debris is repositioned, the abnormal vestibular input is eliminated. Vestibular suppressant medications are also used to decrease abnormal input from the semicircular canal (Table 68–2).

2. **Ménière's disease, labyrinthitis, vestibular neuritis.** Vestibular suppressant medications should be started.

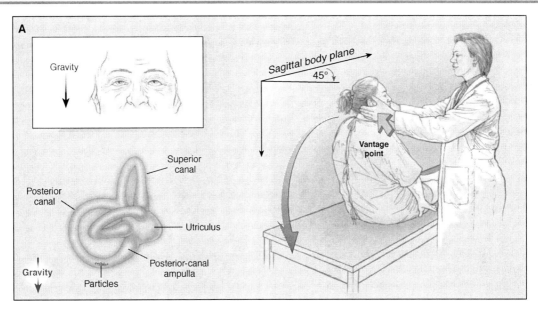

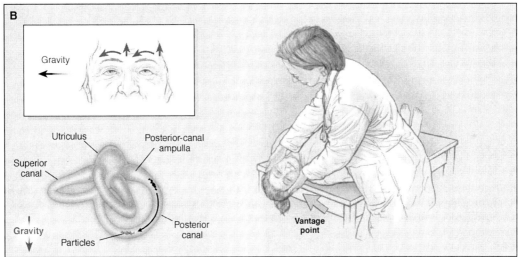

Figure 68–2. Dix-Hallpike test of a patient with BPPV. In Panel A, the examiner stands at the patient's right side and rotates the patient's head 45° to the right to align the right posterior semicircular canal with the sagittal plane of the body. In Panel B, the examiner moves the patient, whose eyes are open, from the seated to the supine right-ear down position and then extends the patient's neck slightly so that the chin is pointed slightly upward. The latency, duration, and direction of nystagmus, if present, and the latency and duration of vertigo, if present, should be noted. The *arrows* in the inset depict the direction of nystagmus in patients with typical BPPV. The presumed location in the labyrinth of the free-floating debris thought to cause the disorder is also shown. Reprinted with permission from NEJM, Vol 341, No. 21, p. 1593, 1999.

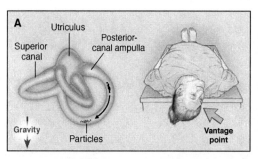

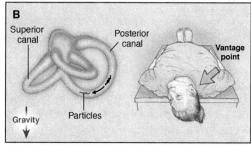

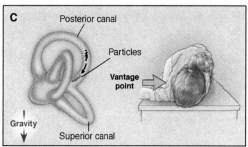

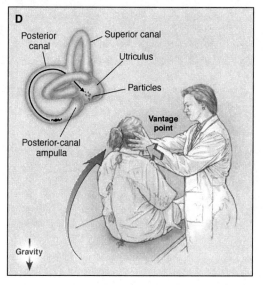

Figure 68–3. Bedside maneuver for the treatment of a patient with BPPV affecting the right ear. Begin with patient in sitting position. A, have the patient lie down with the right ear facing the floor for 30 seconds; B, rotate the head counter-clockwise with the left ear facing the floor for 30 seconds; C, rotate the head counter-clockwise so that the face is toward the floor for 30 seconds; D, have the patient sit up. Repeat until no nystagmus is elicited. Reverse the procedure when the left ear is affected. Reprinted with permission from NEJM Vol. 341, No. 21 p. 1594, 1999.

Table 68–2. Vestibular suppressant therapy.

Class	Medication	Dose
Antihistamine	Meclizine	25 mg PO q 8 hr
Antiemetic	Promethazine	25 mg PO q 6 hr
Benzodiazepines	Diazepam	2–5 mg PO q 8 hr

B. **Central vertigo.** Patients with vertigo from central causes (CNS tumor, bleed, or infarct) should have appropriate neurology or neurosurgical consultation in the ED. Patients suspected of having vertebrobasilar insufficiency should be started on aspirin in consultation with their primary physician.

C. **Presyncope.** Patients with cardiovascular risk factors and presyncope should have an ECG. CBC and electrolytes should be checked. Patients are treated similar to patients with syncope, and may require a telemetry admission to exclude an arrhythmia (see Chapter 18). Patients found to have non-cardiac causes of presyncope, such as dehydration or anemia, are treated accordingly with fluids and/or blood transfusion.

D. **Disequilibrium.** Patients with symptoms consistent with possible decreased visual acuity or peripheral neuropathy can usually be discharged home and follow-up with their primary physician. Vestibular suppressants should never be used in these patients because these drugs can exacerbate symptoms.

E. **Lightheadedness.** More than half of all patients seen in the ED will have no discernible cause for their symptoms. They should undergo a thorough history and physical examination as well as blood studies and an ECG, as dictated by their clinical presentation.

IX. Disposition

A. **Admission.** Patients with central vertigo, focal neurologic findings, a possible cardiovascular cause (arrhythmia, ischemia), an electrolyte abnormality, or anemia should be admitted to the hospital.

B. **Discharge.** Patients with peripheral vertigo, non-specific symptoms without serious comorbidities and a normal ED work-up can be discharged for follow-up with their primary physician.

CASE PRESENTATION

A 70-year-old woman with a history of hypertension and coronary artery disease is brought to the ED by her daughter. The woman is complaining of dizziness. The daughter also notes that her mother complained of having "double vision." She has no associated headache and no nausea or vomiting.

1. *The patient describes the dizziness as the "room spinning." What factors suggest a central cause of her vertigo?*
   · *Age (elderly), atherosclerosis, focal neurologic deficit (diplopia), no nausea or vomiting.*

2. *How will you proceed with the management of this patient?*
   · *CT scan of the head to look for infarct or bleed. She is describing a stroke of the posterior circulation and will require admission.*

SUMMARY POINTS

· *Differentiate true vertigo from other types of dizziness.*
· *Attempt to distinguish peripheral vertigo from central vertigo.*
· *Give vestibular suppressants only to patients with peripheral vertigo.*
· *Consider cerebellar hemorrhage in a patient with acute onset vertigo, ataxia, and headache.*

CHAPTER 69
CEREBROVASCULAR ACCIDENT

I. Defining Features

   A. **Stroke** includes any disruption of blood flow to a focal area of the brain. Etiology may be **ischemic** or **hemorrhagic.**

   B. **Transient ischemic attack** (TIA) refers to a neurologic deficit due to lack of blood flow that usually resolves within 1 hour. The median duration of most TIAs is 10–15 minutes.

II. Epidemiology

   A. Stroke is the 3rd leading cause of death and the number 1 cause of disability in the United States.

   B. Stroke is not just a disease of the elderly—over one third of patients who have a stroke are < age 65.

   C. More than 700,000 strokes and 300,000 TIAs occur in the United States each year.

III. Etiology

   A. **Ischemic stroke** (80%). Due to impaired blood flow to brain tissue from thrombosis or embolism. Thrombosis is the most common cause, occurring in > 80% of incidents. The most common source of embolism is the left atrium in patients with AF. Carotid or vertebral artery dissection is a rare cause of ischemic stroke.

   B. **Hemorrhagic stroke** (20%). Caused by spontaneous bleeding from cerebral vessels. **Intracerebral hemorrhage** is the most common form of hemorrhagic stroke, when bleeding occurs directly into brain parenchyma. The most common areas for intracerebral hemorrhage are the putamen (40%), subcortical white matter (30%), cerebellum (16%), thalamus (10–15%), and pons (5–12%).

   C. **TIA.** TIAs are usually due to a thrombotic process and often precede a thrombotic stroke. Emboli cause TIAs less commonly.

IV. Risk Factors. Atherosclerosis (diabetes, hypertension, elderly), vasculitis, polycythemia, hypercoagulable states, HIV, previous stroke, AF, intracardiac thrombi, valvular heart disease, atrial septal defects, tobacco and alcohol abuse, and African American and Asian ethnicity.

V. Clinical Presentation

A. History

1. History should be obtained from the patient whenever possible. Family, friends, and paramedics should also be used to gather information and establish a timeline of the preceding events. A history of atherosclerotic risk factors, heart disease, or other risk factors (as listed above) should be assessed.

2. The timing of the event is extremely important because some medical centers may use thrombolytic agents to treat acute strokes. If the patient or family is unable to determine when the symptoms began, the time the patient was last symptom-free should be ascertained.

3. New onset headache, weakness, visual, or sensory deficits should be documented. Headaches are more common in hemorrhagic strokes and uncommon in ischemic strokes.

4. Neck pain, trauma, or recent chiropractic manipulation with new onset weakness suggests a **carotid or vertebral artery dissection** as the cause of the stroke.

B. Physical Examination

1. **Vital signs** should be assessed. Hypertension is common during both ischemic and hemorrhagic strokes.

2. **Funduscopic examination** should be performed, looking for papilledema.

3. **Cardiovascular examination** should be performed, looking for signs of atherosclerosis (carotid bruits, pulse deficits), arrhythmias, or murmurs (valvular pathology).

4. **Neurologic examination.** The National Institute of Health Stroke Scale (NIHSS) is a reproducible tool to quantify stroke severity and follow it serially (Table 69–1). LOC (ability to answer simple questions, follow simple commands, and noting the quality of speech), cranial nerves, motor function (pronator drift), sensory function, cerebellar function, and reflexes (upper motor neuron signs of hyperreflexia and Babinski sign) should be assessed. Ischemic strokes often have a typical presentation based on the vascular supply that is affected (Table 69–2).

VI. Differential Diagnosis.
Bell's palsy, Todd's paralysis, DKA, hyperosmolar coma, meningitis, brain tumor, hypertensive encephalopathy, drug toxicity (phenytoin), electrolyte disorders (hyponatremia), Wernicke's encephalopathy, or multiple sclerosis.

RULE OUT

Hypertensive encephalopathy can be confused with an ischemic stroke. Both may have focal neurologic findings and AMS with severely elevated BP and a normal CT scan. Reducing the MAP by 25% over a 30-minute period may resolve the encephalopathy, but should have no effect on a stroke.

VII. Diagnostic Findings

A. Laboratory studies
will aid in making alternative diagnoses. Electrolytes, renal function, CBC, and coagulation studies are considered routine laboratory tests in patients with a stroke.

B. Imaging Studies

1. **Non-contrast head CT scan** is the test of choice to quickly assess for ischemic vs. hemorrhagic stroke. In an ischemic stroke, the CT scan is often

Table 69–1. National Institute of Health stroke scale.

Category	Patient Response	Score
LOC questions	Answers both correctly	0
	Answers one correctly	1
	Answers none correctly	2
LOC commands	Obeys both correctly	0
	Obeys one correctly	1
	Obeys none correctly	2
Beat gaze	Normal	0
	Partial gaze palsy	1
	Forced deviation	2
Best visual	No visual loss	0
	Partial hemianopsia	1
	Complete hemianopsia	2
	Bilateral hemianopsia	3
Facial palsy*	Normal	0
	Minor facial weakness	1
	Partial facial weakness	2
	No facial movement	3
Best motor arm Right _____ Left _____	No drift	0
	Drift < 10 secs	1
	Falls < 10 secs	2
	No effort against gravity	3
	No movement	4
Best motor leg Right _____ Left _____	No drift	0
	Drift < 5 secs	1
	Falls < 5 secs	2
	No effort against gravity	3
	No movement	4
Limb ataxia*	Absent	0
	Ataxia in 1 limb	1
	Ataxia in 2 limbs	2
Sensory	No sensory loss	0
	Mild sensory loss	1
	Severe sensory loss	2
Neglect	Absent	0
	Mild	1
	Severe	2
Articulation	Normal	0
	Mild	1
	Severe	2
Language	Normal	0
	Mild aphasia	1
	Severe aphasia	2
	Mute or global aphasia	3

*Items deleted from the modified NIHSS.[3]

Table 69–2. Ischemic stroke syndromes.

Cerebral Circulation	Vascular Supply	Motor Manifestation	Sensory Manifestation	Speech
Anterior circulation	Anterior cerebral artery	Contralateral weakness of leg > arm (face and hand spared)	Minimal discrimination deficits.	Perseveration
	Middle cerebral artery	Contralateral weakness of face and arm > leg	Contralateral numbness of face and arm > leg	Aphasia, if dominant hemisphere is involved (left in 80% of patients)
Posterior circulation	Posterior cerebral artery (supplies visual cortex)	Minimal motor involvement	Visual abnormalities, light touch, and pinprick affected (patient often unaware of deficits)	
	Vertebral and basilar artery (supplies brain-stem and cerebellum)	Hallmark is crossed deficits (ipsilateral cranial nerve deficits with contralateral motor weakness)		
	Vertebrobasilar artery ischemia	Cranial nerve palsies, limb weakness, diplopia	Dizziness, vertigo, ataxia	Dysarthria
	Cerebellar artery	Drop attack	Vertigo	
Lacunar infarction (4 types)	Penetrating arteries (ischemia of thalamus and internal capsule)			
Motor		Face, arm, and leg		Dysarthria
Sensory			Pure hemisensory deficit	
Clumsy hand dysarthria		Clumsiness of one hand		Dysarthria
Ataxic hemiparesis		Hemiparesis	Ataxia on same side as weakness	

normal initially, followed by edema. Older ischemic strokes appear as hypo-dense areas (Figure 69–1). Hemorrhagic strokes appear as hyperdense (*white*) areas (Figure 69–2).

2. **ECG** is useful to exclude ischemia and atrial fibrillation.

C. **Diagnostic Algorithm**

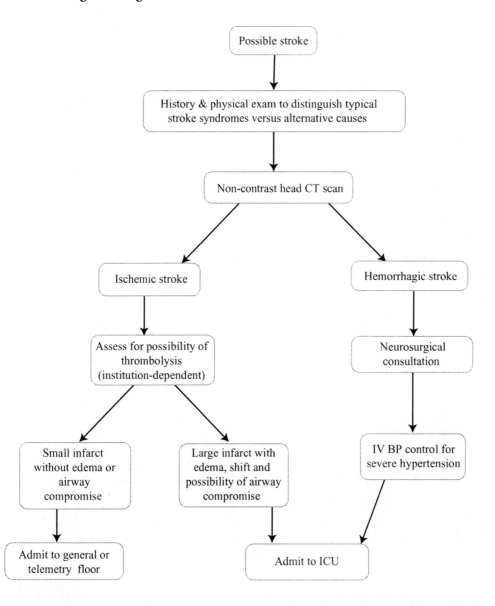

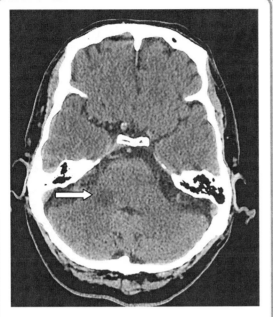

Figure 69–1. CT scan showing ischemic stroke. Note the hypodense area anterior and to the right of the fourth ventricle (*arrow*).

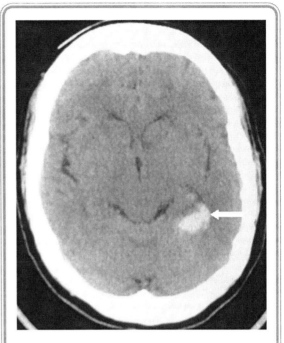

Figure 69–2. CT scan showing hemorrhagic stroke (*arrow*).

VIII. Treatment

A. **Ischemic stroke** patients mainly require supportive care.

  1. **O_2 should be administered for hypoxia. ABCs should be carefully assessed, as some strokes cause airway compromise.**

  2. **BP control** is rarely indicated. Acute elevations typically decline over several days without treatment. Overly aggressive treatment may worsen cerebral ischemia in the area around the stroke (ischemic penumbra) by decreasing the perfusion pressure. Gradual reduction by 15% of the MAP is indicated only when the BP is severe (systolic > 220 mm Hg, diastolic > 120 mm Hg).

  3. **Aspirin** 325 mg should be given to patients with subacute ischemic strokes; this treatment *should not* be started until the CT scan results are available and no hemorrhage is seen.

  4. **Thrombolytics.** Certain patients with acute symptoms of < 3 hours duration may be eligible for IV thrombolysis of the stroke (data supporting this practice is limited).

B. **Intracerebral Hemorrhage (ICH)**

  1. Assess ABCs and perform endotracheal intubation for airway protection if the GCS is < 8.

  2. **Elevated ICP.** Monitoring ICP is indicated in patients with deterioration or a GCS < 9. Treatment measures include elevation of the head of the bed to

30° and mannitol 20% 0.25–0.5 g/kg. Hyperventilation is not employed routinely because it increases cerebral vasoconstriction and worsens ischemia.

3. **Treat coagulopathy.** Obtain coagulation studies and platelet levels. If there is thrombocytopenia or a coagulopathy that may have contributed to the hemorrhage, platelets or FFP should be transfused.

4. **BP control.** BP is treated based on the premise that severe elevations put the patient at a greater risk for extension of the hemorrhage (Table 69–3). However, overly aggressive BP control may result in cerebral hypoperfusion.

5. **Clot evacuation.** An immediate neurosurgical consultation should be obtained. Indications for clot evacuation depend on the patient's age, hemorrhage location, and size of the bleed. Deteriorating patients with lobar hemorrhage or patients with cerebellar hemorrhage > 3 cm are usually evacuated.

C. **TIA.** Administer aspirin 325 mg.

IX. **Disposition**

A. **Admission.** Small ischemic strokes without mass effect or airway compromise are admitted to a general floor. Strokes complicated by possible cardiac ischemia or dysrhythmia such as atrial fibrillation should be admitted to a monitored setting. Patients with large strokes, considerable edema, or mass effect or those with a hemorrhagic stroke of any kind should be admitted to an ICU. Most patients with a TIA should be admitted to a general medical floor for work-up of the etiology. Patients with TIA and any of the following risk factors have a 10% risk of stroke within 90 days: > age 60, diabetes mellitus, symptom duration > 10 minutes, or symptoms involving speech or weakness.

B. **Discharge.** Patients with a clearly defined alternate diagnosis (eg, Bell's palsy) can be discharged home.

Table 69–3. Blood pressure control in hemorrhagic stroke.

Blood Pressure	Recommended Agents
Systolic BP > 230 mm Hg or diastolic BP > 140 mm Hg	Sodium nitroprusside 0.5–10 mcg/kg/min
Systolic BP 180–230 mm Hg Diastolic BP 105–140 mm Hg MAP ≥ 130	Esmolol 500 mcg/kg IV load, then 50–200 mcg/kg/min Labetalol 10–20 mg IV push (repeat every 10 min to max dose of 150 mg) Enalapril 0.625–1.25 mg IV
Systolic BP < 180 mm Hg and diastolic BP < 105 mm Hg	Defer anti-hypertensive therapy

CASE PRESENTATION

A 70-year-old man is brought to the ED by EMS. The man's wife noted that when she awoke this morning her husband was unable to get out of bed. He had slurred speech and could not move the right side of his body, including his face, arm, and leg.

1. *What other historical factors do you want to know?*
   - *Co-morbid illnesses such as diabetes mellitus and hypertension? Previous strokes? Medications (Coumadin)? Trauma?*
2. *What diagnostic studies will you order?*
   - *Bedside glucose, ECG, non-contrast head CT scan.*

SUMMARY POINTS

- *Carefully assess ABCs in patients with a possible stroke.*
- *Order a STAT non-contrast head CT scan in patients with focal neurologic deficits and possible stroke.*
- *Obtain an immediate neurosurgical consultation in patients with cerebellar hemorrhage.*

CHAPTER 70
SEIZURES AND STATUS EPILEPTICUS

I. Defining Features

    A. **Seizure** is abnormal neurologic functioning caused by an inappropriate activation of neurons in the brain.

    B. **Postictal period** is the time following a generalized seizure when the patient slowly returns to normal mental status. This period should last < 1 hour.

    C. **Status epilepticus** classically refers to seizures lasting > 30 minutes, or 2 or more seizures without return to baseline mental status between events. More recently, the definition has changed to seizures lasting 5–10 minutes. This change reflects the importance of initiating treatment early to decrease the risk of neuronal damage from prolonged seizure activity.

    D. Seizures are classified as generalized or partial. **Generalized seizures** are caused by excitation of the entire cerebral cortex. Patients have AMS. The physical manifestation of their seizure activity may be as simple as staring off into space (absence, petit-mal), or it may consist of violent diffuse motor activity (tonic-clonic, grand-mal). **Partial seizures** are caused by a localized neuronal activation that may remain localized or spread to involve other areas of the brain **(partial seizure with secondary generalization)**. Patients with **simple partial seizures** have brief focal motor or sensory manifestations without AMS, whereas **complex partial seizures** are characterized by AMS with mental, psychological, sensory, and motor manifestations (Table 70–1).

II. Epidemiology

    A. Seizures and seizure-related complaints make up about 1% of all ED visits.

    B. The lifetime risk of epilepsy is 3–4%. Incidence is highest among those < age 20 and > age 60.

    C. Status epilepticus has a mortality rate of 10–20%. Half of all patients presenting to the ED in status epilepticus have no prior history of seizures.

III. Etiology

    A. Seizures result from abnormal excitation or lack of inhibition of neurons in the brain. The cause may be **primary** (idiopathic) or **secondary,** with an underlying etiology that may be treatable, such as hypoglycemia.

    B. Alcohol withdrawal seizures usually occur 6–48 hours after a significant reduction in alcohol intake. These seizures must be differentiated from other secondary

Table 70–1. Classification of seizures.

Generalized seizures (always loss of consciousness)
Tonic-clonic seizures (grand mal)
Absence seizures (petit mal)
Myoclonic seizures
Clonic seizures
Atonic seizures
Partial (focal) seizures
Simple partial (no alteration of consciousness)
Complex partial (impaired consciousness)
Partial seizures (simple or complex) with secondary generalization

     causes of seizures that are common in alcoholics, such as head trauma, infections, or metabolic derangements.

   C. There are other medical conditions in which patients may display abnormal movements or behaviors that may be interpreted as seizures, such as syncope.

IV. **Risk Factors.** Certain conditions put an individual at risk of having a seizure. These include febrile illness, alcohol abuse and withdrawal, previous significant head trauma, and family history of epilepsy.

V. **Clinical Presentation**

  A. **History**

    1. Attempt to determine if the event was truly a seizure or something that was mistaken for a seizure. Have the patient or bystanders describe the event. Was it of gradual onset or immediate? Was there a prodrome or aura? Was there a loss of consciousness? Was there diffuse or focal motor activity; if focal, did it then spread or generalize? Was there bowel or bladder incontinence? How long did the event last? Was there a postictal period?

    2. Determine if it was a first seizure or if the patient has a known seizure disorder. If this is a first seizure, is the patient on any medications that cause seizures (tricyclic antidepressants, isoniazid, theophylline)? Was there any headache, trauma, or febrile illness (bleed or meningitis)? Diabetes mellitus or other co-morbid illnesses (hypoglycemia)? Is the patient pregnant (eclampsia)? Is there a history of illicit drug use or alcohol withdrawal? If the patient has a known history of seizures, what medications are they taking and have they missed any doses? Does this fit their normal seizure pattern? Do they

have any concurrent illnesses or are there atypical features (increased frequency despite medication compliance)?

A patient with repetitive seizures who does not return to baseline mental status between events is in status epilepticus and should be treated accordingly.

B. **Physical Examination**
1. Perform a primary survey of the patient assessing ABCs, vital signs, **bedside glucose level,** mental status, and pupils. If the patient is actively seizing, observe the motor activity for focality, generalization, and automatisms (eg, repetitive lip smacking), which may be the only outward sign of seizure activity.
2. Look for physical examination signs of toxidromes (sympathomimetics), trauma (abrasions, contusions, fractures), increased ICP (papilledema or Cushing's response of hypertension and bradycardia).
3. Perform a thorough neurologic examination assessing mental status, cranial nerves, strength, sensation, reflexes, cerebellar function, and gait.

CLINICAL SKILLS TIP

Todd's paralysis *is a transient neurologic deficit that follows a simple or complex focal seizure and resolves within 24 hours. It is an indicator of an underlying pathologic cause for the seizure, such as a mass lesion.*

VI. **Differential Diagnosis**
A. **Primary (idiopathic) seizure disorder** (ie, epilepsy)
B. **Secondary cause of seizure.** Trauma (head), intracranial bleed (SAH, epidural, subdural), infection (meningitis, febrile seizure, sepsis, neurocysticercosis), metabolic (hypoglycemia, hyponatremia, renal failure), toxicologic (cocaine, alcohol withdrawal, isoniazid, theophylline, lidocaine), pregnancy (eclampsia), hypertension (hypertensive encephalopathy), stroke, and mass lesion (tumor, aneurysm).
C. **Conditions mimicking seizures.** Psychogenic pseudoseizures, syncope, myoclonus, cardiac dysrhythmias, cataplexy, dystonias, migraine variants, and hyperventilation syndromes.

RULE OUT

*In patients presenting to the ED with a first time seizure, it is essential to immediately rule out **life-threatening secondary causes.***

VII. **Diagnostic Findings**
A. **Laboratory Studies**
1. First-time seizure patients without co-morbid illnesses and normal history and physical examinations should have glucose and electrolyte levels checked; all females of childbearing age should also have a pregnancy test.
2. Patients with co-morbid illnesses (renal failure) or a history of drug or alcohol abuse should have renal function tests, CBC, drug screen, and calcium, magnesium, and phosphorus levels checked.

3. CPK should be checked in patients with prolonged seizure activity. Rhabdomyolysis is a rare complication.

4. Patients with a known seizure disorder who have had a typical seizure without other complicating factors (trauma, fever, or headache) should have antiepileptic medication levels checked. If a reliable patient admits to not taking the medication for > 1 week, levels do not necessarily need to be assessed as they are presumed to be almost zero.

5. An anion gap metabolic acidosis with elevated lactate is present in patients with a recent generalized tonic-clonic seizure. This may be used to help differentiate a seizure from a seizure mimicker. It resolves within 1 hour of seizure cessation.

B. **Imaging Studies**

1. **Head CT scan.** Most practice guidelines recommend outpatient referral for CT scan in first-time seizure patients with a normal neurologic examination and no identifiable secondary cause for their seizure. Patients with a new focal deficit, persistent headaches, AMS, fever, trauma, cancer, anticoagulant use, or history of immunocompromise (HIV) should have a CT scan performed in the ED (Figure 70–1). Patients with a known seizure disorder and a typical seizure without any new secondary causes identified do not need a CT scan performed in the ED.

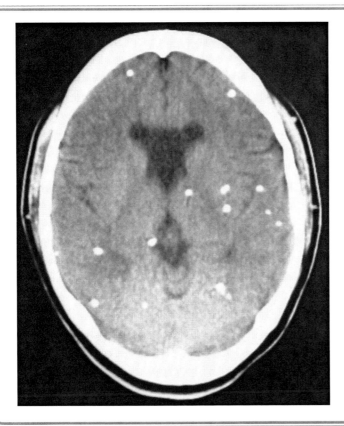

Figure 70–1. Head CT scan of a patient from Mexico who presented to the ED with a first time seizure. CT scan demonstrated multiple calcifications from neurocysticercosis.

C. **Diagnostic Procedures**
   1. **LP** should be considered in patients who present with status epilepticus, persistent AMS, fever, headache, or HIV. LP is *not* a routine part of a first-time seizure work-up.
   2. **EEG** is indicated in the ED when nonconvulsive status epilepticus is suspected or in patients who receive paralytics or phenobarbital, which may mask continued seizure activity.

D. **Diagnostic Algorithm**

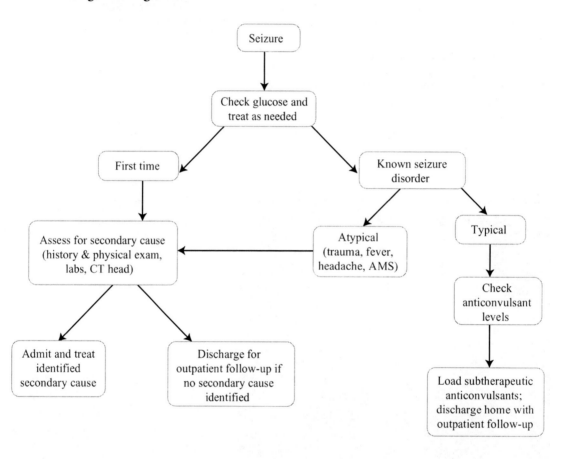

VIII. Treatment

A. **First-Time Seizure, Resolved.** Treatment depends on the underlying cause, if it can be determined. Perform a thorough history and physical examination.

B. **Known Seizure Disorder, Resolved**
   1. Perform a thorough history and physical examination to ensure no atypical features requiring work-up exist.
   2. Obtain anticonvulsant levels.

3. **Phenytoin** is loaded either IV or PO; the dose is 18 mg/kg. IV loading results in therapeutic serum levels within 1 hour. Oral loading results in therapeutic levels in 60% of patients within 12 hours. When administered IV, the rate should be no faster than 50 mg/min, and the patient should be placed on a cardiac monitor. Complications of IV phenytoin administration include skin necrosis if the IV infiltrates or cardiac arrhythmias from the propylene glycol vehicle. In patients with subtherapeutic levels, the correct amount of phenytoin to administer is determined by the formula: phenytoin load (mg) = (0.75 L/kg) × (desired level − current level) × (patient weight in kg). **Fosphenytoin** (20 mg/kg phenytoin equivalents) can be given IM and has fewer side effects, but it is more expensive.

C. **Actively Seizing Patient**
1. Protect the patient from self-harm. Perform ABCs and check vital signs, pulse oximeter, and bedside glucose level.
2. **Benzodiazepines.** Lorazepam 2 mg IV (up to a total dose of 0.1 mg/kg) or diazepam (0.1 mg/kg per dose). Lorazepam is preferred because its anticonvulsant action lasts 12 hours, compared to 20 minutes for diazepam. Other alternatives include diazepam PR (Diastat rectal gel 0.2–0.5 mg/kg) or midazolam IM (0.1 mg/kg). Patients experiencing alcohol withdrawal seizures require benzodiazepines only and do not respond to phenytoin either acutely or chronically.
3. If the seizure does not resolve or the patient does not return to baseline between events, treat for status epilepticus.

D. **Status epilepticus.** Administer medications in a stepwise fashion until the seizure stops.
1. IV benzodiazepines (as above).
2. Phenytoin (18 mg/kg IV load).
3. Phenobarbital (20 mg/kg IV at 100 mg/min). Patient will probably require endotracheal intubation at this time due to respiratory depression from phenobarbital.
4. If seizure continues, consider propofol (3–5 mg/kg bolus followed by an infusion of 1–15 mg/kg/hr) or pentobarbital (5–15 mg/kg bolus, then 0.5–10 mg/kg/hr).
5. Emergent EEG monitoring and neurology consult.
6. If isoniazid toxicity is suspected, administer pyridoxine 1 gram for each gram ingested or 5 gram if unknown.

IX. **Disposition**

A. **Admission.** Patients in status epilepticus should be admitted to an ICU. Patients with a first-time seizure with a secondary cause should be admitted to the hospital. Patients with known seizure disorder and atypical features should undergo ED work-up and possible admission.

B. **Discharge.** Patients with a first-time seizure may be safely discharged home if no secondary cause of the seizure is identified and the patient has returned to a normal mental status. Anticonvulsants are not indicated initially because the risk of a second seizure is only 50%. Give discharge instructions directing the patient not to drive an automobile, swim, or participate in any other activity that may put themselves or others in danger. Primary care or neurology follow-up should be arranged. Patients with a known seizure disorder may be discharged if there are no complicating factors. If they are taking phenytoin and their level is subtherapeutic, they should be loaded IV or orally.

CASE PRESENTATION

A 22-year-old man is brought to the ED by paramedics. En route, the patient began having a generalized tonic-clonic seizure. The paramedics started an IV.

1. *What else do you want to know?*
   - *How long has the patient been seizing? Did the paramedics give any medications in the field? Did the paramedics do a bedside glucose level?*
2. *The glucose level is 110 mg/dL. He has been having a seizure for 5 minutes. What is your first step?*
   - *ABCs and lorazepam 2 mg IV (up to 0.1 mg/kg).*

SUMMARY POINTS

- *Always check a bedside glucose level in seizure patients.*
- *Monitor ABCs in actively seizing patients and intervene when needed.*
- *IV lorazepam is the drug of choice for actively seizing patients.*
- *Search for a secondary cause of seizures in patients with a known seizure disorder who have new or different features.*

SECTION XVI
TRAUMA

CHAPTER 71
TRAUMA PRINCIPLES

I. Defining Features

A. Trauma patients present with a wide range of complex problems.

B. Caring for the trauma patient requires a team approach, involving emergency physicians, trauma surgeons, and virtually every subspecialty.

C. Most trauma care delivery systems utilize the Advanced Trauma Life Support (ATLS) approach developed by the American College of Surgeons.

II. Epidemiology

A. In the United States, trauma is the 4th most common cause of death in all age groups.

B. Trauma is the number 1 cause of death in persons < age 44, and causes more deaths in persons < age 19 than all other diseases combined.

C. Despite the staggering mortality rate associated with trauma, permanent disability is 3 times more likely than death.

D. In the United States, trauma accounts for 40% of all ED visits annually, and the cost of the care delivered exceeds $400 billion.

III. Etiology

A. Trauma is classified as **blunt** (70%) or **penetrating** (30%).

B. Trauma-related death occurs within **minutes** of injury due to catastrophic derangements of system function (ie, apnea secondary to high cervical spine injuries or exsanguination secondary to major vascular lesions); within **minutes to hours** of injury secondary to injuries associated with significant blood loss (ie, splenic laceration, liver laceration, renal pelvis transection, pelvic fractures, or aortic injuries); **days to weeks** after injury secondary to sepsis or multiple organ system failure.

IV. Risk Factors

A. Intoxicants (alcohol and drugs).

B. Lack of safety devices (seat belts, helmets).

C. Elderly. Sensory deficits (hearing, sight, touch), problems with balance, decreased motor strength, problems with coordination, memory deficits.

D. Adverse environmental conditions (road, weather, MVC).

IV. Clinical Presentation

A. History

1. Obtain a brief history using the mnemonic "AMPLE" (allergies, medications, past medical history, last meal, events surrounding injuries).

2. Elicit the following information (when appropriate). **Assault:** Who assaulted you? What were you assaulted with (automobile, gun, knife, fist, club)? When were you assaulted? Where were you hit/shot/stabbed? How many times were you hit/shot/stabbed? **MVC:** How fast was your automobile traveling? Were you wearing a seat belt? Was there significant damage to the car/windshield/steering wheel? Was there a prolonged extrication? Did anyone else in the automobile sustain serious injuries?

3. Patient complaints may guide the physician to the proper diagnosis. **Shortness of breath:** pneumothorax (hemothorax, simple or tension pneumothorax), pulmonary contusion, cardiac tamponade, shock, or neck hematoma. **Chest pain:** cardiac tamponade, pneumothorax (hemothorax, simple or tension pneumothorax), pulmonary contusion, fractures (ribs, sternum), PE, or traumatic aortic rupture. **Abdominal pain:** solid organ or hollow viscus injury. **Extremity pain:** contusion, fracture, neurovascular injury, or compartment syndrome. **Hematuria:** renal, ureteral, bladder, prostatic, or urethral injury.

KEY COMPLAINTS

AMS in the trauma patient suggests the possibility of an intracranial hemorrhage, but other life threats that should be considered first include hypoxia, hypoglycemia, and hemorrhagic shock.

KEY
COMPLAINTS

B. Physical Examination

1. The physical examination of the trauma patient is a 2-step process. Primary survey is a brief survey (< 5 min) where immediate life threats are diagnosed and treated. Secondary survey is a complete head-to-toe examination.

2. The **primary survey** assesses the ABCDEs in a stepwise fashion, *treating any abnormalities before moving on to the next step.*

   a. *A = airway maintenance with cervical spine protection.* Assess the airway for patency (look for foreign bodies, facial, mandibular, or tracheal/laryngeal fractures). If the patient is able to communicate verbally, the airway is usually patent. While assessing the airway, prevent excessive movement of the cervical spine. If the airway is not patent or another reason for airway intervention exists (eg, GCS < 8, combative patient, or shock), the patient should be intubated.

   b. *B = breathing and ventilation.* Expose the chest and look for wounds, contusions, or paradoxical movement. Auscultate breath sounds. The goal is to diagnose immediate life threats such as tension pneumothorax, flail chest, massive hemothorax, or open pneumothorax.

   c. *C = circulation with hemorrhage control.* To rapidly assess hemodynamic stability, note the patient's LOC. Altered LOC is associated with hypovolemia. In addition, ashen, grey, pale skin, thready pulses, and external hemorrhage are associated with hypovolemia. If any of the above conditions are found, stop the hemorrhage (with compression initially) and replenish volume.

d. **D = disability.** A rapid neurologic examination is performed toward the end of the primary survey. This should include LOC, pupil size and reactivity, focal deficits, and GCS.

e. **E = exposure.** The patient is then completely exposed and examined to ensure that no life threats have been missed before covering them with a warm blanket to prevent hypothermia.

3. The **secondary survey** follows once the patient has been stabilized.

a. **Head.** Visualize the head and scalp for lacerations, contusions, and deformities. Check visual acuity and pupil size. Assess the globe for penetration, laceration, or entrapment. Next, examine the mid-face, looking for evidence of fracture (step-offs, facial instability), lacerations, contusions, or septal hematoma. Hemotympanum, periorbital ecchymosis (raccoon eyes), otorrhea, or rhinorrhea frequently heralds basilar skull fracture.

b. **Neck.** Any associated maxillofacial trauma places the cervical spine at higher risk of injury, and it must be protected until appropriate radiologic evaluation can be accomplished. The neck should be evaluated for tenderness, subcutaneous emphysema, tracheal deviation, and laryngeal fracture.

c. **Chest.** Inspect for penetrating injuries, contusions, or paradoxical movement (ie, flail segment). Palpate the ribs, clavicles, and sternum. Auscultate the lungs and heart.

d. **Abdomen and pelvis.** Inspect for penetrations and contusions. Palpate for tenderness, guarding, or rebound. Palpate the pelvis to assess for stability and tenderness. If pelvic instability exists, wrap a sheet tightly around the pelvis to tamponade bleeding.

e. **Perineum.** Look for lacerations, vaginal bleeding, contusions or hematomas. Perform a rectal examination to assess for gross blood, mucosal lacerations, high riding prostate, or abnormal rectal tone. Urethral injury must be ruled out before Foley catheter placement. Findings consistent with urethral injury include scrotal hematoma, blood at the urethral meatus, or a high-riding prostate.

f. **Musculoskeletal.** Note any contusions or deformities. Palpate for tenderness or abnormal movement. Roll the patient and palpate the spine looking for step-offs or tenderness.

g. **Vascular.** Assess the pulses. In penetrating trauma, absent pulses, expanding or pulsatile hematomas, bruits or thrills, and pulsatile hemorrhage are considered "hard" signs of arterial injury. Other findings including a diminished pulse, large hematoma, peripheral nerve injury, and delayed capillary refill are considered "soft" evidence of arterial injury. Patients with soft signs should have an arterial brachial index (ABI) performed. The ABI is the systolic pressure in the affected extremity divided by the systolic pressure in an unaffected arm; ABI < 0.9 is abnormal.

h. **Neurologic.** Perform a comprehensive motor and sensory examination, reevaluate LOC, pupils, and calculate the GCS.

CLINICAL SKILLS TIP

Hypotension in the trauma patient is attributed to hemorrhage, hemorrhage, and hemorrhage—only then are other etiologies of shock considered (ie, spinal, septic, cardiogenic).

VI. **Differential Diagnosis.** Head injury, neck injury, cervical spine injury, thoracic injury, abdominal/back/flank injury, perineal/GU injury, pelvic fracture, extremity injury, spinal injury.

VII. **Diagnostic Findings**

A. **Laboratory Studies**
1. **CBC** obtained serially to follow trends in hemoglobin level and assist in determining the need for transfusion or operative intervention.
2. **Chemistry** obtained to assess renal function prior to imaging studies.
3. **Type and screen or crossmatch,** depending on the anticipated need for blood transfusion.
4. **Urinalysis** used to screen for the presence of GU injuries (hematuria).
5. **Serum lactate level** to assess the response to resuscitation in hypovolemic shock patients. A base deficit can also be used for a similar purpose.
6. **Toxicology screen** to provide possible etiologies for AMS.
7. **Pregnancy test** for all females of child-bearing age.

B. **Imaging Studies**
1. **Plain films** to screen for injuries to the cervical, thoracic, and lumbar spine and chest, pelvis, or long bones.
2. **CT scan** is useful as long as the patient is stable enough to leave the resuscitation room. **Head** to assess intracranial injuries, **chest** to assess major vascular injuries, and **abdomen/pelvis** to assess intra-abdominal and pelvic injuries.
3. **MRI** is useful to investigate spinal cord injuries in the stable trauma patient.
4. **Ultrasound (FAST)** to rapidly assess for cardiac and intra-abdominal injuries requiring surgical intervention.
5. **Angiogram** to assess and delineate arterial injuries within the extremities, neck, chest, or pelvis.

C. **Procedures**
1. Multiple procedures are used in the trauma patient depending on the clinical scenario. Central line placement, chest tube placement (tube thoracostomy), and needle thoracostomy are discussed in Chapters 3 and 7; orotracheal intubation and cricothyrotomy in Chapter 10; emergency thoracotomy in Chapter 74; and diagnostic peritoneal lavage (DPL) in Chapter 75.
2. Other procedures used to treat trauma patients include **urethrogram and cystogram** to determine the presence of injury to the urethra and bladder respectively. These tests are performed in a retrograde fashion by injecting dye into the urethral meatus while obtaining a radiograph (urethrogram), or after injecting 300 cc of dye into the bladder (cystogram). Indications include straddle injury, presence of pelvic fractures, or physical findings (scrotal hematoma, blood at urethral meatus, or high riding prostate).

D. **Diagnostic Algorithm**

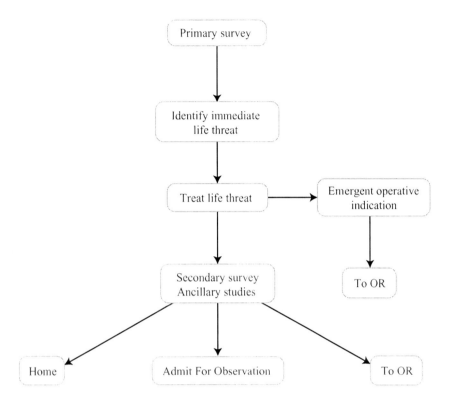

VIII. Treatment

A. Evaluation and treatment often coincide and begin with a primary survey (ABCs).

B. **Airway.** Secured with endotracheal intubation when altered LOC (GCS < 8) or failure to oxygenate or ventilate.

C. **Breathing.** Any clinical evidence of tension pneumothorax should prompt immediate needle thoracostomy in the midclavicular line above the second rib.

D. **Circulation.** Two large bore IV lines or a large bore central line should be placed. Fluids (0.9 NS or LR) are initiated. Blood loss should be estimated based on initial vital signs and clinical presentation (Table 71–1). If vital signs are unstable after giving 2 L bolus, then start blood transfusion with uncross-matched type O blood. Hemorrhagic shock is common in trauma patients. Blood loss may be external (blood lost at the scene of the trauma) or internal (thorax, abdomen, pelvis). The goal of the physician is to rapidly determine the location of blood loss in order to begin definitive treatment.

Table 70–1. Classes of hypovolemic shock.

	Class I	Class II	Class III	Class IV
Blood loss (mL)	Up to 750	750–1500	1500–2000	>2000
Blood loss (% blood volume)	Up to 15%	15–30%	30–40%	> 40%
Pulse rate (beats/min)	< 100	> 100	> 120	> 140
BP	Normal	Normal	Decreased	Decreased
Pulse pressure (mm Hg)	Normal or increased	Decreased	Decreased	Decreased
RR (breaths/min)	14–20	20–30	30–40	> 35
Urine output (mL/hr)	> 30	20–30	5–15	Negligible
CNS/mental status	Slightly anxious	Mildly anxious	Anxious, confused	Confused, lethargic
Fluid replacement (3:1 rule)*	Crystalloid	Crystalloid	Crystalloid and blood	Crystalloid and blood

*Fluid replacement should be 3x the estimated blood loss.

IX. Disposition

A. **Admission.** Most blunt trauma patients are moved to the OR or are admitted for an observation period to rule out occult injuries not found on the primary and secondary survey. Penetrating trauma patients frequently require admission and operative intervention when the implements violate body cavities or cause injury to important structures.

B. **Discharge.** Blunt trauma patients who remain stable may be discharged when only minor injuries are found. In penetrating trauma, patients with stab wounds or missiles that do not violate the body cavities may be discharged, assuming the path of the object does not approximate any other vital structures.

CASE PRESENTATION

The occupant of an automobile involved in a MVC arrives in the ED with cervical spine immobilization and is complaining of abdominal pain. His vital signs are temperature 98.6°F (37°C), pulse 110 beats/min, respirations 16 breaths/min, BP 90/60 mm Hg, GCS 15, and pulse oximeter 98%.

1. What other historical facts do you want to know?

- *AMPLE: allergies, medications, past medical history, last meal. Events surrounding the accident: How fast were you going? Where was the impact? Where were you seated in the vehicle? Did the airbags deploy? Were you wearing a seat belt? What kind of damage was done to the vehicle? Any LOC?*

2. *What ancillary studies will likely assist in the management of this patient?*

  • *CBC, chemistry, urinalysis, type and cross, toxicology screen, pregnancy test. Plain radiographs (cervical spine, chest, and pelvis). Retrograde urethrogram and cystogram if indicated. FAST, CT scan of abdomen and pelvis if patient stabilizes.*

SUMMARY POINTS

• *All trauma patients are assessed the same way—primary survey followed by secondary survey.*

• *Any life threat identified in the primary survey is addressed before moving on to the next step.*

• *Be aware of the capabilities of your institution and begin transfer efforts as soon as you uncover a problem that your hospital cannot accommodate.*

• *Assess patients for hemorrhagic shock and resuscitate with crystalloid and blood when indicated.*

CHAPTER 72
HEAD INJURIES

I. Defining Features

    A. **Traumatic brain injury** (TBI) is classified as **mild, moderate,** and **severe,** based on the patient's GCS (Table 72–1). This classification dictates the workup and ultimate disposition. In patients with mild TBI (GCS 14–15), the goal of the physician is to diagnose patients who have a significant intracranial injury. The prevalence of a positive CT finding in these patients is approximately 10%, with 1% requiring neurosurgical intervention. In patients with moderate (GCS 9–13) and severe (GCS < 9) TBI, the goal of management is to rapidly diagnose injuries and prevent secondary insults that will result in further brain injury.

    B. **Concussion** is a traumatic alteration of neurologic function in the absence of findings on CT scan. Its grade is based on duration of symptoms and the presence of LOC (Table 72–2). Symptoms, including headache, sleep disturbances, and difficulty with concentration, may persist days to months after the injury (post-concussive syndrome).

    C. **Cerebral contusions** are most commonly seen in the frontal, temporal, or occipital regions. When contusions occur at the site of the blunt force and on the opposite side of the brain, they are known as coup and contrecoup injuries, respectively.

    D. **Traumatic subarachnoid hemorrhage** (SAH) is caused by lacerations of the superficial vessels in the subarachnoid space.

    E. **Subdural hematoma** (SDH) is caused by bleeding from bridging veins in the subdural space. It is more common in elderly patients with cerebral atrophy, and may occur in the absence of head trauma.

    F. **Epidural hematoma** (EDH) most often occurs as a result of bleeding from the middle meningeal artery after a blow to the head causes a skull fracture. The arterial pressure acts to dissect the dura away from the skull table, and a crescent-shaped hematoma forms that does not cross the suture lines.

    G. **Diffuse axonal injury** (DAI) is seen when there is a disruption of axonal fibers in the brain due to shearing forces. The patient has persistent AMS, and frequently the CT scan does not reveal evidence of injury.

II. Epidemiology

    A. Injuries are the leading cause of death in persons < age 45, and traumatic brain injuries account for 50% of these deaths.

Table 72–1. Glasgow Coma Scale (GCS).

Eye opening		Best verbal response	
Spontaneous	4	Oriented, converses	5
To verbal command	3	Confused	4
To pain	2	Inappropriate	3
No response	1	Incomprehensible	2
		No response	1
Best motor response			
Obeys commands	6		
Localizes to pain	5		
Withdraws to pain	4		
Abnormal flexion	3		
Abnormal extension	2		
No response	1		

B. In the United States, non-fatal TBI occurs in 1.5 million persons yearly, resulting in 370,000 hospitalizations, and 80,000 cases of residual neurologic disability.

C. In the United States, about 52,000 persons die yearly due to TBI.

D. The annual cost of caring for acute and chronic TBIs is > $4 billion.

III. Pathophysiology

A. TBI results from direct or indirect forces to the brain matter. **Direct injury** is sustained by the force of an object striking the head. **Indirect injury** is caused by acceleration or deceleration forces that result in the movement of the brain inside the skull. Indirect forces create shear injuries as the brain impacts the skull and different parts of the brain move against one another.

B. Regardless of mechanism, the brain sustains an immediate irreversible insult, termed the **"primary injury,"** which is dependent on the cause and severity of the inciting event. A **"secondary injury"** occurs minutes to days later and is the result of neurophysiologic and anatomic changes at the cellular level.

C. Primary and secondary injuries directly damage cells and cause cerebral edema, which increases ICP.

Table 72–2. Grading of concussions.

Grade 1	Grade 2	Grade 3
Transient confusion.	Transient confusion.	Any LOC
Symptoms persist < 15 min	Symptoms persist ≥ 15 min	

D. The calvarium is a closed space with 3 components: blood, CSF, and brain. Increases in the size of any of the 3 components without a corresponding decrease in one of the others result in increased ICP.

E. Decreases in the cerebral perfusion pressure (CPP) lead to ischemia. CPP is decreased by decreases in MAP and increases in ICP (CPP = MAP - ICP).

IV. **Risk Factors.** Infants, young adults, and elderly (due to anatomic and physiologic factors), male gender, and drug and alcohol users (40% more likely to sustain head injury).

V. **Clinical Presentation**

A. **History.** Important historical information to obtain include the patient's baseline mental status, mechanism of injury, condition before and after injury, recent use of intoxicants, presence and length of LOC, vomiting, seizure activity, and anticoagulant use.

KEY COMPLAINTS

In patients with mild TBI and LOC or amnesia, indications for a CT scan include significant mechanism of injury, neurologic deficit (including short-term memory loss), > age 60, intoxication, headache, vomiting, or seizure activity.

B. **Physical Examination**
1. As with all trauma patients, a primary and secondary survey should be performed (see Chapter 71).
2. Vital signs and pulse oximetry should be assessed. Both hypotension (systolic BP < 90 mm Hg) and hypoxia (pulse oximeter < 90%) are associated with worse outcome.
3. Calculate the GCS (see Table 72–1).
4. A dilated pupil in an unconscious patient with head trauma is evidence of transtentorial herniation caused by downward pressure on the uncus and ipsilateral 3rd cranial nerve. Rapid neurologic deterioration may also indicate herniation.
5. "Raccoon eyes" (periorbital ecchymosis), CSF rhinorrhea, hemotympanum, and battle's sign (retroauricular hematomas) are all subtle findings of a basilar skull fracture (Figure 72–1). Step-off deformities of the skull are direct evidence of a skull fracture.

CLINICAL SKILLS TIP

Patients with moderate TBI who are uncooperative or impaired secondary to drugs and alcohol use may require RSI for their own safety and so that diagnostic testing (head CT scan) can be completed.

VI. **Differential Diagnosis.** Illicit drugs and alcohol, hypoglycemia, nontraumatic space occupying lesions (tumor), infectious etiologies, CVA, postictal state, psychiatric disease.

RULE OUT

Cervical spine injury is frequently associated with head trauma. Immobilization is required in patients with traumatic head injuries until a C-spine injury is excluded.

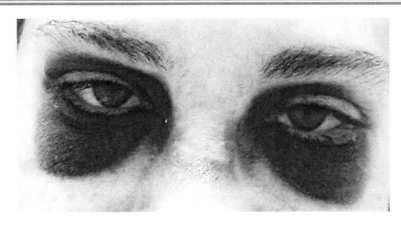

Figure 72–1. Image of patient with "raccoon eyes."

VII. Diagnostic Findings

A. **Laboratory studies.** No laboratory test diagnoses TBI. Routine **blood studies** are often obtained to help rule out the possibilities listed in the differential diagnosis and assess the patient's response to interventions.

B. **Imaging Studies**
1. **Head CT scan** (non-contrast) is the initial study of choice in TBI. Positive findings include skull fractures, cerebral contusion, SDH and EDH, and traumatic SAH (Figure 72–2). Acute blood appears hyperdense (white) on a non-contrast CT scan. As the time from injury to presentation increases, the blood becomes isodense and eventually hypodense. IV contrast may be helpful to diagnose an isodense SDH after a subacute injury (2 days to 2 weeks after injury).
2. **MRI of the brain** is indicated when diffuse axonal injury is suspected, but this test is rarely performed in the acute setting.

C. **Diagnostic Algorithm (see page 441)**

VIII. Treatment

A. In moderate and severe TBI, minimize the risk of further brain injury by treating hypoxia, hypotension, herniation, and seizures.
1. **Hypoxia.** Administer O_2 and maintain PaO_2 > 60 mm Hg (pulse oximeter > 90%). If the GCS is < 8, intubation for airway protection is indicated. In patients with moderate TBI (GCS 9–13), intubation is also appropriate in agitated patients who require diagnostic studies. Laryngeal stimulation during intubation increases ICP; therefore, RSI must be performed using head injury precautions (see Chapter 10).
2. **Hypotension.** Fluid boluses are administered with a goal to maintain systolic BP > 90 mm Hg. A low BP decreases the already compromised CPP via the relationship, CPP = MAP - ICP. The end result is further cerebral ischemia.
3. **Herniation.** Efforts to decrease ICP are instituted. The simplest maneuver is raising the head of the bed. Sedation with airway control should also be

Diagnostic Algorithm

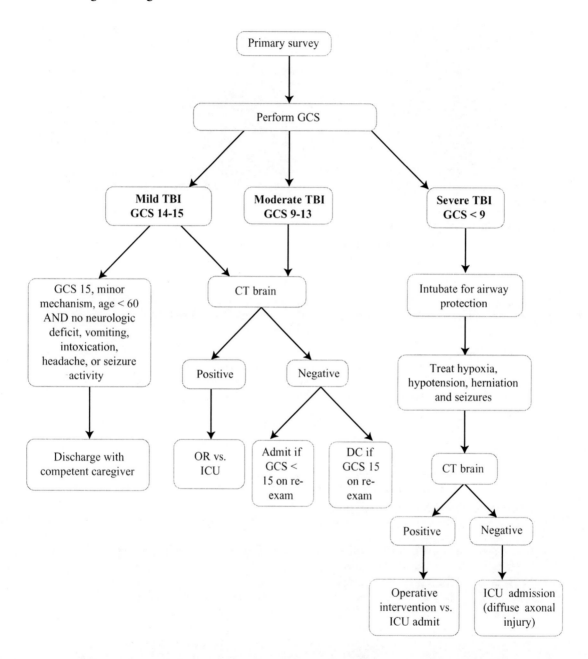

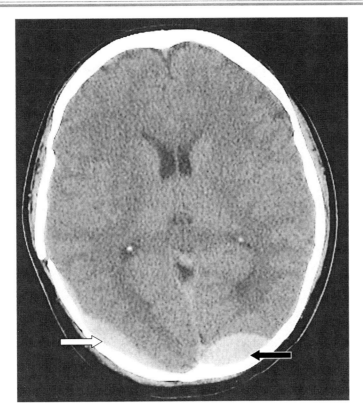

Figure 72–2. CT scan of the head showing an epidural hematoma (*black arrow*) and a subdural hematoma (*white arrow*).

strongly considered. Mannitol (0.25–1 g/kg) will create an osmotic diuresis that decreases ICP within 30 minutes. Hyperventilation, once routinely used in patients with severe TBI, is now reserved only for patients with evidence of herniation. The goal pCO_2 is 30–35 mm Hg. Reduction of the ICP is achieved because of cerebral vasoconstriction. Ultimately, an operative neurosurgical procedure or draining CSF via an external ventricular drain (EVD) may be necessary.

4. **Seizures.** Treat with diazepam (0.1 mg/kg) or lorazepam (0.05 mg/kg) IV every 5 minutes, initially. If seizures persist, administer phenytoin (18 mg/kg). Antiepileptic medications for seizure prophylaxis are indicated to prevent secondary injury in patients with significant injuries on CT scan or a GCS < 8.

B. **Management of specific conditions** varies depending on the injury. Early neurosurgical consultation is recommended in all patients with significant findings.

1. ICP monitoring via an EVD is indicated in patients with severe TBI, hematomas, contusions, or hydrocephalus.

2. Traumatic SAH usually does not require any acute neurosurgical intervention. Patients benefit from nimodipine, a calcium channel blocker that reduces vasospasm, thereby decreasing secondary injury. It should be started as soon as the patient is stable at a dose of 60 mg PO.

3. Patients with SDH and EDH and signs of neurologic dysfunction require clot evacuation.

4. Skull fractures with a depression that is equal to the width of the skull require repair. In addition, patients with basilar skull fractures have a small risk of developing meningitis (< 5%) and, therefore, prophylactic antibiotics should be considered in these patients.

IX. Disposition

A. **Admission.** Admit any patient with a GCS of < 9 or documented injury on CT scan to an ICU. These patients will require ICP and MAP monitoring. Patients with a persistent GCS < 15 should be admitted for observation, even if the CT scan is negative. Admit patients with a basilar skull fracture, depressed or open fractures, or when a linear fracture crosses an arterial or venous groove.

B. **Discharge.** Patients with mild head trauma and a negative CT scan can be discharged home. When a CT scan is deemed unnecessary due to minor mechanism or symptoms, discharge with instructions for post-head injury (return if headaches, vomiting, weakness, or AMS) with a responsible person who can observe the patient for signs of deterioration. Approximately 15% of these patients will suffer from post-concussive symptoms. Athletes with grade 1 concussions may return to play, assuming they have no prior history of head injury. Patients with grades 2 and 3 concussions require referral and should be withdrawn from contact sports for 1 and 2–4 weeks, respectively.

CASE PRESENTATION

A 21-year-old man presents to the ED following an automobile accident. He is moaning and withdraws to painful stimuli, but does not open his eyes.

1. What other historical facts do you want to know?

- *Paramedics' description of the scene, prehospital care, and a brief history.*

2. Once all other immediate life threats have been eliminated, what is the next step in treating this patient?

- *Calculate his GCS. This patient does not open his eyes (1), and withdraws his extremities to painful stimuli (4). He is moaning (2). Thus, his GCS is 7. He has severe TBI.*

- *Secondary survey. Look for signs of head trauma, cerebral herniation, basilar skull fracture, or step-off deformities of the skull or cervical spine.*

- *Intubation, CT head and neurosurgical consultation.*

SUMMARY POINTS

- *The specific management of head injuries depends on the GCS.*
- *Airway control is frequently necessary in patients with moderate and severe TBI.*
- *Consult the neurosurgeon early and aggressively treat hypoxia, hypotension, herniation, and seizures to avoid secondary (preventable) injuries.*

CHAPTER 73
CERVICAL SPINE INJURIES

I. Defining Features

A. The cervical spine is made up of 7 vertebrae. The first 2 cervical vertebrae are unique, while the remaining cervical vertebrae are fundamentally similar. The atlas (C1) has no body and consists of a bony ring upon which the occipital condyles of the skull articulate. The axis (C2) has a small anterior body, which continues superiorly to form a protuberance called the dens. The dens articulates with the anterior portion of C1. The remainder of the cervical vertebrae are composed of a body anteriorly and a vertebral arch posteriorly. The spinal canal is between the body and the arch.

B. A series of ligaments serve to maintain the alignment of the spinal column. The anterior and posterior longitudinal ligaments run along the vertebral bodies anteriorly and posteriorly. Surrounding the vertebral arch are the ligamentum flavum and the supraspinous and interspinous ligaments (Figure 73–1).

C. External forces can cause the cervical spine to move in directions that go beyond normal mobility, resulting in ligamentous disruption, bony fracture, dislocation, and ultimately, spinal cord injury.

II. Epidemiology

A. There are approximately 10,000 new spinal cord injuries in the United States each year. About 55% of cases occur in the group aged 16 to 30 years.

B. Most patients with spinal cord injury are the victims of vehicular trauma, followed by victims of assault.

C. The most common site of fracture in the cervical spine is C2 (24%).

D. Dislocations occur most commonly at C5–C6 and C6–C7.

E. Children and the elderly usually sustain injury to the upper cervical spine (C1–C3), whereas teenagers to middle-aged adults usually sustain injury to the lower spine (C6-T1).

III. Etiology

A. For purposes of classification of injury, the cervical spine can be divided into anterior and posterior columns, divided by the posterior longitudinal ligament attached to the posterior vertebral body.

B. **Flexion injuries** cause compression of the anterior column and distraction of the posterior column. This results in crush injury to the anterior vertebral body

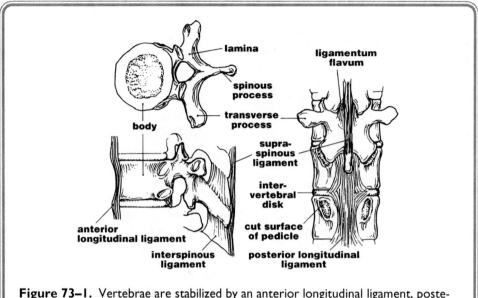

Figure 73–1. Vertebrae are stabilized by an anterior longitudinal ligament, posterior ligament, and interspinous ligament.

and ligamentous disruption of the posterior ligaments. Examples of flexion injuries include simple wedge fractures, unilateral facet dislocations, flexion teardrop fractures, and bilateral facet dislocations. These injuries are classified as stable (simple wedge, unilateral facet dislocation) or unstable fracture/dislocations.

C. **Extension injuries** cause distraction of the anterior column and compression of the posterior column. There is disruption of the anterior ligaments and crush injury to the posterior spinal elements. Extension injuries include the "hangman's fracture" and the extension teardrop fracture, both of which are unstable.

D. **Axial load injuries** cause compression of the anterior and posterior columns. These forces result in the vertebral body shattering outward, causing a "burst fracture." A C1 burst fracture results from an axial load mechanism and is an extremely unstable fracture.

E. Most spinal cord injuries are complete. However, some patients present with a specific neurologic syndrome corresponding to a specific cord lesion.
   1. **Central cord syndrome.** Hyperextension injury resulting in predominantly upper extremity distal motor weakness.
   2. **Anterior cord syndrome.** Hyperflexion injury resulting in loss of sensory and motor function below the level of the injury with preserved position and vibration sense (posterior columns).
   3. **Brown-Séquard syndrome.** Also known as hemisection of the cord, usually the result of penetrating injury. Physical findings include contralateral loss of pain and temperature sensation with ipsilateral motor paralysis and loss of position and vibration sense.

IV. **Risk Factors.** MVC, pedestrian hit by automobile, alcohol intoxication, failure to use seat belt, victim of assault, recreational sporting activities, fracture in another part of the spine.

V. **Clinical Presentation**
   A. **History**
      1. ABCs should be assessed, addressing any immediate life threats. In the event that the patient does not present with the cervical spine already immobilized, a cervical collar should be applied. A thorough primary and secondary survey is performed (see Chapter 71).
      2. Presence of neck pain, weakness, numbness, or burning should be ascertained.

KEY COMPLAINTS

Past medical history may be important as certain preexisting conditions may put the patient at risk for a C-spine injury. Rheumatoid arthritis and ankylosing spondylitis both cause decreased spine mobility and ligamentous rupture with minimal trauma.

   B. **Physical Examination**
      1. Mental status should be assessed. Any alteration makes examination of the neck unreliable when attempting to rule out serious injury.
      2. Inspect the spine for any gross deformities or ecchymosis. Palpate the spine noting any focal tenderness.
      3. Assess the patient for any distracting painful injuries that may make the spinal examination unreliable (fractures, burns, significant soft tissue injury).
      4. Perform a detailed neurologic examination, including motor strength, sensation (light touch and proprioception), reflexes, and rectal tone.

CLINICAL SKILLS TIP

The bulbocavernosus reflex can be assessed in patients with a spinal deficit to determine complete vs. incomplete injury. With one finger inserted in the rectum, apply gentle squeezing pressure to the glans or clitoris. This should elicit an involuntary contraction of the anal sphincter. A negative reflex suggests complete cord injury.

   VI. **Differential Diagnosis.** Cervical strain, blunt carotid or vertebral artery injury, spinal cord injury without radiologic abnormality (SCIWORA), spinal shock.

RULE OUT

***SCIWORA** is a syndrome of neurologic injury without evidence of fracture or dislocation seen on x-ray or CT scan. It is most common in children due to the flexibility of their ligaments and bones. Patients with neurologic complaints after trauma and normal initial imaging should undergo further testing with MRI.*

   VII. **Diagnostic Findings**
      A. **Laboratory studies.** No laboratory test aids in the detection of cervical spine injuries.
      B. **Imaging Studies**
         1. **C-spine radiographs.** Initial test to evaluate the cervical spine. Three views of the spine (AP, lateral, open mouth) are the standard and have a sensitivity ranging from 83–98%. Sensitivity varies due to the quality of x-rays and er-

rors in interpretation. See Table 73–1 and Figures 73–2 through 73–7 for keys to interpreting cervical spine films. Indications for radiography are based on the NEXUS (National Emergency X-Radiography Utilization Study) criteria. Patients must meet 5 criteria to be classified as having a low probability of injury and therefore do not require x-rays: no midline cervical tenderness, no focal neurologic deficit, normal alertness, no intoxication, and no painful distracting injury.

2. **C-spine CT scan.** About 95–100% sensitive for bony injuries. Indicated in patients who are intubated, have initially abnormal or inadequate x-rays, or have a high clinical suspicion of injury or persistent pain despite normal x-rays.

3. **MRI.** Indicated for patients with any neurologic deficit, and for suspicion of ligamentous injury despite normal x-ray or CT scan.

C. **Diagnostic Algorithm**

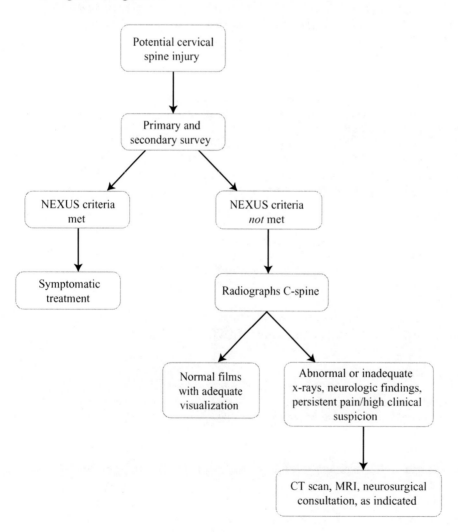

Table 73–1. Key to interpretation of cervical spine radiographs.

Radiograph	Alignment	Bones	Cartilage	Soft Tissue
Lateral (Figure 73–2)	Anterior middle and posterior arcs, posterior laminal line and predental space (Figures 73–3 and 73–4)	Vertebrae and spinous process uniformity and height	Intervertebral disk space and height	Prevertebral soft tissue width. (Figure 73–5)
AP	Spinous processes should be in a straight line (Figure 73–6)	Interspinous process distance should be equal (Figure 73–6)		
Open mouth (odontoid)	Lateral margins of C1 should align with lateral margins of C2 (Figure 73–7)	Space on each side of odontoid should be equal. Inspect odontoid for fractures		

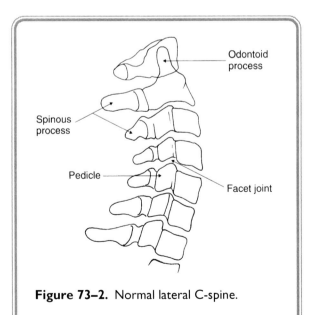

Figure 73–2. Normal lateral C-spine.

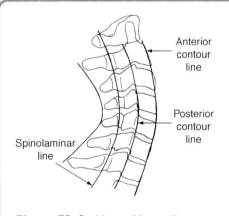

Figure 73–3. Normal bony alignment of the lateral C-spine. The anterior and posterior vertebral bodies should line up to within 1 mm. The spinolaminar line can be traced through the base of the spinous process of each vertebra.

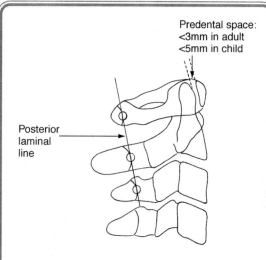

Figure 73–4. The predental space demonstrated on a lateral C-spine. The posterior laminal line should be drawn from the base of the spinous process of C1 to C3. The base of the spinous process of C2 should be within 2 mm. This can help rule out pseudo-subluxation of C2 on C3, commonly seen in children.

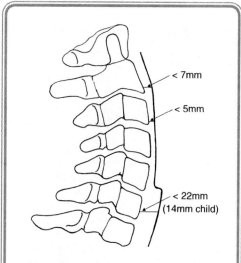

Figure 73–5. The normal prevertebral soft tissue distance on the lateral C-spine. Increased distance indicates soft tissue swelling and possible associated fracture or ligamentous injury.

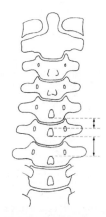

Figure 73–6. AP C-spine. Note the unequal distance between the spinous processes. This indicates a C-spine fracture.

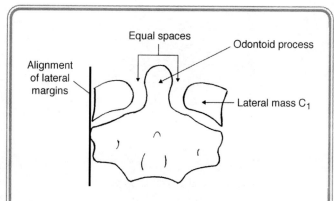

Figure 73–7. Odontoid view. Note the alignment of the lateral masses of C1 and C2.

VIII. Treatment

A. Rigid cervical collar in the supine position on a gurney. If the patient is to be removed from a spine board, at least 3 persons skilled in spine precautions are needed.

B. If intubation is required, either keep the cervical collar in place or have a second person perform in-line manual stabilization during intubation.

C. Patients with normal x-rays without other findings or who meet the NEXUS criteria should have collar removed. Treat symptomatically with oral pain medications (eg, ibuprofen)

D. Patients with abnormal radiographs or neurologic findings should undergo emergent MRI to assess the spinal cord. Neurosurgery should be consulted.

E. Steroids are indicated for patients with known or suspected blunt spinal cord injury. They should be started within 8 hours of injury to provide benefit. When started within 3 hours of injury, the duration of treatment is 24 hours; when started 3–8 hours post injury, the duration of treatment is 48 hours. Contraindications include penetrating injury, isolated nerve root involvement, and cauda equina syndrome. Dosing: bolus 30 mg/kg over a 15-minute period, with continuous infusion of 5.4 mg/kg/hr for 24–48 hours.

IX. Disposition

A. **Admission.** All patients with spinal cord injury should be admitted to an ICU setting, preferably a neurosurgical ICU (transfer to a facility specializing in spinal cord injuries should be considered). Patients with unstable C-spine fractures without cord injury should also be admitted to an ICU setting, pending operative fixation by neurosurgery.

B. **Discharge.** Patients who meet the NEXUS criteria may be discharged. Patients with normal imaging studies or without persistent pain or high clinical suspicion may be discharged. Patients with stable C-spine fractures (anterior wedge, spinous process) should only be discharged after consultation with a neurosurgeon.

CASE PRESENTATION

A 13-year-old boy is brought to the ED by EMS after he dove into a shallow pool and hit his head on the bottom. He is "boarded and collared." His pulse is 75 beats/min and his BP is 120/70 mm Hg.

1. What else do you want to know?

 • *How was he removed from the pool? Pupillary examination? Movement of extremities? Spinal examination looking for deformity? Presence of rectal tone, bulbocavernosus reflex?*

2. The patient is awake and alert. He has complete motor paralysis and no bulbocavernosus reflex. What are your next steps?

 • *Administer steroids. CT scan followed by MRI of C-spine. Neurosurgical consultation.*

SUMMARY POINTS

• *Patients who meet the NEXUS criteria do not require C-spine imaging.*

• *3 views of the C-spine have sensitivities as low as 80% for spinal fractures. Have a low threshold to obtain a C-spine CT scan.*

• *Be aware of SCIWORA, especially in children. Patients with neurologic abnormalities despite normal imaging should undergo an MRI.*

• *Administer steroids to patients with blunt spinal cord injuries within 3 hours of their injury.*

CHAPTER 74
THORACIC TRAUMA

I. Defining Features

A. Thoracic trauma causes injuries to the chest wall, lungs, great vessels, and heart. It is clinically divided into blunt and penetrating injuries.

B. **Blunt Thoracic Injuries**
1. **Blunt aortic injury (BAI)** is also referred to as traumatic rupture of the aorta (TRA). BAI occurs when rapid deceleration shears the aorta, resulting in aortic rupture. Survival is rare unless the tear is partial or there is containment of rupture (pseudoaneurysm).
2. **Blunt myocardial injury** should be considered in any patient with significant mechanism of injury (eg, MVC > 30 mph). Rarely, significant blunt myocardial injury results in hypotension or dysrhythmia.
3. **Pulmonary contusions** are hemorrhage and edema of the lung in the absence of a pulmonary laceration. Their severity peaks at 48–72 hours.

C. **Penetrating Thoracic Injuries**
1. **Penetrating cardiac injury** should be considered in any patient with a gunshot or stab wound whose path may involve the heart. If blood is trapped in the pericardium, a pericardial tamponade will result.
2. **Pneumothorax and hemothorax** are common after penetrating trauma but may also occur following blunt trauma, where a fractured rib acts as the "penetrating" implement. **Open pneumothorax** is present when air is allowed to communicate from outside the chest wall to within the pleural space. **Tension pneumothorax** occurs when an air leak acts as a 1-way valve, allowing air to enter the pleural cavity on inspiration and not escape on expiration. This causes lung collapse, progressive mediastinal shift, impairment of venous return, and shock. **Hemothorax** is the accumulation of blood in the pleural space that occurs due to injuries of the chest wall, lung, or heart.

II. Epidemiology

A. Thoracic trauma is responsible for 16,000 deaths in the United States yearly, which accounts for approximately 25% of all trauma-related deaths.

B. Significant blunt chest trauma is due to MVC in 80% of cases.

C. About 80% of patients with BAI die in the field. Of patients that reach the hospital, 50% die within the first 24 hours and 75% die within 1 week.

D. Blunt myocardial injury requires treatment in only 3% of cases in which it is diagnosed.

III. Etiology

A. **Blunt thoracic injuries.** The thoracic aorta is mobile anteriorly and fixed in the descending portion by the ligamentum arteriosum and intercostal arteries. With rapid deceleration, shearing forces within the thoracic aorta cause a tear between the mobile anterior aorta and the fixed descending aorta, resulting in *BAI*. Rupture is most common immediately distal to the ligamentum arteriosum. When the tear affects all 3 layers of the vessel wall (intima, media, and adventitia), death will result. If the adventitia is spared, containment in a pseudoaneurysm may allow for initial survival and treatment. *Blunt myocardial injury* results in subendocardial hemorrhage and edema when the heart becomes contused by rapid deceleration or when an object strikes the chest. *Pulmonary contusion* is caused by compression-decompression injuries of the chest (eg, MVC).

B. **Penetrating thoracic injuries.** *Penetrating cardiac injury* is usually due to a stab or gunshot wound. Bleeding causes pericardial tamponade (intact pericardium) or hemothorax (injured pericardium). *Pneumothorax* reduces vital capacity and increases intrathoracic pressure. The net result is decreased venous return to the heart. During inspiration, negative intrathoracic pressure may force air into the pleural space through a wound in the chest wall. *Hemothorax* occurs due to bleeding from intercostal vessels, lung parenchyma, intrathoracic vessels, or the heart. Each hemithorax can hold about 40% of circulating blood volume. Massive hemothorax is defined as 1500 mL of blood. Hemothorax is deleterious because of blood loss, hypoxia caused by collapsing lung tissue, and compression on the vena cava that diminishes venous return.

IV. Risk Factors.
High-speed MVCs, falls, gang activity, hunting, and riding a motorcycle.

V. Clinical Presentation

A. **History**
1. A thorough history is frequently deferred until the primary survey is complete.
2. **Mechanism of injury** is important to obtain in MVCs. BAI is most common in patients with rapid deceleration after front or side impact. Falls from > 3 stories or vehicle decelerations of > 30 mph are generally required to result in BAI. If the speed is not known, ask the paramedics about the condition of the vehicles involved or whether the airbags were deployed.
3. Use of seat belts, steering wheel or dashboard deformity, or death of other occupants should be ascertained.
4. For penetrating injury, number of gunshots heard or details of stabbing (weapon used, trajectory) should be obtained.

KEY COMPLAINTS

Patients who fall from > 3 stories or deceleration injuries at > 30 mph should be evaluated for blunt aortic injury.

B. **Physical Examination**
1. **Vital signs.** Sinus tachycardia is common and may reflect pain, myocardial injury, or shock. Pulse oximetry will detect hypoxia due to pulmonary contusion, hemothorax, or pneumothorax.

2. **Neck.** Distended neck veins are present in patients with pericardial tamponade or tension pneumothorax. Deviation of the trachea suggests tension pneumothorax.

3. **Chest wall.** Palpate the chest for tenderness or crepitus. Look for penetrating wounds on the anterior chest, axilla, and back. A wound in the "cardiac box" or 2 wounds that transect the box are most likely to involve the heart and require a work-up. The **anterior cardiac box** is defined by the suprasternal notch superiorly, the xiphoid process inferiorly, and the nipples laterally (Figure 74–1). The **posterior cardiac box** is defined by the superior border of the scapulae superiorly, the costal margin inferiorly, and the medial borders of the scapulae laterally (Figure 74–2). Asymmetry with paradoxical movement of the chest during respiration suggests a **flail chest.**

4. **Cardiac examination.** Pericardial friction rub or an S3 may be heard in patients with blunt myocardial injury. Decreased heart sounds are consistent with a pericardial effusion.

5. **Lung examination.** Listen for decreased breath sounds that may indicate a pneumothorax or hemothorax. Rales may be present in patients with a significant pulmonary contusion.

6. **Abdomen.** Patients with significant thoracic trauma frequently have abdominal injuries. This is especially true in patients with lower rib fractures who are at risk for splenic and liver lacerations. Abdominal examination in these patients is not reliable to rule out injury.

7. **Extremities.** Asymmetric pulses suggest disruption of the aorta, although this finding is not sensitive.

CLINICAL SKILLS TIP

Fractures of ribs 8–12 should raise the suspicion of associated abdominal injuries.

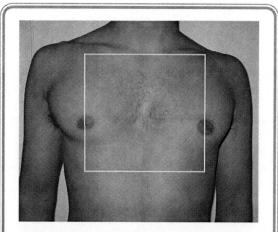

Figure 74–1. Anterior cardiac box. The anatomic borders that make up this box include the suprasternal notch, xiphoid process, and nipples.

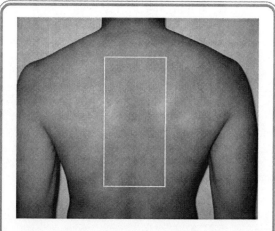

Figure 74–2. Posterior cardiac box. The anatomic borders that make up this box include the superior border of the scapulae, the costal margin, and the medial borders of the scapulae.

VI. Differential Diagnosis

A. **Blunt thoracic injuries.** Rib and sternal fracture, pneumothorax and hemothorax, flail chest, pulmonary contusion, blunt cardiac injury, blunt aortic injury, and diaphragmatic injuries.

B. **Penetrating thoracic injuries.** Pneumothorax and hemothorax, tracheobronchial injuries, diaphragmatic injuries, cardiac injuries (including pericardial tamponade), esophageal injuries, great vessel injuries.

RULE OUT

Flail chest occurs when 3 or more adjacent ribs are fractured in 2 or more places. In a spontaneously breathing patient, the segment is seen to move paradoxically (inward rather than out with inspiration) with the remainder of the chest because of negative intrathoracic pressure during inspiration. Flail chest by itself does not compromise ventilation, but the injury signals a significant mechanism with a high likelihood of other injuries that will adversely affect respiration (pulmonary contusion).

VII. Diagnostic Findings

A. **Laboratory studies.** CBC, electrolytes, renal function, serum and urine toxicology screen, base deficit, and lactate level are commonly obtained.

B. **Imaging Studies**

1. **CXR. Rib fractures** are often difficult to visualize. Approximately 50% will not be seen on the initial CXR, with fractures to the anterior and lateral portions of the first 5 ribs being particularly difficult to diagnose. Any penetrating wound to the thorax will require a CXR to look for **pneumothorax** or **hemothorax.** A negative initial film is followed with a CXR repeated in 6 hours to rule out a delayed presentation. Hemothorax can be visualized on an upright film when > 200–300 mL blood is present. On a supine film, massive hemothorax appears as haziness of the entire hemithorax. **Pulmonary contusions** appear as areas of opacification that occur within 6 hours of blunt trauma. CXR is used to screen for **BAI.** Findings consistent with BAI include widened superior mediastinum (> 8 cm), indistinct or obscured aortic knob, rightward NG tube, or apical pleural cap (Figure 74–3). The sensitivity of CXR ranges between 90% and 95%; therefore, a completely normal CXR cannot be relied upon to exclude BAI.

2. **ECG.** This is the best screening tool for blunt myocardial injury. Findings include conduction abnormalities, new ST depression or elevation, T wave inversion, or dysrhythmias. Nonspecific findings may also be present. A normal ECG is an excellent negative predictor for complications.

3. **Echocardiography** (ECHO). This is the initial test of choice for patients with penetrating thoracic injuries that include the cardiac box. Transthoracic echocardiogram can be performed in minutes, and a qualified ultrasonographer can detect as little as 20–50 mL of blood in the pericardial sac.

4. **Chest CT angiogram.** Spiral CT is employed to diagnose BAI in stable patients (Figure 74–4). Indications include significant mechanism (MVC > 30 mph or fall > 3 stories) plus an abnormal CXR or evidence of thoracic trauma on physical examination. A normal CT scan excludes the diagnosis with 100% sensitivity.

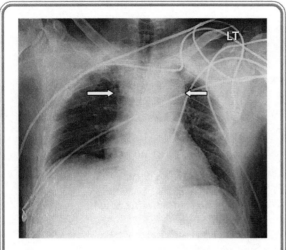

Figure 74–3. Chest x-ray showing widened mediastinum in a patient with a traumatic rupture of the aorta (*arrows*).

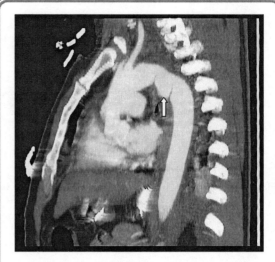

Figure 74–4. CT angiogram of a patient with a traumatic rupture of the aorta (*arrow*).

     5. **Aortography.** Traditionally, aortography has been considered the gold standard for diagnosing blunt aortic injury, although it now has been largely replaced by CT angiography.

  C. **Procedures**

    1. **Needle and tube thoracostomy** (see Chapter 7).

    2. **Emergency thoracotomy** is performed in trauma patients without vital signs when signs of life were present initially (in the field or in the ED). The survival rate is low overall but highest after penetrating trauma, especially stab wounds. The procedure involves making an incision on the left side of the chest, along the 4th or 5th interspace (inferior to the nipple) from the sternum to the gurney. The intercostal muscles are cut and the ribs are retracted. The pericardium is identified by moving the lung out of the way. Pericardial tamponade, if present, will be apparent. Incise the pericardium and identify sites of cardiac injury. Treatment of cardiac wounds includes direct pressure, staples, sutures, or wound occlusion with a Foley catheter balloon.

  D. **Diagnostic Algorithm (see page 457)**

VIII. **Treatment**

  A. ABCs, primary survey, followed by a secondary survey (see Chapter 71).

  B. **Blunt Thoracic Injuries**

    1. **Blunt aortic injury.** Reduce the systolic BP to 100–120 mm Hg, which decreases the shearing effect of the pulse pressure and reduces the likelihood of rupture. The best agents are esmolol and nitroprusside, used in combination. Definitive treatment options include emergency repair, endovascular stenting, or BP control with delayed repair.

    2. **Blunt myocardial injury.** Clinically significant injuries requiring treatment are rare. Hemodynamically stable patients with a normal ECG can be safely

Diagnostic Algorithm

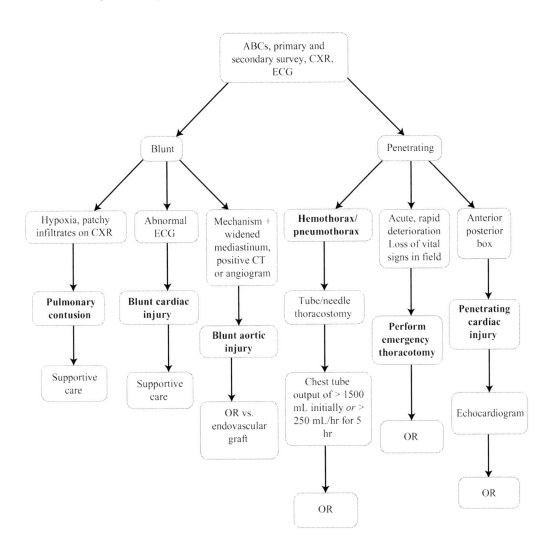

discharged home. Patients with an abnormal ECG who are otherwise stable should be monitored for 12–24 hours in a telemetry unit to assess for worsening arrhythmia or cardiogenic shock.

3. **Pulmonary contusions** are treated with supportive care to maintain adequate oxygenation. Administer O_2 via a nonrebreather mask. Avoid excessive hydration that can precipitate pulmonary edema. Intubation is necessary in patients with respiratory failure.

C. **Penetrating Thoracic Injuries**

1. **Penetrating cardiac injury.** Patients with loss of vital signs in the field or ED should have an emergency thoracotomy. Pericardial tamponade from a stab wound has the highest likelihood of survival. In stable patients with pericardial fluid seen on ECHO, options include an operative pericardial window or thoracotomy. In unstable patients, ultrasound-guided pericardiocentesis may be considered.

2. **Pneumothorax and hemothorax.** Tension pneumothorax requires immediate treatment, with needle thoracostomy followed by tube thoracostomy. Tube thoracostomy is required for most patients with pneumothorax and hemothorax. A small pneumothorax (< 1 cm on CXR) or an occult pneumothorax (seen on CT only) without hemothorax can be observed without tube thoracostomy. Operative repair following hemothorax is required in only 5% of cases. Indications include > 1500 mL blood evacuated initially, > 150–200 mL/hr over the first 2–4 hours, or if persistent blood transfusions are required to maintain hemodynamic stability.

IX. **Disposition**

A. **Admission.** Most patients with thoracic trauma require admission to the hospital. Patients with an isolated pneumothorax can be admitted to a regular hospital bed after tube thoracostomy. Patients with pulmonary contusions and blunt myocardial injury will require an ICU setting, while patients with penetrating cardiac injury or blunt aortic injury will need operative repair followed by ICU admission.

B. **Discharge.** When the mechanism of injury is minor or the work-up is negative, the patient can be discharged. Patients with penetrating chest wounds require a CXR repeated at 6 hours to exclude a delayed pneumothorax.

CASE PRESENTATION

A 25-year-old woman presents to the ED after being stabbed in the chest during a fight. She is awake, talking, and denies any other injuries. The patient states that she is short of breath. Her pulse oximetry is 92%. The wound is located 2 cm above and medial to the right nipple, and breath sounds are diminished on the right. Her BP is normal. Her neck veins are not distended.

1. *What tests will you order?*

   • *CXR (hemothorax or pneumothorax). Echocardiogram (pericardial fluid).*

2. *CXR reveals a hemothorax on the right, and echocardiography performed at bedside reveals a moderate amount of fluid around the heart. What should be the next step in treating this patient?*

   • *Tube thoracostomy on the right. Consult trauma and cardiothoracic surgeon. Prepare to transfer patient to the operating room.*

SUMMARY POINTS

- *Thoracic trauma is a leading cause of trauma death.*
- *Consider blunt aortic injury in patients with significant deceleration injuries, even when the CXR is normal.*
- *A significant amount of blood can be lost into the hemithorax. In the supine patient, a large hemothorax results in generalized haziness on the CXR.*
- *In patients with penetrating thoracic trauma and loss of vital signs in the field or ED, an emergency thoracotomy may be lifesaving, especially following a stab wound.*

CHAPTER 75
ABDOMINAL TRAUMA

I. Defining Features

A. Abdominal trauma can result in injuries that are intraperitoneal and retroperitoneal. Retroperitoneal organs include the kidneys and GU tract, the duodenum, and the pancreas. Intraperitoneal injuries occur to the solid and hollow organs and the diaphragm.

B. Abdominal trauma is divided into blunt and penetrating mechanisms. **Blunt abdominal trauma** involves a crushing force that causes disruption of solid viscera (spleen or liver) or hollow viscera (intestine). These injuries are most common after falls or MVCs. **Penetrating abdominal trauma** occurs most commonly due to stab wounds (SW) and gunshot wounds (GSW) that enter the intraperitoneal cavity. Skin wounds may be seen over the surface of the abdomen, but other wounds (lower chest, pelvis, back, or flank) can cause intraperitoneal injury, depending on their trajectory.

C. There are 4 anatomic zones of the abdomen. Penetrating trauma that occurs in one of these zones suggests what organs might be injured. **Anterior abdomen** is defined by the anterior axillary lines, costal margins, and inguinal ligaments (Figure 75–1). **Thoracoabdominal** area includes the area defined by the nipple line and inferior scapular borders superiorly and the inferior costal margins inferiorly (Figure 75–2). Wounds in this location are at an increased risk of injuring the diaphragm. This is important because small injuries are difficult to diagnose and may go undetected until the contents of the bowel herniate into the chest months to years later. **Flank** is located between the anterior and posterior axillary line between the inferior costal margins and iliac crests. **Back** is defined by the inferior scapular tips and the iliac crests, posterior to the posterior axillary line. SWs in this location have only a 10% chance of inflicting significant intra-abdominal injury.

II. Epidemiology

A. Death due to penetrating trauma is greatest in African Americans and Hispanics aged 15–34.

B. GSWs to the abdomen account for 90% of deaths from penetrating abdominal trauma. The most commonly injured organs are the small bowel, colon, and liver.

C. SWs are less likely to penetrate the peritoneal cavity and cause significant injury. The most commonly injured organ is the liver. Laparotomy is required in only 25–33% of patients.

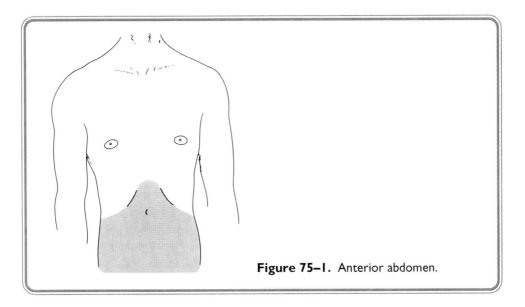

Figure 75–1. Anterior abdomen.

III. Pathophysiology

A. Blunt abdominal trauma causes injury by direct energy transmission that disrupts solid or hollow organs. Injury is more common in areas of transition from a fixed to mobile position. Examples include the ligament of Treitz or at the junction of the small bowel and right colon.

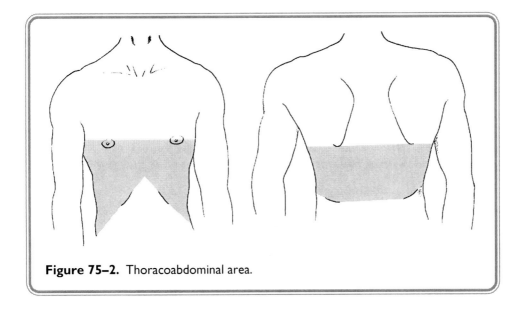

Figure 75–2. Thoracoabdominal area.

B. GSWs impart a large amount of energy to the tissues and have a high rate of causing a significant intra-abdominal injury. Missile velocity, stability, and distance all affect the amount of energy imparted.

C. Shotguns differ in that the velocity of the pellets decreases with increasing distance traveled. The greater the distance, the larger the pellet spread on the victim. Wounds with a pellet spread of 10–25 cm occurred at a distance of 3–7 yards and have enough energy to penetrate the peritoneum.

IV. **Risk Factors.** Young, male, African American or Hispanic, gang activity, alcohol or drug use, low socioeconomic status.

V. **Clinical Presentation**

A. **History**
1. Thorough history is delayed until ABCs are assessed.
2. Talk to the paramedics about the scene.
3. AMPLE history (allergies, medications, past medical history, last meal, and events).
4. The presence of abdominal pain, vomiting, or hematemesis should be ascertained. Hematemesis is an indication for laparotomy.
5. MVCs. Inquire about damage to the vehicle, presence of seat belt, airbag deployment, or injuries to other occupants.
6. GSWs. Ask about the number of shots fired or the type of weapon involved.

KEY COMPLAINTS

Kehr's sign. *Pain in the shoulder that is not associated with tenderness or pain with shoulder ROM suggests that blood is present under the diaphragm, causing referred pain to the shoulder. This commonly occurs from a splenic or liver laceration.*

KEY
COMPLAINTS

B. Physical Examination
1. **Vital signs.** Abnormal vital signs suggest hypovolemic shock and require aggressive resuscitation. When bleeding is occurring in the abdomen, laparotomy is indicated.
2. **Abdominal examination.** Inspect for abrasions, ecchymosis, or wounds. Lap-belt ecchymoses are suspicious for hollow organ injuries or vertebral fractures. In penetrating trauma, carefully note the location of all wounds and determine the zone of injury. Local wound exploration may be useful if the depth of the wound is easily determined. Evisceration or a retained implement is an indication to proceed to laparotomy. Palpation of the abdomen should occur in all 4 quadrants. Peritonitis is an indication for operation in both penetrating and blunt trauma. *Abdominal examination is not sensitive enough to diagnose all patients with significant injuries requiring operative intervention.*
3. **Rectal examination** to assess for gross blood. In abdominal trauma, the presence of gross blood is an indication to perform laparotomy.

VI. **Differential Diagnosis**

A. **Blunt abdominal trauma.** Splenic laceration, liver laceration, pancreatic injury, bowel perforation, duodenal hematoma, diaphragmatic injury, retroperitoneal hematoma, GU injury (bladder rupture, renal laceration), extra-abdominal trauma (rectus sheath hematoma, muscle strain or contusion).

B. **Penetrating abdominal trauma.** Injury to any structure or organ may occur. The most common injuries are to the liver and bowel, due to the relative size of these organs within the abdomen.

VII. Diagnostic Findings

A. **Laboratory studies.** CBC, electrolytes and renal function, lactate or base deficit, type and cross, toxicology screen, urinalysis and urine pregnancy.

B. **Imaging Studies**

1. **Plain radiographs (abdominal and chest).** The presence of a missile may help define its trajectory. Placing markers (eg, ECG leads) on the skin at the location of the wound will also aid in determining the missile tract. On the CXR, bowel seen in the chest cavity is evidence of a diaphragmatic injury. Free air under the diaphragm is evidence of a hollow organ rupture.

2. **Abdominal CT scan.** Useful in stable patients after blunt abdominal trauma to detect solid visceral injury and hemoperitoneum (Figure 75–3). CT scan is indicated in patients with an unreliable (distracting pain or AMS) or equivocal examination. In penetrating injuries to the back and flank, abdominal CT scan with PO, IV, and rectal ("triple") contrast is used to diagnose retroperitoneal injuries. In SWs, CT scan may be useful in determining the presence of peritoneal penetration. However, CT scan has limited sensitivity to diagnose small diaphragmatic injuries and isolated hollow viscus injury.

C. **Procedures**

1. **FAST** (see Chapter 8). The examination can be performed within 5 minutes, and identifies blood in the abdomen with a sensitivity that increases with

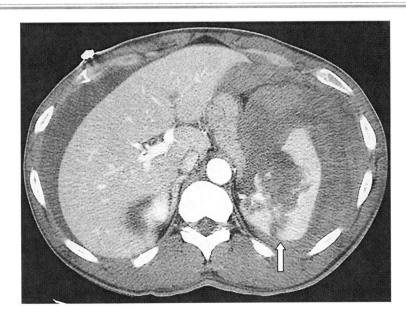

Figure 75–3. CT scan demonstrating a splenic laceration (*arrow*). Note the free fluid around the liver.

increasing amounts of blood present. FAST can diagnose as little as 100 mL of fluid and, most importantly, when enough intraperitoneal blood is present to cause hemodynamic instability in the patient, the sensitivity is very high.

2. **Deep peritoneal lavage** (DPL). This test is used to diagnose the presence of intraperitoneal blood after penetrating abdominal trauma. The technique involves introducing a catheter into the peritoneum via the Seldinger technique. One liter NS is introduced into the abdomen, and the fluid is then removed. The number of RBCs/mm^3 is determined by the laboratory. A count > 100,000 RBC/mm^3 suggests that approximately 20 mL of blood is present in the abdomen and is sensitive for detecting visceral injury and the need for laparotomy. When diaphragmatic injuries are suspected (thoracoabdominal wounds), a count of 5000–10,000 RBC/mm^3 is used to ensure that no injuries go undetected.

D. **Diagnostic Algorithm (see pages 465 and 466)**

VIII. **Treatment**

A. Initial treatment includes ABCs, 2 large IV lines, and high flow O_2.

B. *Unstable patients with blunt or penetrating abdominal trauma require laparotomy.* The source of bleeding (abdomen, thorax, or pelvis) must be determined as rapidly as possible using physical examination and diagnostic tests (FAST, DPL, plain radiographs). When multiple possible sources for hypotension are present (ie, positive FAST examination and hemothorax), further care should be arranged in close consultation with a trauma surgeon.

C. In hemodynamically stable patients, indications for laparotomy include peritonitis, free air, diaphragmatic injury, gross blood from stomach or rectum, evisceration, positive diagnostic test, retained stabbing implement, or any non-tangential GSW (intra-peritoneal penetration) (see VII D, diagnostic algorithm).

D. The work-up for stable patients with penetrating abdominal trauma and no immediate operative indication is **anterior abdomen:** DPL is positive with > 100,000 RBC/mm^3 (SWs) or > 10,000 RBC/mm^3 (tangential GSWs); **thoracoabdominal:** DPL is positive with > 10,000 RBC/mm^3; and **back and flank:** CT scan with PO, IV, and rectal contrast. If equivocal, DPL is positive with > 10,000 RBC/mm^3.

E. Solid organ injury is managed operatively in the unstable patient, and may be managed nonoperatively in hemodynamically stable patients. Nonoperative management of liver injuries has a failure rate of 10%, vs. 20% for patients with splenic injuries. The use of angiography with embolization of bleeding vessels can also be employed and decreases the need for laparotomy.

IX. **Disposition**

A. **Admission.** Patients who require laparotomy or hemodynamically stable patients with a splenic or liver injury identified on CT scan require admission.

B. **Discharge.** Patients with SWs or tangential GSWs that do not penetrate the peritoneum (based on a negative work-up) can be discharged, assuming that no other traumatic injuries are present. In blunt abdominal trauma, a normal CT scan has a negative predictive value of 99.6%. In the absence of other injuries, these patients can be safely discharged.

Diagnostic Algorithm

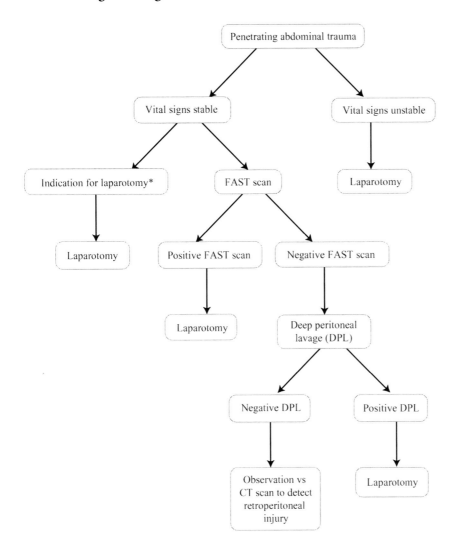

CASE PRESENTATION

A 34-year-old man presents to the ED after falling off a ladder. Witnesses say the man was painting a second-story window. He is unconscious on arrival. There is a contusion to his scalp and his abdomen.

1. *What do you want to do first?*

   • *ABCs. He will require intubation for airway protection. Check vital signs. If the patient is hypotensive, the work-up will proceed differently. Examination and plain films (CXR, lateral C-spine, pelvis, extremities).*

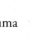

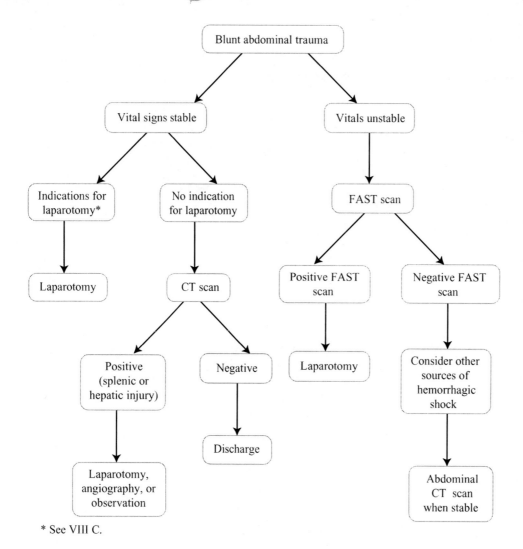

* See VIII C.

2. *BP is 120/80 mm Hg with HR of 110 beats/min. What do you do now?*
   * *Initiate IV fluids. He will need CT scan of the head, C-spine, and abdomen as long as his vital signs remain stable. Abdominal examination will not be reliable to detect significant injury in this unconscious and intubated patient.*

SUMMARY POINTS

* *Physical examination is unreliable in patients with abdominal trauma.*
* *Patients with abdominal trauma and hemodynamic instability should undergo a laparotomy.*
* *A GSW with an obvious trajectory into the abdomen requires an emergency laparotomy because of the high likelihood for significant injury.*
* *In patients with blunt abdominal trauma, a negative CT scan rules out significant injury.*

CHAPTER 76
BURNS

I. Defining Features

A. Burns are caused by **thermal, chemical,** or **electrical injuries.** Thermal burns are due to scalding or flame injuries. Chemical burns are secondary to alkali or acids. Electrical burns are caused by the flow of current through tissue.

B. Burns are classified as first, second, or third-degree. **First-degree** burns involve only the most superficial epidermal layers (eg, sunburn). **Second-degree** burns are further subdivided into superficial and deep partial thickness. Superficial partial-thickness burns heal well without scarring, while deep partial-thickness burns require skin grafting. **Third-degree** burns are also referred to as full-thickness burns. In this type of burn, dermal structures, including nerve endings, are destroyed.

II. Epidemiology

A. The American Burn Association estimates that there are 700,000 visits to the ED, 45,000 hospitalizations, and 4,500 deaths annually due to burns. The most common location for a death caused by burn is the home, followed by automobiles, then aircraft.

B. Chemical burns account for 5–10% of burn admissions.

C. There are 125 specialized burn centers in the United States that account for half of all admissions.

D. The average size of a burn injury in a patient admitted to a burn center is 14% of the total body surface area (TBSA).

E. About 20% of pediatric burns are caused by abuse or neglect.

III. Pathophysiology

A. The skin functions to reduce evaporative water loss in addition to creating a barrier to infection and a control of body temperature.

B. Deep partial-thickness burns result in damage to deeper layers of the dermis, hair follicles, sweat glands, and sebaceous glands, while these structures are spared in superficial partial-thickness burns.

C. Burns may result in **hypovolemic shock** due to increased peripheral blood flow, capillary leak, decreased cardiac output, and third spacing of fluids.

467

D. Inhalational injury occurs when smoke particulate matter reaches the terminal bronchioles and initiates an inflammatory response that leads to bronchospasm and edema.

IV. **Risk Factors.** Morbidity and mortality is increased in patients with greater severity of the burn (size and depth), presence of inhalational injury, associated injuries, extremes of age, co-morbid illnesses, and acute organ system failure.

V. **Clinical Presentation**

A. **History**

1. In any child with a burn, a careful history should be obtained from the parents or caretakers in an attempt to exclude child abuse or neglect.
2. The burning agent may provide a clue to the degree of burn sustained. A scald injury usually results in a partial-thickness burn. Flame injury is more likely to result in full-thickness burns. Deeper injuries should be suspected in patients with electrical or chemical burns.
3. A patient who has been in a house fire or any closed-space fire should be suspected of having inhalational injury or CO or cyanide poisoning. Cyanide is formed when nitrogen-containing polymers (eg, wool, silk, polyurethane, vinyl) burn.

B. **Physical Examination**

1. **Vital signs** may reveal hypotension, although an accurate BP reading may be difficult to obtain if there are circumferential burns to the extremities. Tachycardia usually represents pain or volume depletion.
2. Airway evaluation should include assessment for evidence of inhalational injury, including carbonaceous sputum, singed facial hairs, stridor, wheezing, cough, dysphonia, or tachypnea.
3. A **complete physical examination** is essential because burn patients often have concomitant traumatic injuries. The patient must be fully undressed.
4. **Circulation distal to circumferential burns** must be evaluated for evidence of decreased blood flow.
5. **Skin examination**
   a. **First-degree burn.** The skin is red, painful, and tender. There are no blisters.
   b. **Second-degree burn, superficial partial thickness.** The skin is red and blistering. The exposed dermis is moist, and there is good capillary refill.
   c. **Second-degree burn, deep partial thickness.** The skin may be blistered, but the exposed dermis is pale white to yellow. Capillary refill is absent.
   d. **Third-degree burn, full thickness.** These burns may be difficult to distinguish from deep partial-thickness burns. In general, the skin is leathery, pale, painless, and may be charred.
   e. Calculate the %TBSA, not including first-degree burns, using the "rule of nines" (Figure 76–1).

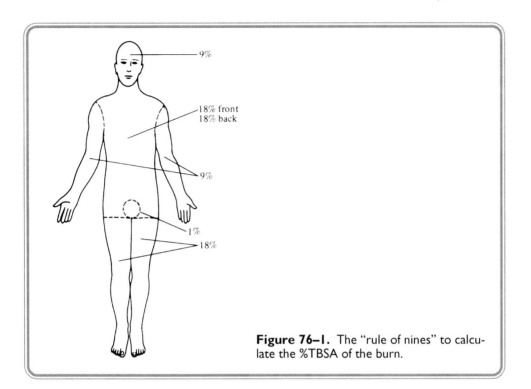

Figure 76–1. The "rule of nines" to calculate the %TBSA of the burn.

VI. Differential Diagnosis

A. Thermal injury. **Flame** or **scald** (grease or oil).

B. Chemical burn. **Acids:** hydrofluoric acid, acetic acid (hair-wave neutralizer), chromic acid, hydrochloric and sulfuric acid. **Alkalis:** sodium hydroxide (lye), calcium hydroxide (lime), cement, airbag deployment (sodium hydroxide).

C. Electrical burn.

RULE OUT

Immersion burns (circumferential margins, flexor surface sparing) in a child are considered abuse until proven otherwise.

VII. Diagnostic Findings

A. **Laboratory Studies**
   1. **CBC**
   2. **Electrolytes and renal function.** Metabolic acidosis suggests shock or cyanide toxicity.
   3. **CPK** in electrical injury to exclude rhabdomyolysis.
   4. **ABG** when CO poisoning is suspected.

B. **Imaging studies. CXR,** initially may be normal even with significant inhalational injury. ARDS is common in intubated burn patients, but is not present acutely.

C. **Procedures**

    1. Emergency escharotomy is indicated in patients with circumferential burns and compromise of distal circulation or respiration due to an inflexible eschar and increasing edema.

    2. The procedure is most commonly performed by a surgeon, but can be performed by the emergency physician if necessary. The incision is made on the lateral side of the limb and extends to the fingers. For thoracic burns, the incision is at the anterior axillary line. The incision should extend down to the subcutaneous fat.

D. **Diagnostic Algorithm**

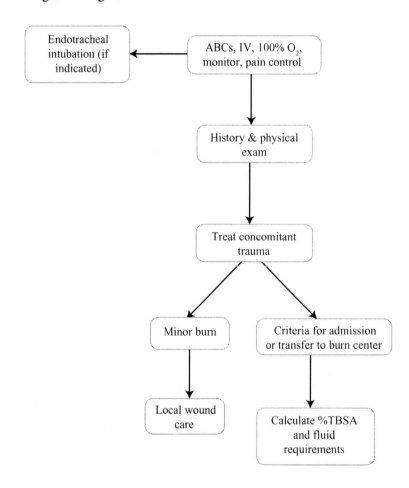

VIII. **Treatment**

    A. ABCs, fully undress patient, immobilize as needed, and consider associated traumatic injuries.

    B. **Airway management.** Administer O_2 via nonrebreather. Indications for endotracheal intubation include full-thickness burns of the face or perioral region,

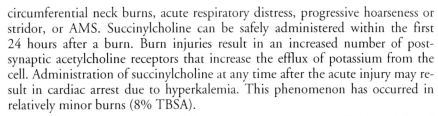

circumferential neck burns, acute respiratory distress, progressive hoarseness or stridor, or AMS. Succinylcholine can be safely administered within the first 24 hours after a burn. Burn injuries result in an increased number of post-synaptic acetylcholine receptors that increase the efflux of potassium from the cell. Administration of succinylcholine at any time after the acute injury may result in cardiac arrest due to hyperkalemia. This phenomenon has occurred in relatively minor burns (8% TBSA).

C. **Fluid resuscitation.** Patients with burns > 15% TBSA receive fluids (LR) based on the Parkland formula (4 mL/kg x %TBSA over 24 hr with 50% given in first 8 hr). Goal is to achieve urine output of 0.5–1 mL/kg/hr. Give less fluid to patients with renal insufficiency or heart failure.

D. **Pain control.** Morphine 0.1 mg/kg titrated IV to pain relief.

E. **CO poisoning.** Treat, as discussed in Chapter 51. If there is a persistent acidosis with a normal CO level and adequate fluid administration, treat for cyanide toxicity.

F. **Local burn wound care.** For patients with chemical burns, copious irrigation and removal of clothing is the primary concern. Sterile dressing if the patient is to be hospitalized. Nonadherent dressings for superficial partial-thickness burns. For deeper burns, debride necrotic tissue, dress with a topical agent (silver sulfadiazine, DuoDerm, Biobrane, OpSite, and Inerpan) and cover with gauze and stockinette. Change dressings twice a day. Definitive treatment for deep partial-thickness or full-thickness burns is early excision and grafting.

IX. Disposition

A. **Admission.** Criteria for admission or transfer to a burn center are listed in Table 76–1.

B. **Discharge.** Patients with minor burns may be discharged with follow-up in 24–48 hours.

Table 76–1. Criteria for admission or transfer to a burn center.

• Partial-thickness burns > 10% TBSA
• Burns involving face, hands, feet, genitalia, perineum, or major joints
• Third-degree burns
• Electrical burns (including lightning)
• Chemical burns
• Inhalational injury
• Patients with preexisting medical disorders that could complicate management
• Children, where the originating hospital does not care for children

CASE PRESENTATION

A 14-year-old boy is brought to the ED, via paramedics, after being found on the front lawn of his home. The child received burns to 60% of his body in a house fire and is unconscious. The paramedics are ventilating him with a BVM. They were unable to establish an IV line.

1. *What do you want to do first?*
   · *Maintain precautions for C-spine injury. Continue BVM while preparing for endotracheal intubation.*
2. *Intubation is successful and an IV is established. How much fluid should be administered in the first 24 hours, assuming a weight of 50 kg?*
   · *4 mL/kg x 50 kg x 60%TBSA = 12,000 mL LR solution, 6 L in the first 8 hours. Goal is to achieve urine output of 0.5–1.0 mL/kg/hr.*

SUMMARY POINTS

· *Administer high flow O$_2$ and check CO level in all burn victims, especially patients burned in a house fire.*
· *Endotracheal intubation is best performed early in patients with evidence of significant inhalation injury.*
· *Concomitant trauma should not be overlooked in burn patients.*
· *Emergency escharotomy may be necessary if the constrictive eschar is causing respiratory difficulty or limb ischemia.*
· *Consider abuse or neglect in a burned child.*

SECTION XVII
ORTHOPEDIC EMERGENCIES

CHAPTER 77
UPPER EXTREMITY INJURIES

I. Defining Features

A. **Shoulder**

1. **Shoulder dislocation.** Anterior dislocations account for 95% of all shoulder dislocations (Figure 77–1). Axillary nerve injury is present in 12% of cases, and is noted by testing sensation over the deltoid muscle and strength of abduction. Posterior dislocations are less common (5%) and present with inability to abduct and externally rotate. The classic mechanism of injury is a seizure.

2. **Shoulder separation.** This is a soft tissue injury to the acromioclavicular and coracoclavicular ligaments, which provide stability to the acromioclavicular joint. Injuries are divided into first, second, and third-degree. **First-degree** injuries are sprains of the acromioclavicular ligament. **Second-degree** injuries are the result of complete disruption of the acromioclavicular ligament, but an intact coracoclavicular ligament. When both ligaments are disrupted, a **third-degree** injury is present.

B. **Humerus fracture.** These fractures occur anywhere on the shaft of the humerus (Figure 77–2). Distal third fractures are associated with radial nerve injuries in 5–15% of cases.

C. **Forearm fractures.** There are several types of forearm fractures. **Nightstick fracture** is an isolated fracture of the ulnar shaft that occurs most frequently when a patient is protecting the body from a blow to the upper torso or head. **Both bone forearm fractures** (radius and ulna) are common in children after a fall. A **Galeazzi fracture-dislocation** is a distal radius fracture with dislocation of the ulna at the distal radioulnar joint (wrist). A **Monteggia fracture-dislocation** is a proximal ulna fracture with dislocation of the radial head at the proximal radioulnar joint (elbow). Both injuries require surgical reduction.

D. **Wrist and Hand**

1. **Distal radius fractures** (Figure 77–3). There are several types of distal radius fractures, including **Colles'** (extra-articular metaphyseal fracture with dorsal angulation), **Smith's** (extra-articular metaphyseal fracture with volar angulation), **Barton's** (fracture of the volar or dorsal rim of the distal radius with subluxation of the carpals), and **Hutchinson's** (fracture of the radial styloid).

2. **Scaphoid fracture.** Of the 8 carpal bones, the scaphoid accounts for 60–80% of all fractures (Figure 77–4). A fracture to this bone is significant

475

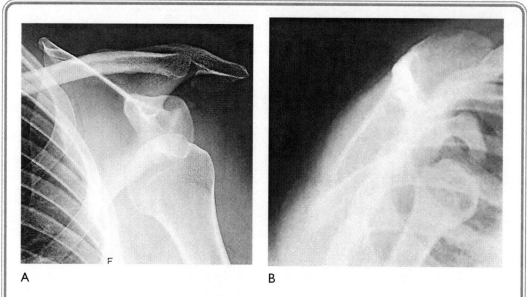

Figure 77–1. Anterior shoulder dislocation. A, AP view; B, scapular Y view.

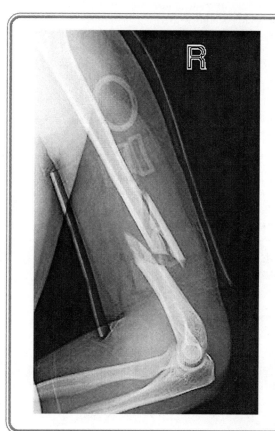

Figure 77–2. Humerus fracture. This fracture is described as a spiral, distal-third humerus fracture, with comminution, 100% displacement, and no angulation.

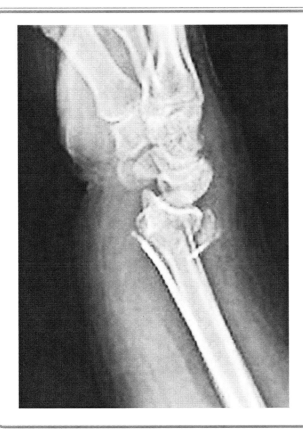

Figure 77–3. Distal radius fracture is an example of a Colles' fracture.

because the blood supply is such that the more proximal the fracture the more frequently avascular necrosis will occur. The false-negative rate of plain radiographs is as high as 20%, making conservative treatment in patients with tenderness over the scaphoid (anatomical snuffbox) appropriate.

3. **Metacarpal fracture.** These fractures may occur in the base, shaft, neck, or head of the bone. The most common is a fracture to the neck of the 4th and/or 5th metacarpal, called a **boxer's fracture** (Figure 77–5). Angulation is acceptable if it is < 40°. For fractures of the metacarpal shafts of the 2nd and 3rd metacarpal necks, less angulation (10–20°) is acceptable because healing with significant angulation in these more anatomically fixed metacarpals will inhibit function.

4. **Carpal dislocation.** Injury to the ligaments of the wrist produces several patterns of injury observed on plain radiographs. Progressive ligamentous injury results in scapholunate dissociation, perilunate dislocation and, finally, lunate dislocation. **Scapholunate dissociation** occurs when the interosseus ligament between the scaphoid and lunate is injured. On the AP radiograph, the joint space between the scaphoid and lunate is > 3 mm, a finding termed the Terry Thomas sign. The other two patterns are best seen on the lateral radiograph. On this view, a line drawn through the center of the radius should

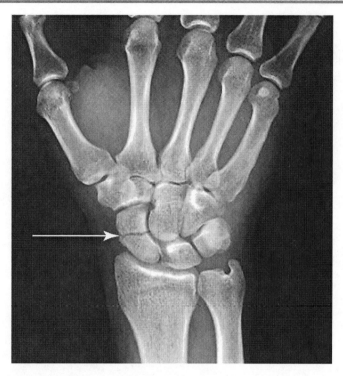

Figure 77–4. Scaphoid fracture (*arrow*).

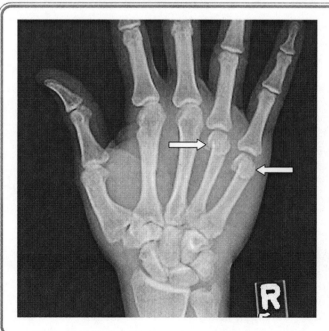

Figure 77–5. Fracture of the neck of the 4th and 5th metacarpals—boxer's fracture (arrows).

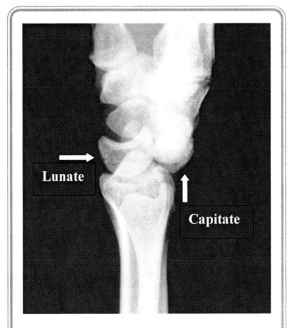

Figure 77–6. Perilunate dislocation. Note that the lunate still articulates with the radius (*horizontal arrow*) but the capitate is dislocated dorsally (*vertical arrow*).

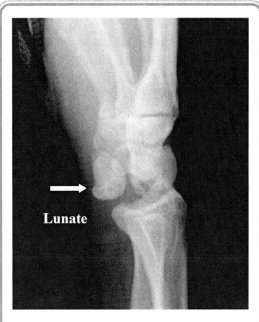

Figure 77–7. Lunate dislocation. The lunate (*arrow*) is volarly dislocated and no longer articulates with the radius.

transect the lunate and capitate. Following a **perilunate dislocation,** the capitate located dorsally (Figure 77–6). In a **lunate dislocation,** the lunate is in an anterior position and is tipped over like a "spilled teacup" (Figure 77–7).

5. **Tendon injuries.** Tendon lacerations are common following lacerations of the hand. Examination should include testing the movement and strength of the digit, as well as inspection of the tendon through its full ROM. Flexor tendons are tested by noting flexion at the distal interphalangeal joint (flexor digitorum profundus) and the proximal interphalangeal joint (flexor digitorum superficialis). **Mallet finger** is a closed extensor tendon injury due to forced flexion of an extended distal phalangeal joint. This injury occurs commonly when a person attempts to catch a ball. The injury may be associated with an avulsion fracture.

II. Epidemiology

A. Distal radius fractures account for up to 15% of upper extremity fractures.

B. The glenohumeral joint of the shoulder is the most commonly dislocated joint in the body, accounting for 50% of all major dislocations seen in the ED.

III. Etiology

A. **Fall.** The most common mechanism is a fall on an outstretched hand (**FOOSH**).

B. **Blunt force.** The nightstick fracture of the ulna is an example of an injury due to blunt force.

C. **Shoulder separations** occur after a fall with direct impact onto the shoulder.

D. **Shoulder dislocations** occur most commonly when the arm is abducted, externally rotated, and extended and a posterior directed force is applied to the humerus.

IV. **Risk Factors.** Elderly, contact athletic activities, trauma.

V. **Clinical Presentation**

A. **History**
1. The physician should inquire about other more urgent injuries (eg, head, torso) prior to focusing attention on the extremity.
2. The mechanism of injury is useful in determining the type of injury present.

KEY COMPLAINTS

A patient with wrist pain and anatomical snuffbox tenderness should have the wrist splinted and treated as a scaphoid fracture, even if radiographs are negative.

B. **Physical Examination**
1. A neurovascular assessment including pulses, skin color, capillary refill, and nerve function.
   a. *Radial nerve.* Motor: wrist extension. Sensory: dorsal web space between the first and second digits.
   a. *Ulnar nerve.* Motor: spread the digits apart. Sensory: 5th digit.
   c. *Median nerve.* Motor: opposition of the thumb and 5th digit. Sensory: 3rd digit.
2. Evaluate for gross deformity and swelling.
3. Note any lacerations that could represent open fractures.
4. Palpate areas for tenderness and "tenseness" of the tissues that might suggest compartment swelling.

VI. **Differential Diagnosis** (see I)

RULE OUT

Compartment syndrome *should be considered in patients with upper extremity injuries, significant swelling, and pain unresponsive to narcotic medications.*

VII. **Diagnostic Findings**

A. **Laboratory studies** usually are unnecessary.

B. **Imaging Studies**
1. **Plain radiographs** are all that are necessary in most cases of upper extremity trauma. It is imperative to obtain both an AP and lateral view of the bone to fully understand and describe the fracture. Viewing the joint above and below the fracture is also important, because frequently there are associated injuries.

2. Fractures are described based on their **pattern** (spiral, transverse, oblique), **location,** degree of **angulation,** percentage of **displacement,** and the level of **comminution** (see Figure 77–2). Intra-articular involvement is also an important feature and frequently impacts the definitive treatment plan.

3. **Shoulder radiographs** consist of AP films in internal and external rotation, a scapular "Y" view, and an axillary view. The axillary and "Y" view allow for evaluation of dislocation.

4. **Wrist radiographs** consist of AP, lateral, and oblique views. The carpal bones are scrutinized on the AP radiograph. Overlap of the bones suggests a carpal dislocation (ie, lunate or perilunate). The lateral view is best for detecting carpal dislocations and fractures of the distal radius and triquetrum. The oblique view allows for better visualization of the first metacarpal and the distal scaphoid. The scaphoid view, an AP view with the wrist ulnar deviated, will increase the sensitivity for detecting scaphoid fractures.

5. **Other imaging techniques** are sometimes useful. CT scan and MRI provide a higher sensitivity to detect fractures of the scaphoid.

C. **Procedures.** A shoulder dislocation can be reduced by several techniques. The external rotation maneuver, scapular manipulation, and Stimson are 3 of the most common methods.

1. **External rotation maneuver.** The patient is seated upright or at 45°. The patient's elbow is supported by one hand and the other hand is used to slowly and gently externally rotate the arm. The shoulder may reduce spontaneously. If not, the arm is slowly abducted and the humeral head is lifted into the socket.

2. **Scapular manipulation maneuver.** The inferior portion of the scapular tip is pushed medially, while the superior aspect is rotated laterally. This movement shifts the glenoid inferiorly toward the humeral head, allowing it to reduce spontaneously.

3. **Stimson technique.** Place the patient prone and hang the arm with 10- to 15-lb weights. The humerus will often reduce within a period of 20–30 minutes.

D. **Diagnostic Algorithm** (see page 482)

VIII. Treatment

A. **General Principles**

1. Splint the joint above and below an injury.
2. Ice 3 to 4 times daily for 20 minutes during the initial 72 hours after injury.
3. Elevate the involved extremity.
4. Compress with an elastic bandage. Be careful not to induce compartment syndrome by wrapping the bandage too tightly.
5. Narcotic drugs are indicated following fractures. NSAIDs may inhibit bone healing and therefore are not recommended for pain control after fractures. NSAIDs are appropriate following soft-tissue injuries.

B. **Shoulder**

1. **Shoulder dislocation.** Reduction as described, followed by a sling or shoulder immobilizer. The patient should be instructed to avoid external rotation of the arm. Early ROM is frequently recommended for patients with shoulder injuries, especially the elderly.

Diagnostic Algorithm

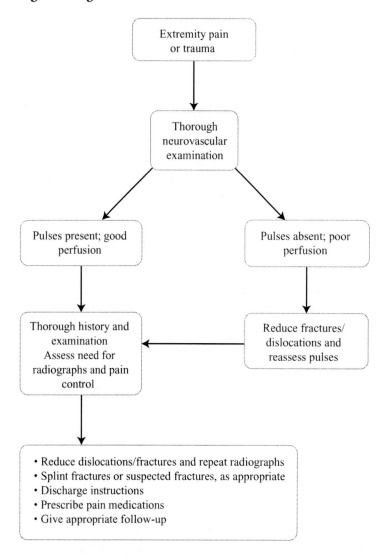

2. **Shoulder separation.** Initial treatment of a first, second, or third- degree injury is with a sling.

C. **Humerus fracture.** Treatment of these fractures includes a coaptation splint and
referral. Management of radial nerve injuries is conservative in most cases.

D. **Forearm fractures.** Both bone forearm fractures can be successfully reduced in a
closed manner in children; however, in adults, these injuries require open reduction and internal fixation (ORIF). Fracture-dislocations require ORIF. These
fractures are associated with a high incidence of compartment syndrome.

E. **Wrist and Hand**
1. **Distal radius fracture.** Closed reduction is recommended for displaced fractures, followed by a sugar tong splint.
2. **Scaphoid fracture.** Thumb spica splint.
3. **Metacarpal fracture.** Reduction when there is significant angulation, followed by a radial or ulnar gutter splint.
4. **Carpal dislocation.** Volar splint and orthopedic consultation for operative reduction.
5. **Mallet finger.** Splint the distal interphalangeal joint in extension for 6 weeks. Instruct the patient that the splint should not be removed for any reason.
6. **Tendon injury.** Treatment of open tendon injuries in the ED includes thorough wound irrigation, laceration repair (skin), and prophylactic antibiotics. Extensor tendon injuries should be splinted in extension and flexor tendon injuries are splinted in flexion. Complete open tendon injuries require referral to a hand surgeon for repair within a 7-day period.

IX. Disposition

A. **Admission** is required after orthopedic consultation for irreducible fractures or dislocations, open fractures, when compartment syndrome is suspected, or for operative repair.
B. **Discharge** is acceptable in most patients after proper splinting and pain medications. Discharge instructions should cover the signs and symptoms of compartment syndrome.

CASE PRESENTATION

A 63-year-old man is working on a fence when a post falls on his left shoulder. He is unable to use the shoulder and presents to the ED. Examination reveals that the humeral head cannot be palpated in its usual position. Radiographs confirm an anterior shoulder dislocation.

1. *What other examination findings should be documented?*
   · *Distal pulses, capillary refill, and axillary nerve function.*
2. *Following successful reduction, what else should be done?*
   · *Reassess pulses and neurologic function. Obtain a post-reduction radiograph to ensure proper reduction and absence of new fractures. Place the arm in a sling and instruct him not to externally rotate the arm. Provide orthopedic follow-up.*

SUMMARY POINTS

· *When assessing an extremity, vascular compromise must be excluded before proceeding further.*
· *A patient who has fallen on an outstretched hand and has tenderness in the anatomical snuffbox of the wrist and a negative radiograph should have a thumb spica splint placed until a scaphoid fracture is definitively excluded.*
· *Avoid NSAIDs after fractures. These medications inhibit bone healing.*
· *Patients with tense swelling of the upper extremity with pain unresponsive to narcotic pain medications should have compartment syndrome excluded.*

CHAPTER 78
LOWER EXTREMITY INJURIES

I. Defining Features

A. **Hip**

1. **Hip fracture.** The most common hip fractures are of the femoral neck and between the trochanters (intertrochanteric) (Figure 78–1). These fractures are more common in the elderly and in women. The most common mechanism of injury is a fall. Patients with displaced fractures present with leg shortening and external rotation. Femoral neck fractures are at risk for avascular necrosis.

2. **Hip dislocation.** These injuries generally require a high-energy mechanism. The dislocation is posterior in > 90% of cases. The most common mechanism of injury is when the knee strikes the dashboard during an MVC.

B. **Femur fractures** are generally the result of a high-energy trauma. Bleeding into the thigh after such a fracture can be as high as 1–1.5 L in an adult.

C. **Knee**

1. **Tibial plateau fractures** are intra-articular fractures of the proximal tibia. They are classified based on their location (medial or lateral) and the presence of depression of the fragments.

2. **Knee dislocations** are due to high-energy (MVC) and low-energy trauma (fall). An anterior dislocation (tibia is positioned anterior to the femur) is most common. Dislocations of the knee are considered orthopedic emergencies because an associated popliteal artery injury is present in a third of cases.

3. **Meniscal injury.** The knee has a medial and lateral meniscus. Medial meniscal injuries are more common because the meniscus is more securely attached to bony and ligamentous structures. Once an injury has occurred, healing is limited because the menisci are relatively avascular. Patients with meniscal injuries present with joint line pain and joint effusion. Locking occurs in 30% of patients.

4. **Ligamentous injury.** The ligaments of the knee include the anterior and posterior cruciate and the lateral and medial collateral ligaments. Patients with ligamentous injuries of the knee often report hearing a "pop" or "snap" at the time of injury. Up to three fourths of patients with a complete tear of a ligament will be ambulatory at the time of evaluation. An acute hemarthrosis suggests a tear of the anterior cruciate ligament (ACL). Further examination should include stress testing (Table 78–1).

D. **Tibia fracture.** The tibia is the weight-bearing bone of the lower leg. A fracture will result in an inability to ambulate. These fractures are associated with a high incidence of compartment syndrome.

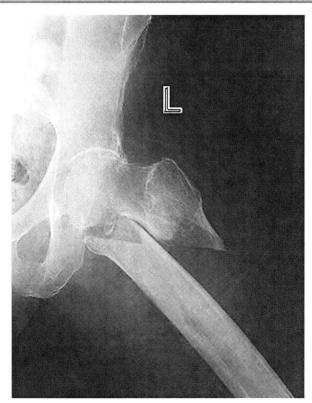

Figure 78–1. A displaced intertrochanteric fracture of the hip.

Table 78–1. Stress testing the ligaments of the knee.

Ligament	Stress Test	Description
Anterior cruciate ligament (ACL)	Lachman	Knee flexed to 30°, pull tibia forward; anterior displacement is positive
Posterior cruciate ligament (PCL)	Posterior drawer	Knee flexed to 90°, tibia pushed backwards; posterior displacement is positive
Medial collateral ligament (MCL)	Valgus stress test	Knee flexed 30° and hanging off lateral aspect of bed; valgus force applied to leg while palpating the MCL
Lateral collateral ligament (LCL)	Varus stress Test	Knee flexed 30° and hanging off lateral aspect of bed; varus force applied to leg while palpating the LCL

E. **Ankle**

1. **Ankle sprains.** Three quarters of all injuries to the ankle are sprains. Sprains are due to forced inversion or eversion of the ankle, usually while the ankle is plantar flexed. Ankle sprains are categorized as first, second, or third-degree injuries, according to the clinical presentation and the instability demonstrated by stress testing. **First-degree** sprains involve stretching without rupture of the lateral ligamentous structures (anterior talofibular, calcaneofibular, and posterior talofibular ligaments). **Second and third-degree** sprains are partial and complete tears of the ligaments of the lateral ankle. These sprains are difficult to distinguish acutely due to significant swelling and pain.

2. **Ankle fractures.** The most common ankle fracture is a distal fibula (lateral malleolar) fracture. An ankle fracture of the distal fibula and distal tibia (medial malleolus) is referred to as a **bimalleolar** fracture (Figure 78–2). When the posterior malleolus (posterior distal tibia) is involved also, the injury is called a **trimalleolar** fracture. A **Maisonneuve** fracture occurs when the fibula is fractured proximally, in combination with a medial malleolus fracture (or deltoid ligament rupture) and disruption of the tibial-fibular syn-

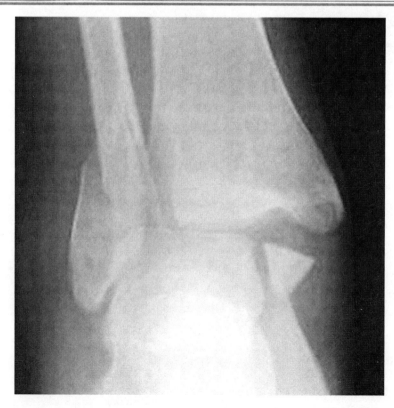

Figure 78–2. A bimalleolar fracture of the ankle.

desmosis. A **pilon** fracture is a fracture of the distal tibia. It is due to an axial load mechanism. This fracture is usually comminuted and involves the intra-articular surfaces.

3. **Achilles tendon rupture.** This injury is more common in men aged 30 to 50 who participate in recreational sports.

F. **Foot**

1. **Calcaneus fractures.** The mechanism of injury is an axial load, usually after a fall from a height. Because of this mechanism, more than 50% of patients with calcaneal fractures will have other associated extremity injuries or vertebral fractures. Most calcaneus fractures are intra-articular (involving the subtalar joint between the talus and calcaneus) and depressed. These fractures may be complicated by compartment syndrome.

2. **Metatarsal fractures.** The most common location for a metatarsal fracture is the base of the 5th metatarsal. These fractures are divided into 2 clinically important types: **Jones** and **tuberosity avulsion** fractures. Tuberosity avulsion fractures are more common, accounting for approximately 90% of all cases (Figure 78–3). These fractures heal well, and treatment with a posterior splint or hard-soled shoe is appropriate. A Jones fracture exists when the fracture line extends to the joint space between the 4th and 5th metatarsals.

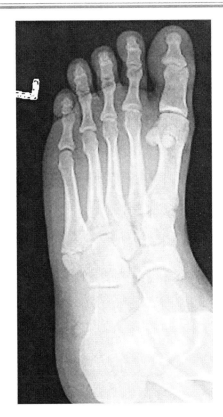

Figure 78–3. Fracture of the base of the 5th metatarsal. This fracture is an avulsion fracture of the tibial tuberosity. Note that it does not involve the joint space between the 4th and 5th metatarsals. In contrast to the Jones fracture, these fractures are more common and have a low rate of nonunion.

Because of a tenuous blood supply, these fractures heal poorly and require immobilization with non-weight bearing status.

3. **Lisfranc fracture-dislocation.** This is an injury to the bones and ligaments of the tarsometatarsal joint. It is heralded by fracture and dislocation of the metatarsals from the midfoot (ie, cuneiforms and cuboid).

II. Epidemiology

A. Ankle injuries account for 30% of athletic injuries and 12% of all traumatic injuries seen in the ED.

B. Fractures of the calcaneus represent 2% of all fractures. The calcaneus is the most commonly fractured bone in the foot, representing 60% of foot fractures.

III. Etiology

A. Meniscal injuries occur frequently in patients with sudden rotary or extension-flexion motions. In older patients with degenerative disease of the menisci, a simple twist or squatting motion may result in a tear.

B. Ankle fractures occur due to rotational forces or axial loading of the tibia.

C. The most common mechanism to sustain a calcaneus fracture is a fall from a significant height where the weight of the body is absorbed by the heel. In most individuals, a height of > 8 feet is needed to produce such a fracture but in older, osteoporotic patients, falls from shorter distances can produce these injuries.

IV. Risk Factors. MVCs, elderly, athletic activity.

V. Clinical Presentation

A. **History**
1. The physician should inquire about other injuries (head, torso) prior to focusing attention on the lower extremity.
2. The mechanism of injury is useful in determining the type of injury present.
3. Significant pain despite narcotic pain medications may suggest a compartment syndrome.

KEY COMPLAINTS

*Patients with a ruptured Achilles tendon report a sudden onset of pain and the sensation that they were struck or kicked in the back of the leg. An audible snap may be heard. **This condition is misdiagnosed in 20–30% of cases because of insignificant pain or an incomplete examination.***

B. **Physical Examination**
1. **Knee.** Apley's test is the most reliable test for detecting **meniscal tears** and is performed on a prone patient with the knee flexed. The examiner gradually extends the leg while it is externally rotated. This maneuver is repeated, first while providing distraction and then compression. If the pain is worse with compression, the test is positive, indicating the possibility of a medial meniscus tear. Stress testing of the knee will assist in excluding ligamentous injury (see Table 78–1). Frequently, pain and swelling in the knee make these tests unreliable following an acute injury.
2. **Ankle and foot.** The examiner should note tenderness over the malleoli and base of the 5th metatarsal. Pain when squeezing the leg or tenderness of the

proximal fibula suggests injury to the interosseus ligament or a Maisonneuve fracture, respectively. The calf-squeeze test is performed to detect rupture of the Achilles tendon. While the patient lies supine on the examining table with feet hanging off the edge, the calves are squeezed bilaterally and the foot is observed for plantar flexion. If a complete rupture is present, little or no foot movement will occur.

VI. Differential Diagnosis (see I)

RULE OUT

Compartment syndrome. Tibia and calcaneus fractures are the most common causes of compartment syndrome. The incidence of compartment syndrome after tibia shaft fractures is 4.3%. Compartment syndrome is present in 10% of patients with calcaneus fractures.

VII. Diagnostic Findings
- A. **Laboratory studies** are usually unnecessary after lower extremity trauma.
- B. **Imaging Studies**
  1. **Plain radiographs** are all that are necessary in most cases of lower extremity trauma.
  2. **Hip radiographs.** AP, internal, and external rotation views. Approximately 4% of hip fractures are occult on plain radiographs.
  3. **Knee radiographs.** AP, lateral, and oblique views are usually adequate in demonstrating fractures.
  4. **Ankle radiographs.** Routine films include AP, lateral, and mortise views. The mortise view is an AP view with 20° of internal rotation. **Lateral talar shift** on the AP or mortise views suggests deltoid ligament rupture. It is present when the space between the medial malleolus and talus is greater than the talar dome (superior aspect of the talus) and tibial plafond (inferior aspect of the tibia) (Figure 78–4).
  5. **Foot radiographs**
     a. In the setting of a calcaneus fracture, the lateral view allows for an assessment of Böhler's angle. ***Böhler's angle should be calculated to help identify subtle fractures and measure the degree of fracture depression.*** This angle is calculated by measuring the intersection of 2 lines: from the superior margin of the posterior tuberosity of the calcaneus through the superior tip of the posterior facet, and from the superior tip of the anterior facet to the superior tip of the posterior facet. Normally, this angle is 20–40° (Figure 78–5). If the angle is < 20°, an occult depressed fracture should be suspected.
     b. The first 3 metatarsals should align with the 3 cuneiforms and the 4th and 5th metatarsals should align with the cuboid. In addition, the medial portion of the middle cuneiform should align with the medial aspect of the 2nd metacarpal. Any disruptions in this alignment suggest a **Lisfranc injury.**
  6. **Other imaging techniques** such as bone scan, CT scan, or MRI are occasionally useful when an occult fracture is suspected. CT scan and MRI will detect hip fractures that are occult on plain films. CT scan is also used to

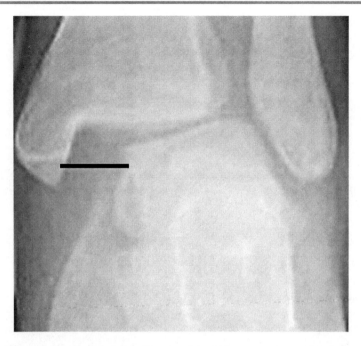

Figure 78–4. Lateral talar shift indicating deltoid ligament disruption (*arrows*).

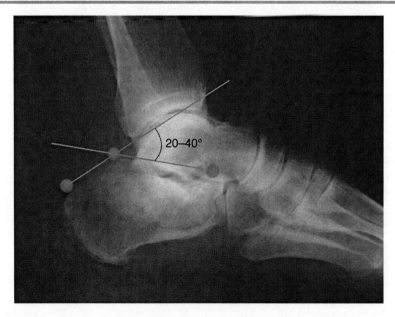

Figure 78–5. The normal Böhler's angle is between 20° and 40°.

plan operative management in patients with fractures of the calcaneus and tibial plateau.

C. **Diagnostic Algorithm (see Chapter 77, page 482)**

VIII. Treatment

A. **General Principles**
1. **RICE:** rest, ice, compression, elevation.
2. Most patients are kept non–weight bearing with the use of crutches.
3. Splint suspected fractures even if the plain radiographs are negative.
4. Narcotic pain medications for fractures. NSAIDs for soft-tissue injuries.

B. **Hip**
1. **Hip fracture.** Patients with either femoral neck or intertrochanteric hip fractures should be kept non-weight bearing and require admission of operative reduction and internal fixation (ORIF).
2. **Hip dislocation.** Patients require early reduction to limit the risk of avascular necrosis. Results are best if reduction is achieved within 6 hours.

C. **Femur fracture.** A splint should be applied in the pre-hospital setting. Treatment is with operative reduction and internal fixation with an intramedullary rod. Operative repair within 24 hours of injury reduces the incidence of fat embolism syndrome.

D. **Knee**
1. **Tibial plateau fracture.** Patients are put in a long leg posterior splint and given crutches. Follow-up with an orthopedist in 24–48 hours is appropriate. Surgery is frequently indicated. Associated ligamentous injuries are common.
2. **Knee dislocation.** When signs of poor perfusion remain after reduction, operative repair is indicated. If perfusion is intact, a course of observation vs. angiography is acceptable to rule out the possibility of occult vascular injury.
3. **Meniscal and ligamentous injury.** Patients with acute injuries should be kept non-weight bearing. Initial management includes a compression dressing or knee immobilizer, ice, crutches, and elevation.

E. **Tibia fracture.** These fractures should be immobilized with a long leg posterior splint. Admission is required in most cases because of the high association of compartment syndrome. The degree of comminution, mechanism of injury, and soft tissue injury all play an important role in the selection of definitive therapy. Options include cast or brace immobilization, external fixation, or intramedullary nailing.

F. **Ankle**
1. **Ankle sprain.** Treatment of first-degree sprains consists of RICE with early mobilization. Patients with second and third-degree sprains should be immobilized in a short leg splint in a neutral ankle position.
2. **Ankle fractures.** An isolated distal lateral malleolus fracture is a stable fracture and should be immobilized (short leg posterior splint) and referred to an orthopedist. The other fracture patterns are unstable and frequently require reduction in the emergency department before immobilization (posterior splint and a "U" shaped splint on the sides of the leg). Unstable fractures require operative fixation.
3. **Achilles tendon rupture.** Treatment includes ice, analgesics, and immobilization in the "gravity equinus position," with the ankle plantar flexed to a

comfortable position. The patient should be given crutches and instructed not to bear weight. Surgical treatment is frequently preferred in younger or more active patients.

G. **Foot**

1. **Calcaneus fracture.** The emergency management of these fractures includes ice, elevation, and immobilization in a bulky compressive dressing with a posterior splint.

2. **Metatarsal fractures.** Metatarsal fractures should be immobilized in a posterior leg splint and referred.

3. **Lisfranc fracture-dislocation.** These injuries require operative repair. Admission is warranted because of the high incidence of compartment syndrome.

IX. **Disposition**

A. **Admission** is required in patients with the potential for compartment syndrome or fat embolism (tibia and femur fractures). Mechanically or hemodynamically unstable patients with pelvic fractures require admission to an ICU.

B. **Discharge** is appropriate for most patients with lower extremity injuries. If non–weight-bearing status is required, the patient must be able to ambulate with crutches or have assistance in the home.

CASE PRESENTATION

A 28-year-old man presents to the ED with a painful right knee following an MVC. The patient denies any other trauma. Vital signs are normal. A dislocation of the knee is noted on physical examination.

1. *What further examination should be performed to assess vascular supply?*

 • *Presence of distal pulses, ankle brachial index, capillary refill, and skin color.*

2. *Distal pulses are absent. What is required in the treatment of this patient?*

 • *Immediate reduction of the dislocation, reassessment of pulses, and an angiogram to exclude a popliteal artery injury.*

SUMMARY POINTS

• *If a hip fracture is suspected clinically but plain radiographs are negative, obtain a CT scan or MRI.*

• *Delay in the reduction of a hip dislocation increases the likelihood of avascular necrosis of the femoral head.*

• *Patients who have sustained dislocations of the knee are at a high risk for popliteal artery injury.*

CHAPTER 79
LOW BACK PAIN

I. Defining Features

  A. Low back pain is caused by many conditions, ranging from benign muscle strain to more severe conditions that can result in permanent neurologic disability.

  B. The goal of the emergency physician is to detect and treat the minority of patients with conditions that threaten neurologic function (cauda equina syndrome, spinal infection, vertebral malignancy, or fracture) and provide symptomatic relief for most patients with benign, self-limiting illness.

  C. A **herniated intravertebral disk** occurs when the nucleus pulposus protrudes through the outer annulus fibrosis. The most frequent location for the herniation is posterolaterally, causing compression of a peripheral nerve root and a radiculopathy. Herniation is most common in the 3rd through the 5th decades of life and is uncommon after the 5th decade. Herniation at the L5 or S1 disk spaces accounts for 95% of all cases.

  D. **Cauda equina syndrome** is a neurosurgical emergency secondary to compression of the spinal nerves within the cauda equina. The most common etiology is a large central disk herniation. Other causes include epidural abscess, hematoma, trauma, malignancy, and spinal surgery. Diagnosis and treatment within 48 hours decreases the likelihood of irreversible neurologic injury.

  E. **Spinal infections** include epidural abscess and vertebral osteomyelitis. Risk factors for spinal infections include immunocompromise, IV drug use, elderly, and recent bacterial infection. **Epidural abscess** presents with the classic triad of fever, back pain, and neurologic deficits in only 13% of cases. Patients in one half to two thirds of cases have a fever. Patients with **vertebral osteomyelitis** (spondylitis) have a fever in 25–50% of cases.

  F. **Vertebral malignancy** is 25 times more likely to be due to metastasis than to primary malignancy such as multiple myeloma. The malignancies that most commonly metastasize to bone can be remembered by the mnemonic "**BLT** with **K**osher **P**ickle": breast, lung/lymphoma, thyroid, kidney, prostate.

  G. **Vertebral body fractures** occur in the setting of trauma, and include wedge (compression) and burst fractures (Figure 79–1). A **wedge fracture** occurs in older patients and is described based on the percentage of height lost in the anterior vertebral body compared to the normal posterior vertebral body. A **burst fracture** is present when the posterior portion of the vertebral body is also compressed.

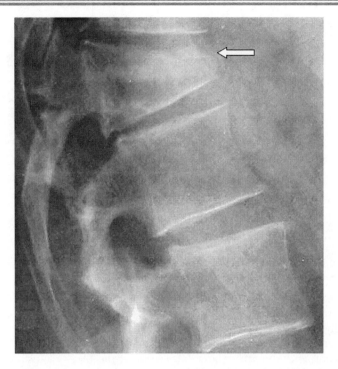

Figure 79–1. T12 compression fracture. Note the decreased height of the anterior portion of the vertebral body. A CT scan would better delineate whether this fracture involves the posterior column (ie, burst fracture).

II. Epidemiology

A. Low back pain occurs in 60–90% of the population at some point during their lifetime. About 90% will have resolution of symptoms within 6 weeks, but recurrences are common.

B. No definitive diagnosis can be made in most patients.

III. Etiology

A. **Acute.** Herniated intravertebral disk, fracture, spinal infection (epidural abscess and vertebral osteomyelitis), muscle strain.

B. **Subacute.** Vertebral malignancy, spinal stenosis, spondylolisthesis, ankylosing spondylitis.

C. **Non-thoracolumbar etiology.** AAA, pancreatitis, pyelonephritis, nephrolithiasis, ectopic pregnancy.

IV. Risk Factors. Trauma (fracture), immunocompromise (fracture, spinal infection), fever (spinal infection), IV drug use (spinal infection), bowel/bladder incontinence/retention (cauda equina syndrome), bilateral leg pain (cauda equina syndrome), pain worse at night/rest (vertebral malignancy, spinal infection), duration > 6 weeks (vertebral malignancy), > age 50 (vertebral malignancy, AAA), history of malignancy or unexplained weight loss (vertebral malignancy).

V. Clinical Presentation

A. **History**

1. Assess for the presence of risk factors for serious diagnoses.
2. A patient with a herniated disk presents most frequently with a radiculopathy, commonly of the L5 or S1 nerve root. Pain radiates down the leg, usually past the knee, and may be more severe than the back pain. Pain is worse with movement, sitting, or Valsalva maneuver (ie, coughing).
3. Bilateral leg pain or bowel or bladder dysfunction suggests cauda equina syndrome.
4. Pain worse at night or at rest suggests malignancy or spinal infection.

B. **Physical Examination**

1. **Straight leg raise (SLR) test** is positive when pain radiates down the leg and past the knee when the affected leg is raised. The sensitivity is 80% and the specificity is 40% for an intravertebral disk herniation. The **crossed SLR test** is positive when raising the unaffected leg produces pain in the contralateral, affected leg. This test is less sensitive (25%), but more specific (90%).
2. An L5 radiculopathy presents with decreased sensation between the 1st and 2nd toes and decreased strength of great toe/ankle dorsiflexion.
3. An S1 radiculopathy presents with decreased sensation on the lateral aspect of the foot and decreased strength of ankle plantarflexion. Loss of Achilles tendon reflexes may also be present.
4. Findings consistent with cauda equina syndrome include decreased sensation to light touch and pinprick of the inner thighs and perineum—saddle anesthesia (sensitivity 75%), decreased rectal tone (sensitivity 60–80%), and urinary retention with a post-void residual > 100 mL (sensitivity 90%).
5. Physical examination should also include pulse examination and abdominal palpation for an aortic aneurysm.

VI. Differential Diagnosis (see III)

VII. Diagnostic Findings

A. Laboratory Studies

1. An elevated WBC count may indicate a spinal infection.
2. ESR is elevated in the setting of spinal infections. An ESR > 20 mm/hr is 98% sensitive for diagnosing epidural abscess.

B. Imaging Studies

1. **Plain films** of the lumbar spine are indicated in patients with low back pain only in certain circumstances (Table 79–1). In addition to fractures, other plain radiographic findings include spondylolisthesis (slippage of one vertebral body on another). This condition is most commonly associated with degenerative disease and is asymptomatic in two thirds of patients.
2. **CT scan** is frequently indicated in the setting of trauma to differentiate a wedge fracture from a burst fracture. Up to 20% of burst fractures appear as a wedge fracture if plain radiography is used alone. This is significant because 65% of patients with burst fractures have or will develop a neurologic deficit.
3. **MRI** is best for evaluating the spinal canal when there is concern for spinal cord compression (ie, cauda equina syndrome) or when there is suspicion of spinal infection. If there is suspicion of vertebral malignancy, an MRI is indicated emergently when there are neurologic deficits and urgently (within 24 hours) when no neurologic deficits exist.

C. Diagnostic Algorithm

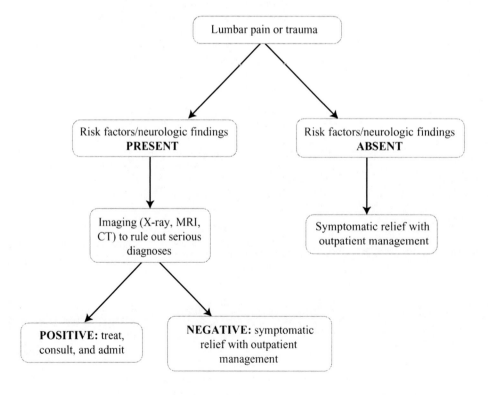

Table 79–1. Indications to obtain plain radiographs in patients with low back pain.

- Extremes of age (< age 18 and > age 50)

- History of malignancy or unexplained weight loss

- History of fever, immunocompromise, IV drug use

- Neurologic deficits or other findings of cauda equina syndrome
---
- Duration of symptoms > 6 weeks

VIII. Treatment

A. Treatment depends on the underlying cause.

B. **Muscle strain.** Treat with NSAIDs; if pain is severe, treat with a muscle relaxant. Patients should avoid heavy lifting and should begin a rehabilitation program when symptoms abate.

C. **Disk herniation** (back pain with a radiculopathy). Treatment is usually conservative (as above) because most patients recover without surgery.

D. **Burst fractures** and **cauda equina syndrome** require emergent surgical intervention. Consultation with a neurosurgeon is required.

E. **Spinal infections** are treated with antibiotics aimed at coverage of *Staphylococcus aureus,* as 90% of infections are caused by this bacterium. Patients with an epidural abscess require neurosurgical decompression and drainage.

F. **Vertebral malignancy** with new neurologic deficits suggests tumor compression on the spinal cord. After MRI confirmation, these patients should receive emergent radiation treatment to shrink the tumor and relieve impingement on the cord. Steroids (dexamethasone 10 mg IV) are also routinely administered.

IX. Disposition

A. **Admission** is necessary for patients with serious diagnoses (fracture, cauda equina syndrome, spinal infection). Patients suspected of vertebral malignancy should receive an urgent MRI if there are no neurologic deficits or radiculopathy.

B. **Discharge** is appropriate for patients without risk factors for serious diagnoses and who have a history and physical examination consistent with muscle strain or disk herniation.

CASE PRESENTATION

A 50-year-old man with low back pain that started acutely the day before comes to the ED.

1. *What historical features are important?*

   · *History of malignancy, immunocompromise, fevers, or trauma.*

2. *The patient states that he has a history of prostate cancer. What physical examination findings suggest spinal cord compression?*

   · *Radiculopathy, decreased rectal tone, urinary retention, and saddle anesthesia.*

SUMMARY POINTS

- *Musculoskeletal back pain is a diagnosis of exclusion and should not be made until more serious diagnoses have been considered and excluded.*
- *Cauda equina syndrome is a neurosurgical emergency that presents with bilateral leg pain, saddle anesthesia, decreased rectal tone, or urinary retention.*
- *Only 50% of patients with a spinal infection (epidural abscess and vertebral osteomyelitis) will present with fever.*

CHAPTER 80
COMPARTMENT SYNDROME

I. Defining Features

    A. Compartment syndrome occurs when the pressure and volume increase within a confined myofascial space, resulting in muscle and nerve ischemia.

    B. If this condition goes undiagnosed, the end result is muscle contractures, termed **Volkmann's ischemic contractures.**

II. Epidemiology. The exact incidence of compartment syndrome is unknown. The diagnosis should be considered in any patient with extremity pain and either trauma, infection, or vascular occlusion.

III. Pathophysiology

    A. Increased pressure in a closed tissue space compromises the blood supply to the muscles and nerves within the compartment. As cellular elements are injured, further swelling occurs due to the release of osmotically active substances, which attract more fluid into the confined space.

    B. After 8 hours of ischemia, muscle and nerve damage is irreversible.

IV. Risk Factors

    A. Fractures (75% of cases), crush injury, constrictive dressings or casts, seizures or chronic exertion, IV infiltration, burns, prolonged immobilization, snakebites, infection, or acute arterial occlusion.

    B. Patients taking anticoagulants (Coumadin) or those with hemophilia are at increased risk of developing compartment syndrome due to excessive bleeding after minor trauma.

V. Clinical Presentation

    A. **History**

        1. Compartment syndrome has occurred in every muscle compartment in the body. The most commonly affected compartments are those of the arm and leg. Other affected compartments include those in the hand, forearm, shoulder, back, buttocks, thigh, abdomen, and foot.

        2. The earliest symptom is disproportionate pain.

        3. The patient may complain of paresthesias.

Patients with compartment syndrome will complain of significant pain that may seem out of proportion to the original injury.

KEY
COMPLAINTS

    B. **Physical Examination**
        1. Pain with passive stretching of the muscles within the compartment is the most sensitive sign.
        2. Sensory loss is the second most sensitive sign. The physician should check for diminished 2-point discrimination.
        3. The muscles within the compartment will feel "tense" due to increased pressure.
        4. Late findings include pallor and pulselessness.

VI. **Differential Diagnosis**

    A. The pain secondary to a compartment syndrome must frequently be distinguished from the pain caused by the underlying etiologic reason for the compartment syndrome (eg, fracture, crush injury).

    B. Rhabdomyolysis may be present if significant injury to the muscles has occurred.

VII. **Diagnostic Findings**

    A. **Laboratory Studies**
        1. There are no laboratory studies that are diagnostic of compartment syndrome.
        2. If significant muscle injury has occurred, a CPK level will aid in the diagnosis of rhabdomyolysis.

    B. **Imaging studies.** Plain radiographs will assist in the diagnosis of fractures.

    C. **Procedures.** Compartment pressures are most often measured with a Stryker STIC device (Figure 80–1).

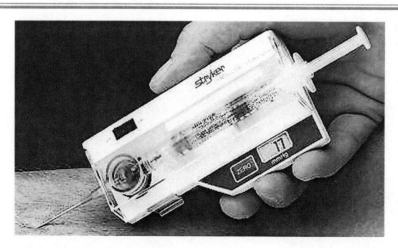

Figure 80–1. Stryker STIC device.

D. **Diagnostic Algorithm**

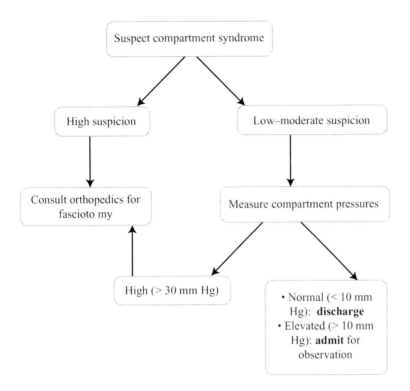

VIII. Treatment

A. Circumferential bandages and casts should be removed immediately.

B. Fasciotomy should be performed as soon as possible once compartment syndrome is diagnosed.

IX. Disposition

A. **Admission.** Patients with compartment syndrome should be admitted to the hospital for operative fasciotomy. When there is concern that a compartment syndrome may develop following an injury, admission for observation is recommended.

B. **Discharge.** If the compartment pressure is normal and the underlying injury has been treated appropriately, the patient can be discharged. It is important to give thorough discharge instructions to patients sustaining extremity trauma to return to the ED if they develop worsening swelling, numbness, or pain that is not responsive to pain medications.

CASE PRESENTATION

A 7-year-old girl falls off a swing and lands on her outstretched arm. Radiographs reveal a supracondylar fracture of the humerus.

1. *What features of the history and physical examination will lead you to suspect compartment syndrome in this child?*
   - *Pain unresponsive to narcotic pain medications, tense swelling of the arm, pain with passive movement of the muscles within the compartment, and sensory deficits distal to the injury.*

SUMMARY POINTS

- *Consider compartment syndrome in patients with pain that seems unresponsive to narcotic pain medications or is disproportionate to the injury.*
- *Delay in diagnosis and treatment results in Volkmann's ischemic contractures in up to 10% of cases.*

CHAPTER 81
SEPTIC ARTHRITIS

I. Defining Features

    A. Of all causes of arthritis, **joint infection** is of greatest concern to the emergency physician, because missing the diagnosis may lead to rapid joint destruction and irreversible loss of function.

    B. Septic (infectious) arthritis is classified as gonococcal or nongonococcal. **Nongonococcal septic arthritis** is most frequently due to *Staphylococcus aureus* (50%), but it is also caused by *Streptococcus pneumoniae, Streptococcus pyogenes* (25%), and gram-negative bacilli (20%). **Gonococcal arthritis** represents 5% of cases. Other rare causes include mycobacteria, fungi, and viruses.

    C. The knee is involved in almost half of all cases, and there is polyarticular involvement in 10%.

II. Epidemiology

    A. Acute arthritis is a common complaint evaluated in the ED.

    B. The incidence of septic arthritis is 2–10 cases per 100,000 persons in the United States.

    C. Septic arthritis has a mortality rate of 10% in adults.

    D. Residual joint damage occurs in 30% of patients.

III. Pathophysiology

    A. In most cases of septic arthritis, bacteria reach the joint by hematogenous spread. Contiguous spread from a soft tissue infection or after a penetrating extremity injury may also occur.

    B. Once bacteria enter the closed joint space, an inflammatory response is triggered and an influx of inflammatory cells results in purulence. Cytokines and proteases lead to cartilage degradation if the infection is not treated early.

IV. Risk Factors. Immunosuppression (eg, diabetes mellitus), injection drug use, remote focus of infection, bacteremia, elderly, prosthetic material within the joint (ie, joint replacement), previous joint injury (eg, rheumatoid arthritis), recent joint surgery.

V. Clinical Presentation

    A. **History**
        1. Onset of septic arthritis is usually acute, occurring within hours to 1 week.
        2. History of similar attacks suggests an alternate diagnosis.

3. Systemic symptoms and a "toxic" appearance may be present, but should not be relied upon. Fever is present in only half of patients with septic arthritis.
4. The patient will report exquisite pain in the affected joint(s) and worsening pain with subtle movement.
5. Patients with gonococcal arthritis may report pelvic pain or discharge, in addition to arthritis.

KEY COMPLAINTS

Patients with septic arthritis will present with marked inability to move the joint through normal range of motion.

B. **Physical Examination**
1. Erythema, warmth, and effusion are present in all patients with septic arthritis.
2. Tenderness is localized to the joint.
3. Range of motion is severely limited and painful. This is in contradistinction to periarticular conditions, like bursitis, in which pain is less severe with passive range of motion and with joint distraction.

CLINICAL SKILLS TIP

Arthrocentesis is an essential skill to obtain synovial fluid for cell count, crystal analysis, Gram stain, and culture. There are several important principles to successful arthrocentesis: sterile technique, comparison with the unaffected extremity to obtain landmarks, gentle distraction of the extremity to increase the joint space, entrance through extensor surfaces to avoid important neurovascular structures, and slight flexion (10–20°) of the joint.

VI. **Differential Diagnosis.** Crystal-induced arthropathy (gout, pseudogout), hemarthrosis, osteoarthritis, rheumatoid arthritis, spondyloarthropathy (ankylosing spondylitis), systemic lupus erythematosus, periarticular disease (ie, bursitis, tendinitis)

RULE OUT

Septic arthritis is the "rule out" diagnosis. Crystals found on fluid analysis suggests a diagnosis of gout; however, these conditions may coexist. Up to 3% of patients with gout have a positive culture.

VII. **Diagnostic Findings**
A. **Laboratory Studies**
1. **CBC.** Peripheral leukocytosis is generally not helpful, as it is elevated in only half of cases.
2. **ESR** > 30 mm/hr is 96% sensitive but lacks specificity.
3. **Synovial fluid analysis** (Table 81–1). Synovial fluid leukocyte count lacks sensitivity and specificity for detection of septic arthritis; however, a count > 50,000/mm^3 should be considered infectious until proven otherwise. In 10% of patients with septic arthritis, the synovial fluid leukocyte count is < 10,000/mm^3. Gram stain is positive in approximately 60–80% of cases. Culture is positive in most cases, but the results are not reported for several days and therefore, are not helpful in the ED.

Table 81–1. Typical synovial fluid laboratory findings in patients with acute monoarthritis.

Condition	Appearance	WBC/mm³	Crystals	Culture/Gram stain
Normal	Clear	< 200	None	Negative
Osteoarthritis	Straw-colored	< 400	None	Negative
Acute gout	Turbid	> 2,000–100,000	Present	Negative
Rheumatoid arthritis	Turbid	> 2,000–100,000	None	Negative
Septic arthritis	Purulent/turbid	> 5,000–100,000	None	Positive

B. **Imaging Studies.** Plain films usually are not helpful unless the diagnosis is in question or the patient reports a history of trauma or prior joint surgery.

C. **Procedures**

1. **Arthrocentesis.** Perform to remove synovial fluid for laboratory analysis (Figure 81–1). In most cases, the emergency physician performs this procedure. Sterile technique is essential to avoid causing a joint infection.

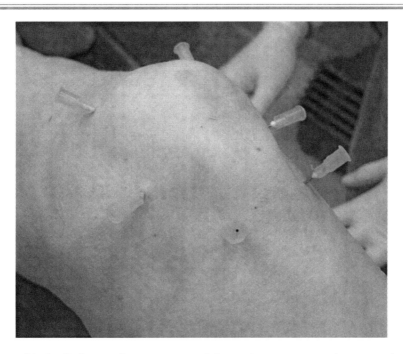

Figure 81–1. Cadaveric demonstration of the six locations to perform an arthrocentesis of the knee (suprapatellar, parapatellar, and infrapatellar).

2. Orthopedic consultation for arthrocentesis should be sought for hip arthrocentesis, due to a high rate of complications, and in a patient with prosthetic material in the joint. Arthrocentesis performed through infected soft tissues should be avoided.

D. **Diagnostic Algorithm**

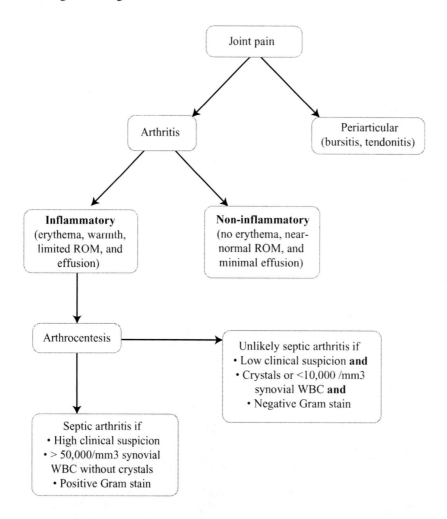

VIII. Treatment

A. Empiric treatment should include a penicillinase-resistant penicillin (eg, nafcillin) and a third-generation cephalosporin (eg, ceftriaxone). Patients who are allergic to penicillin or who have recently been hospitalized should be given vancomycin. When gonococcal arthritis is likely, ceftriaxone is the agent of choice.

B. The extremity should be elevated and splinted for comfort.

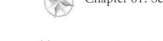

C. Orthopedic consultation should be obtained for possible operative irrigation ("wash out") of the joint.

IX. Disposition

A. **Admission.** All patients with suspected septic arthritis should be admitted to the hospital for IV antibiotics.

B. **Discharge.** Patients determined to have crystalline arthropathies or patients who are unlikely to have septic arthritis, as determined above, may be discharged. In unclear cases, however, orthopedic consultation is recommended.

CASE PRESENTATION

A 65-year-old man presents with a painful joint. How do you approach this patient?

1. What historical questions do you want to ask?

• *How long have the symptoms been present? Similar symptoms in the past? Trauma? Fever or other constitutional symptoms?*

2. On examination, what findings support the diagnosis of septic arthritis?

• *Erythema, warmth, limited range of motion, effusion, fever.*

SUMMARY POINTS

• *Septic arthritis is a difficult diagnosis to make but an important one, because it is associated with mortality and residual joint damage if left untreated.*

• *Arthrocentesis should be performed in patients with clinical suspicion of septic arthritis (acute onset of erythema, warmth, and severely limited ROM).*

• *In patients with suspected septic arthritis, admission for IV antibiotics is frequently necessary until culture results are negative.*

CHAPTER 82
SPLINTING

I. Indications

A. A fracture is immobilized to permit healing, relieve pain, and to stabilize an unstable fracture. Most injuries in the ED are immobilized with a splint so that swelling following the injury will not cause a significant increase in tissue pressure.

B. Not all fractures require splinting, and in some situations, prolonged immobilization can be deleterious and cause contractures and prolonged immobility.

C. Splints are indicated for most fractures and some soft tissue injuries (eg, after reduction of a dislocation). A splint is also indicated when there is clinical evidence of a fracture, yet the plain radiographs are equivocal or negative. In some cases, fractures remain occult on the initial radiograph and will appear days to weeks later.

D. In most cases, the extremity is placed in the position of function before immobilization. One joint above the fracture and one joint below the fracture are immobilized.

E. **Posterior leg splint** (Figure 82–1). This splint extends along the posterior aspect of the leg from the toes to just below the knee (short leg) or to the middle of the thigh (long leg). Fractures at the knee (ie, tibial plateau) will require a long leg splint, while ankle fractures require a short leg splint. With particularly unstable ankle fractures, a U-shaped splint is added for additional support. It should extend from the medial aspect of the leg just below the knee, around the heel, to the same height on the lateral aspect of the leg.

F. **Coaptation splint** (Figure 82–2). The coaptation splint is the preferred splint for fractures of the humeral shaft. This splint extends from above the shoulder joint down the lateral aspect of the arm, around the elbow, and then up the medial aspect of the arm to the axilla.

G. **Sugar-tong splint** (Figure 82–3). This splint gets its name because it is shaped like the tongs that grab a cube of sugar for coffee or tea. With the elbow positioned at 90°, this splint extends from the dorsal aspect of the hand at the metacarpophalangeal (MCP) joints, around the elbow, and to the flexor crease of the palm. This splint is useful for distal radius fractures and fractures of the radial and ulnar shafts.

H. **Gutter splint (radial and ulnar)** (Figure 82–4A-F). These splints are positioned on either the radial or ulnar portion of the hand and forearm and extend two

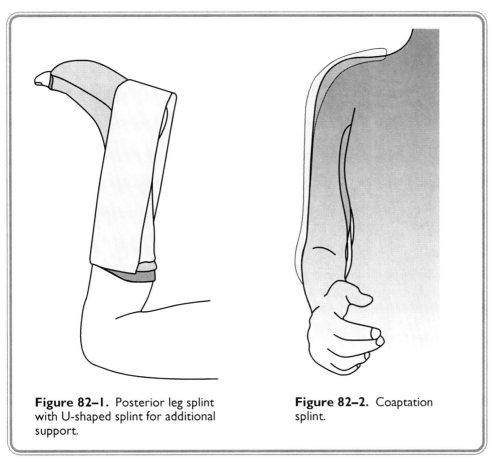

Figure 82–1. Posterior leg splint with U-shaped splint for additional support.

Figure 82–2. Coaptation splint.

thirds of the way up the forearm. Both splints include the fingers (4th and 5th digits for an ulnar gutter, and the 2nd and 3rd digits for a radial gutter). For the radial gutter splint, a hole is cut out for the thumb. ***Do not immobilize the digits in full extension.*** If the digits are immobilized in full extension, the collateral ligaments of the joints will contract, resulting in stiffness. The ideal position of the

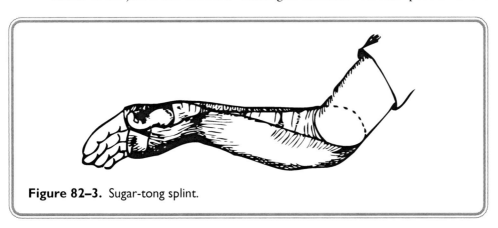

Figure 82–3. Sugar-tong splint.

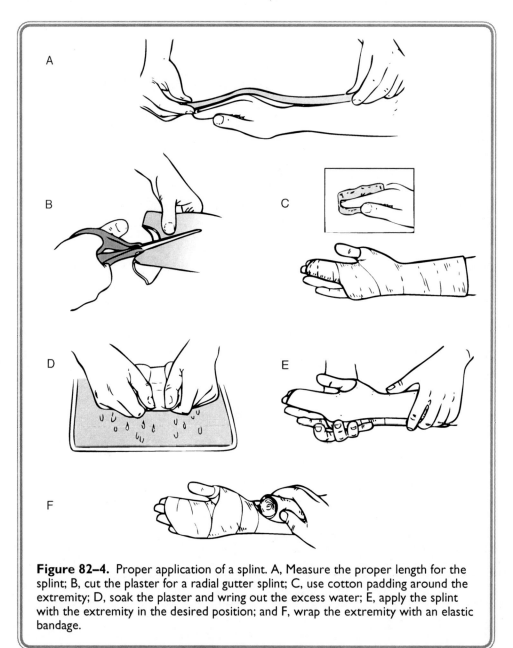

Figure 82–4. Proper application of a splint. A, Measure the proper length for the splint; B, cut the plaster for a radial gutter splint; C, use cotton padding around the extremity; D, soak the plaster and wring out the excess water; E, apply the splint with the extremity in the desired position; and F, wrap the extremity with an elastic bandage.

digits is 50–90° of flexion of the MCP joints and 15–20° of flexion of the proximal interphalangeal (PIP) and distal interphalangeal (DIP) joints. The wrist should be in approximately 15° of extension. This position is referred to as the "wine glass position of the hand," because the hand appears as if the patient were holding a glass of wine. These splints are useful for fractures of the metacarpals and phalanges of digits 2 through 5.

I. **Dorsal splint with extension hood ("clam digger").** This splint is applied to the dorsal aspect of the hand and forearm and extends the length of the digits. The hand is cupped in such a way that when the splint is applied, the patient has the appearance that they could "dig for clams on the beach." The hand is kept in the "wine glass position," as described above. This splint is useful for fractures of multiple bones of the hand.

J. **Thumb splint** is applied for phalangeal fractures of the 1st digit or ulnar collateral ligament injuries (gamekeeper's thumb). A thumb splint is applied with a single plaster slab that extends from the distal aspect of the thumb to two thirds of the way up the forearm.

K. **Thumb spica splint** is used to immobilize the thumb, 1st metacarpal, and the scaphoid. First, a thumb splint is applied, followed by an additional plaster slab placed on the volar aspect of the forearm from the palmar crease to proximal forearm. Extending the splint to above the elbow prevents pronation and supination of the forearm and provides further immobilization of the scaphoid (Figure 82–5).

L. **Finger splints.** This splint can be rapidly placed on a digit using commercially available malleable padded materials. These splints are used to protect the digits after phalangeal fractures. Alternatively, when a minor ligamentous sprain occurs at the PIP joint, a dynamic finger splint is used. This functional splint is applied by taping the proximal and middle phalanx of the injured digit to an uninjured neighboring digit.

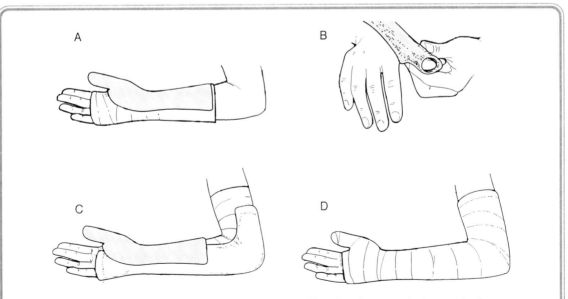

Figure 82–5. Thumb splint and thumb spica splint. A, Thumb splint is applied over the forearm; B, the thumb splint extends over the interphalangeal joint and around the thumb; C, a thumb spica splint is created by adding a second volar splint that extends above the elbow; and D, an elastic bandage is wrapped around the plaster splints.

II. **Contraindications.** There are no absolute contraindications to splinting. Wound care is required before a splint is applied in the event of lacerations or open fractures. In this situation, the splint will need to be removed to inspect for subsequent wound infection.

III. **Equipment.** Stockinette, cotton padding, plaster rolls or slabs (widths of 3, 4, and 5 inches), fiberglass splint material (alternative), scissors, warm water and a bucket, elastic bandages.

IV. **Procedure** (see Figure 82–4)

 A. A stockinette is placed on the extremity covering both the proximal and distal ends where the splint will be applied (optional).

 B. Approximately 10 sheets of plaster are cut or torn to the proper length. For the radial gutter splint, a hole is cut for the thumb.

 C. Several layers of cotton padding are applied to the extremity in a circumferential manner. Special care is taken to apply extra padding to bony protuberances (ie, malleoli) where excessive pressure might cause skin necrosis. Padding should also be placed between digits that will be involved in the splint.

 D. The plaster is briefly soaked in warm water. The water reacts with the calcium sulfate in the plaster, resulting in heat, which the patient will notice after the splint is applied.

 E. Excess water is removed by wringing the plaster together between the hands. Then, holding the plaster up on one end with one hand, the thumb and index finger of the other hand are used to smooth out the plaster.

 F. The splint is applied to the extremity as required based on the fracture.

 G. An additional layer of cotton padding is placed over the plaster (optional). This will prevent the next layer (elastic bandage) from adhering to the drying plaster.

 H. An elastic bandage is wrapped circumferentially around the extremity, and the splint is checked to make sure that it is still in the desired position. ***This layer should not be wrapped too tight to avoid creating a compartment syndrome.***

 I. The patient is instructed to avoid moving the extremity until the splint has dried (5–10 minutes).

V. **Complications**

 A. **Compartment syndrome.** Circumferential bandages, especially if they are applied too tight, may produce a compartment syndrome. The patient should be instructed to return to the ED if pain worsens or there is numbness or tingling of the extremity.

 B. **Thermal injury.** As the plaster dries, heat is produced. If sufficient cotton padding is not used, thermal injury can occur.

SECTION XVIII

DERMATOLOGIC EMERGENCIES

CHAPTER 83
LIFE-THREATENING DERMATOSES

I. Defining Features

A. Cutaneous lesions can be the first clinical sign of a serious systemic illness. It is important to recognize and treat these illnesses early.

B. Life-threatening dermatoses can be grouped into 3 distinct categories: diffuse red rashes, vesiculobullous lesions, and hemorrhagic lesions.

II. Diffuse Red Rashes

A. **Staphylococcal Scalded Skin Syndrome** (SSSS)
 1. **Clinical presentation.** SSSS generally begins on the face (perioral area) as red patches that are warm and tender. The erythema spreads and becomes flaccid bullae, which then desquamate in large sheets. The mucous membranes usually are not involved. Nikolsky's sign is positive and can be elicited when gentle stroking of the skin produces peeling. Only the superficial layer of the epidermis is shed; therefore, healing occurs within 10–14 days.
 2. **Epidemiology.** SSSS is most common in children and neonates; 98% of patients are < age 6.
 3. **Etiology.** Exotoxin is produced by coagulase-positive *Staphylococcus aureus.*
 4. **Treatment.** Systemic antibiotics (eg, nafcillin), hydration, and admission.

B. **Toxic Shock Syndrome** (TSS)
 1. **Clinical presentation.** TSS is a diffuse red macular rash associated with fever, hypotension, and involvement of at least 3 organ systems. It was originally diagnosed in menstruating women using tampons, but can also be seen in patients with surgical wounds and nasal packings. The patient may present with a strawberry-appearing tongue, red conjunctiva, and edema of the face, hands, and feet. The rash fades within 72 hours and is followed by acral desquamation within 1–2 weeks.
 2. **Epidemiology.** About 10–20 cases per 100,000 persons.
 3. **Etiology.** TSS is caused by *Staphylococcus aureus,* which produces an exotoxin (TSST-1). *Streptococcus pyogenes* exotoxin A and B are also causative.
 4. **Treatment.** IV immunoglobulin G (IVIG) has been shown to be effective in neutralizing the TSS toxin and aids in recovery. Systemic antibiotics (eg, nafcillin) and ICU admission.

C. **Kawasaki Disease**
 1. **Clinical presentation.** Clinical diagnosis of Kawasaki disease includes fever > 39.4 °C (103.5°F) of 5 days' duration, plus 4 of 5 of the following criteria:

515

bilateral conjunctival injection; mucous membrane involvement (strawberry tongue, cracked lips); erythema, edema of hands and/or feet, or desquamation; diffuse maculopapular rash; and cervical lymphadenopathy (usually > 1.5 cm and unilateral).

2. **Epidemiology.** About 3,000 hospital admissions annually. Usually appears in children < age 5, with a peak incidence in children 18 to 24 months. Epidemics occur primarily in the late winter and spring. About 20% develop cardiovascular complications. The most common cause of death is MI. Coronary aneurysm may develop 2–8 weeks after fever.

3. **Etiology.** An immunologic disorder triggered by infection or toxin, leading to a generalized vasculitis.

4. **Treatment.** High-dose aspirin, IVIG, and hospital admission.

III. Vesiculobullous Lesions

A. **Erythema Multiforme** (EM)

1. **Clinical presentation.** The typical lesion of EM is the "target lesion," described as erythematous plaques with dusky centers and bright red borders resembling the "bull's eye" of a target (Figure 83–1). As the name implies, many types of lesions may present simultaneously, including macules, papules, and bullae. The lesions are symmetric and are usually found on the

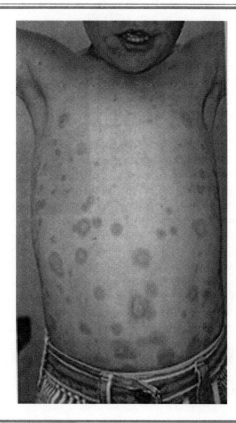

Figure 83–1. Target lesions of erythema multiforme.

extremities, palms, and soles, and may also involve the oral mucosa. A burning sensation is present, and pruritus is notably absent.

2. **Epidemiology.** Accounts for as many as 1% of dermatological outpatient visits and is more common in spring and fall.

3. **Etiology.** EM is a hypersensitivity reaction precipitated by medications, infections, sarcoidosis, collagen vascular diseases, or malignancies. About 50% of cases are idiopathic.

4. **Treatment.** EM is generally a benign, non-pruritic, self-limited rash that generally resolves within 2–4 weeks. It requires no specific treatment except cool compresses and an attempt to identify and remove the precipitating cause.

B. **Toxic Epidermal Necrolysis** (TEN)

1. **Clinical presentation.** The skin is painful with hot red blisters and large areas of sloughing. TEN affects > 30% of the skin. There is usually mucous membrane involvement. It may be a more severe form of EM with constitutional symptoms of fever, malaise, and myalgias.

2. **Epidemiology.** About 1 case per 1 million persons occurs annually. Adults are most commonly affected. TEN desquamates the entire thickness of the epidermis; therefore, mortality rates are 30–40%.

3. **Etiology.** TEN is caused by drugs such as phenytoin, sulfas, penicillins, and NSAIDs. Onset is usually within the first 8 weeks of therapy.

4. **Treatment.** Similar to burns (fluid resuscitation, cover skin with petroleum gauze, admission to burn unit).

C. **Stevens-Johnson's Syndrome** (SJS)

1. **Clinical presentation.** SJS is a more severe form of EM and involves blistering of 2 or more mucosal surfaces such as eyes, lips, mouth, urogenital area, or anus (Figure 83–2). Blistering of < 10% of the skin is also characteristic. Fever, malaise, myalgias, and arthralgias are common. Lesions begin on the dorsal surfaces of the hands and feet and spread centrally. SJS can progress to TEN, with large bullae and sloughing of epidermis in sheets.

2. **Epidemiology.** Up to 6 cases per 1 million persons annually.

3. **Etiology.** Similar to EM but medications are more commonly associated with SJS.

4. **Treatment.** Fluids and debridement of large bullae in a burn unit. Treat any underlying infection. Steroids are *not* indicated.

D. **Pemphigus Vulgaris** (PV)

1. **Clinical presentation.** PV is characterized by flaccid bullae that begin in the mouth and spread to involve the skin. Almost all patients have mucosal lesions. The bullae rupture easily, so the patient may present with painful erosions.

2. **Epidemiology.** About 3 cases per 100,000 persons. Peak age of onset is 50–60.

3. **Etiology.** Autoimmune blistering disease characterized by autoantibodies directed against keratinocyte cell surfaces. Some cases are drug-induced.

4. **Differential diagnosis.** Bullous pemphigoid (BP) is a similar autoimmune blistering disease, but it usually only affects the elderly. Unlike PV, the bullae of BP are tense rather than flaccid, and oral involvement is uncommon.

5. **Treatment.** Fluid resuscitation, systemic corticosteroids, and admission.

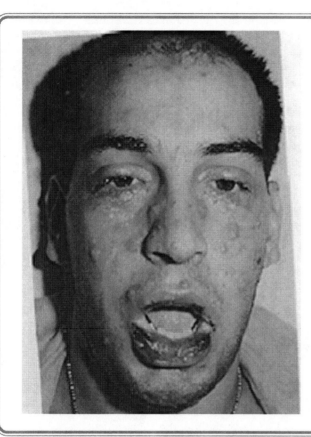

Figure 83–2. Stevens-Johnson syndrome. Mucosal surface involvement of the face resulting in thick, hemorrhagic crusts on the lips.

IV. Hemorrhagic Lesions

A. **Disseminated Gonococcal Infection** (DGI)
  1. **Clinical presentation.** The patient is usually a young, sexually active woman with fever, skin lesions, arthritis, arthralgias, or migratory tenosynovitis. Lesions are described as hemorrhagic gray necrotic pustules on an erythematous base, numbering between 10–30, and appearing on the extremities and resolving rapidly.
  2. **Epidemiology.** DGI occurs following approximately 1% of gonococcal genital infections.
  3. **Etiology.** *Neisseria gonorrhoeae:* certain subtypes are more likely to lead to disseminated infection.
  4. **Treatment.** Ceftriaxone IV. Admission for systemically ill patients or those with involvement of weight-bearing joints.

B. **Meningococcemia**
  1. **Clinical presentation.** The classic rash can be petechial or macular, with pale gray vesicular centers, and may progress to a confluent hemorrhagic rash (Figure 83–3). Fever, headache, and vomiting are present. Meningitis may or may not be present.

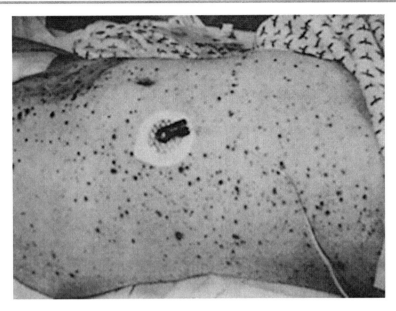

Figure 83–3. Meningococcemia. Diffuse petechia in a patient with meningococcemia.

2. **Epidemiology.** About 2 cases per 100,000 persons annually, although sporadic outbreaks with higher prevalence occur frequently. Mortality rate is approximately 10%.
3. **Etiology.** *N. meningitidis.*
4. **Treatment.** The patient can deteriorate quickly over several hours, leading to hypotension, shock, renal failure, ARDS, and DIC. Treatment consists of high-dose IV antibiotics and ICU admission.

CASE PRESENTATION

An 18-year-old woman presents to the ED complaining of rash, fever, and myalgias. The patient was seen 8 days ago for a nose bleed and had an anterior nasal pack placed to stop the bleeding. Her skin is diffusely red and painful. Her hands, face, and feet are swollen. Vital signs are temperature 39.5°C (103.2°F), pulse 138 beats/min, BP 80/50 mm Hg, and RR 22 breaths/min.

1. *How would you begin treatment?*
   - *IV fluids, O₂, monitor, antipyretics. Remove nasal packing and irrigate with water. IV antibiotics.*
2. *What is your diagnosis and disposition?*
   - *TSS. Admission to the ICU.*

SUMMARY POINTS

- *Rapid identification of life-threatening rashes and immediate treatment can be life saving.*

CHAPTER 84
ALLERGIC REACTIONS

I. Defining Features

A. **Urticaria,** or "hives," is an IgE-mediated hypersensitivity reaction that results in red raised wheals that itch and sting.

B. **Angioedema** is nonpitting edema of the deeper layers of the skin. It is not pruritic but can cause burning, numbness, or pain.

C. **Anaphylaxis** is a severe systemic allergic reaction that can present rapidly with hypotension, bronchospasm, or laryngeal edema.

II. Epidemiology

A. **Urticaria.** Urticaria is one of the most common skin lesions seen in the ED in both young and older patients. About 20% of the population experiences at least 1 attack of urticaria in a lifetime.

B. **Angioedema.** Approximately 94% of cases of angioedema presenting to the ED are drug induced. Most drug-induced angioedema occurs in patients taking ACE inhibitors. About 0.1–0.2% of the 35 million patients in the United States being treated with ACE inhibitors develop angioedema.

C. **Anaphylaxis.** About 500–1000 persons in the United States die every year due to anaphylaxis. Approximately 1 in 5,000 parenteral doses of a penicillin or cephalosporin antibiotic cause anaphylaxis.

III. Pathophysiology

A. **Urticaria** is most commonly caused by an IgE-mediated hypersensitivity to an allergen. Circulating antibodies bind the allergen and IgE receptors on mast cells. In response, mast cells release inflammatory substances (histamine, bradykinin), which result in increased vascular permeability.

B. **Angioedema** is due to several different mechanisms. **IgE-mediated angioedema** is similar to urticaria and frequently urticaria and angioedema appear together. **Hereditary angioedema** is an autosomal dominant disorder caused by a deficiency of C1 esterase inhibitor (C1-INH), which leads to the formation of bradykinin. **Acquired angioedema** is characterized by normal C1-INH that becomes bound to circulating antibodies that inactivate it. **ACE inhibitor-induced angioedema** is due to decreased degradation of bradykinin because of inhibition of the enzyme kininase II.

C. **Anaphylaxis** is IgE mediated and results from release of histamine, leukotrienes, and prostaglandins from inflammatory cells. The result is a systemic increase in vascular permeability, vasodilatation, and smooth muscle contraction.

IV. **Risk Factors**

A. **Urticaria.** Medications (eg, aspirin, NSAIDs, antibiotics), foods (eg, peanuts, seafood), insect bites, latex exposure, infections, heat or cold, exercise, malignancy, pregnancy.

B. **Angioedema.** Similar to urticaria, plus
1. Patients with C1-INH deficiency.
2. Patients taking an ACE inhibitor. ACE inhibitor-induced angioedema can occur with use of all types of ACE inhibitors, but lisinopril and enalapril are more common offenders than is captopril. African Americans have a 3 to 5-fold increased incidence. Recent initiation of therapy (20–60% within the first week, although it should be noted that ACE inhibitor-induced angioedema has been reported in patients taking ACE inhibitors for as many as 5 years).

C. **Anaphylaxis.** Prior history of urticaria or angioedema. Foods, drugs, vaccines, blood products, contrast media, pollens, and insect venoms.

V. **Clinical Presentation**

A. **History**
1. Patients with urticaria present with transient, pruritic, well-circumscribed lesions that are erythematous, nonpitting plaques (wheals) surrounded by an erythematous ring (flare) (Figure 84–1).
2. Patients with angioedema present with swelling of the face, lips, tongue, eyelids, distal extremities, or genitalia. The swelling is nonpitting and may occur with urticaria. ACE inhibitor-induced angioedema has a predilection for the face (Figure 84–2).
3. Patients with anaphylaxis present with a sensation of impending doom or lump in the throat followed by shortness of breath, chest pain, hypotension, nausea, vomiting, or diarrhea. More than 90% of patients have urticaria or angioedema.
4. If the patient is stable, try to identify the inciting factors. Ask about medications, exposures, contacts, underlying illness, allergies, diet, and family history of allergic reactions.

B. **Physical Examination**
1. Initial evaluation should focus on ABCs.
2. Airway obstruction is evidenced by swelling (lips, tongue, uvula), hoarseness, stridor, wheezing, or respiratory distress.
3. In patients with ACE inhibitor-induced angioedema, the face is involved in 86% of cases. Laryngeal involvement is present in 9%, while the tongue is affected in 39% of cases.
4. Once a patient is hemodynamically stable, a more detailed physical examination should be performed.
5. Examine the skin while the patient is undressed and describe the rash. Important features include type (macular, papular, vesicular), size, shape, number, and color.

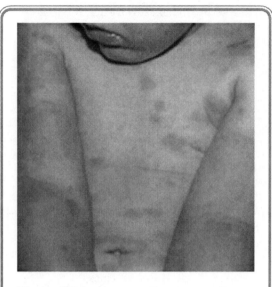

Figure 84–1. Urticaria. Transient, well-circumscribed, erythematous, annular plaques are characteristic of urticaria.

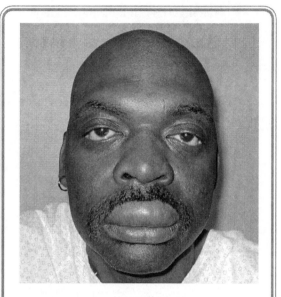

Figure 84–2. Photograph of angioedema of the upper lip of a man taking an ACE inhibitor.

VI. Differential Diagnosis

    A. **Urticaria.** Viral rash, erythema multiforme, bullous pemphigoid, and vasculitis.

    B. **Angioedema.** Infection (cellulitis), contact dermatitis (insect bites), and renal or liver disease.

    C. **Anaphylaxis.** PE, acute MI, acute asthma, airway obstruction, sepsis, and TSS.

VII. Diagnostic Findings

    A. **Diagnosis of urticaria, angioedema, and anaphylaxis is based on clinical symptoms, and no specific laboratory or imaging tests are necessary.**

    B. **Diagnostic Algorithm (see page 523)**

VIII. Treatment

    A. **General.** Initial stabilization consists of ABCs, cardiac monitoring, O_2, and IV fluids. Treatment depends on the severity and extent of the reaction. ***When the airway is threatened, intubation is lifesaving.*** All offending agents or exposures should be eliminated.

    B. **Epinephrine.** Indicated in patients with angioedema when the airway is compromised or in patients with bronchoconstriction or hypotension from anaphylaxis. **Normotensive:** 0.3 mg SQ (0.3 mL of 1:1000 solution). **Hypotensive:** 0.1–0.2 mg IV (1–2 mL of 1:10,000 solution diluted in 10 mL NS given slowly over 3–5 minutes).

Diagnostic Algorithm

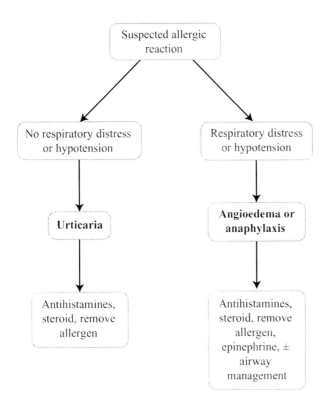

C. **Antihistamine.** H1 blocker (diphenhydramine 25–50 mg PO or IM for mild to moderate reaction or 1–2 mg/kg IV in more severe reactions). H_2 blocker in combination with an H_1 blocker for patients with severe urticaria, angioedema, or anaphylaxis. Famotidine 20 mg IV, *or* ranitidine 50 mg IV, *or* cimetidine 300 mg IV.

D. **Corticosteroids.** For patients with severe urticaria, angioedema, or anaphylaxis. Onset of action is not immediate. Prednisone 60 mg PO or methylprednisolone 125 mg IV

E. **Albuterol.** Indicated if bronchospasm is present; 2.5 mg in 3 mL saline nebulized.

F. **Hereditary and ACE inhibitor-induced angioedema.** Patients with hereditary and ACE inhibitor-induced angioedema are usually refractory to treatment with SQ epinephrine, antihistamines, and steroids. However, it is difficult to distinguish these from angioedema due to an IgE-mediated reaction, which may respond to these therapies. In the presence of an acutely ill patient, treatment of a presumed hypersensitivity reaction is necessary while considering other etiologies and treatments. Discontinuing the ACE inhibitor leads to resolution within 24–48 hours. Administering FFP replaces the enzyme (kininase II) that breaks down excess bradykinin. When the airway is threatened, 2–4 units of FFP may reverse angioedema within a few hours. Prophylactic intubation or cricothyrotomy should be performed when edema is progressive and there is evidence of airway compromise.

IX. Disposition

A. **Admission.** Patients with systemic symptoms or potential airway compromise that does not resolve must be hospitalized.

B. **Discharge.** Patients with resolution of symptoms may be discharged after several hours of ED observation. Refer to an allergist or immunologist, prescribe antihistamines and steroids for 3 days, and if the reaction was severe, prescribe an EpiPen. Patients with known triggers should be advised about strict avoidance of those triggers. Patients taking an ACE inhibitor should be instructed to discontinue the medication and avoid angiotensin receptor blockers.

CASE PRESENTATION

A 60-year-old man who was stung by a bee complains of swelling of his lower lip and throat of 2 hours' duration. He describes some difficulty breathing and throat tightness.

1. *What would you look for on physical examination?*
   - *Drooling or tongue swelling, hoarseness, stridor, wheezing, hypotension, or tachycardia.*
1. *How would you treat this patient?*
   - *IV or SQ epinephrine, IV diphenhydramine, IV steroids, IV H_2 blocker, prepare airway supplies.*

SUMMARY POINTS

- *Administer epinephrine, antihistamines, and steroids for life-threatening reactions that are accompanied by laryngeal edema, hypotension, or wheezing.*
- *Urticaria may be the first sign of what might progress to angioedema or anaphylaxis.*
- *For patients with respiratory symptoms or throat swelling, perform a rapid assessment of the airway and intubate early.*
- *Attempt to determine and then discontinue the inciting agent.*

INDEX

ABBREVIATIONS

AAA   abdominal aortic aneurysm
ABC   airway, breathing, circulation
ABG   arterial blood gas
ACE   angiotensin-converting enzyme
ACS   acute coronary syndrome
AF   atrial fibrillation
ALS   amyotrophic lateral sclerosis
AMS   altered mental status
APAP   acetaminophen
ARDS   acute respiratory distress syndrome
BID   twice a day
BP   blood pressure
BUN   blood urea nitrogen
BVM   bag-valve-mask
CAD   coronary artery disease
CBC   complete blood count
CCU   coronary care unit
CHF   congestive heart failure
CK (CPK)   creatine kinase (creatine phosphokinase)
CNS   central nervous system
CO   carbon monoxide
COHb   carboxyhemoglobin
COPD   chronic obstructive pulmonary disease
CPR   cardiopulmonary resuscitation
CSF   cerebrospinal fluid
C-spine   cervical spine
CT   computed tomography
CVA   costovertebral angle or cerebrovascular accident
CXR   chest x-ray
DIC   disseminated intravascular coagulation
DKA   diabetic ketoacidosis
DVT   deep venous thrombosis
ECG   electrocardiogram
ED   emergency department
EDH   epidural hematoma
EEG   electroencephalogram
EMS   emergency medical services
ESR   erythrocyte sedimentation rate
ET or ETT   endotracheal tube
FAST   focused assessment with sonography for trauma
FFP   fresh frozen plasma
GI   gastrointestinal
GCS   Glasgow Coma Scale
GERD   gastroesophageal reflux disease
GU   genitourinary
Hb   hemoglobin
HR   heart rate
HPV   human papillomavirus
HSV   herpes simplex virus
ICP   intracranial pressure
ICU   intensive care unit
I&D   incision and drainage
IM   intramuscular
IV   intravenous, intravenously
IVF   intravenous fluids
IVIG   intravenous immunoglobulin
JVD   jugular venous distension
LBBB   left bundle branch block
LDH   lactate dehydrogenase

LLQ   left lower quadrant
LMA   laryngeal mask airway
LMW   low molecular weight
LOC   level of consciousness
LP   lumbar puncture
LR   lactated Ringer's solution
LUQ   left upper quadrant
LVH   left ventricular hypertrophy
MAP   mean arterial pressure
MI   myocardial infarction
MRI   magnetic resonance imaging
MS   multiple sclerosis
MVC   motor vehicle collision
NG   nasogastric
NGT   nasogastric tube
NS   normal saline solution
NSAID(s)   nonsteroidal anti-inflammatory drug(s)
OR   operating room
OTC   over-the-counter
PA   posteroanterior
PCI   percutaneous coronary intervention
PEA   pulseless electrical activity
PID   pelvic inflammatory disease
PO   per os (by mouth)
PPI   proton pump inhibitor
PUD   peptic ulcer disease
q   every
QD   once a day
QID   four times a day
RBBB   right bundle branch block
RBC   red blood cell
RLQ   right lower quadrant
ROM   range of motion
ROSC   return of spontaneous circulation
RR   respiratory rate
RSI   rapid sequence intubation
RUQ   right upper quadrant
SAH   subarachnoid hemorrhage
SBI   serious bacterial infection
SCD   sudden cardiac death
SDH   subdural hematoma
SIADH   syndrome of inappropriate antidiuretic hormone
SQ   subcutaneously
SVC   superior vena cava
TB   tuberculosis
TIA   transient ischemic attack
TID   three times a day
TSS   toxic shock syndrome
TTP   thrombotic thrombocytopenic purpura
UA   urinalysis
URI   upper respiratory infection
US   ultrasound
UTI   urinary tract infection
VBI   vertebrobasilar insufficiency
VF   ventricular fibrillation
V/Q   ventilation-perfusion
VT   ventricular tachycardia
WBC   white blood cell

CPSIA information can be obtained at www.ICGtesting.com
Printed in the USA
BVOW060547170712

295196BV00007B/2/P

9 780071 463881